AN ORAL HISTORY OF NEUROPSYCHOPHARMACOLOGY

THE FIRST FIFTY YEARS

Peer Interviews

Volume Two: Neurophysiology

Thomas A. Ban (series editor)
AN ORAL HISTORY OF NEUROPSYCHOPHARMACOLOGY

Max Fink (volume editor)
VOLUME 2: Neurophysiology

Library of Congress Cataloging-in-Publication Data
Thomas A. Ban, Max Fink (eds):
An Oral History of Neuropsychopharmacology: The First Fifty Years, Peer Interviews
Includes bibliographical references and index
ISBN: 1461161452
ISBN-13: 9781461161455

1. Electroencephalography and neurophysiology 2. Pharmaco-EEG
3. Sleep EEG 4. Cerebral blood flow 5. Brain metabolism
6. Brain imaging

Publisher: ACNP
ACNP Executive Office
5034A Thoroughbred Lane
Brentwood, Tennessee 37027
U.S.A.
Email: acnp@acnp.org
Website: www.acnp.org

Cover design by Jessie Blackwell; JBlackwell Design www.jblackwelldesign.com

AMERICAN COLLEGE OF NEUROPSYCHOPHARMACOLOGY

AN ORAL HISTORY OF NEUROPSYCHOPHARMACOLOGY
THE FIRST FIFTY YEARS
Peer Interviews

Edited by
Thomas A. Ban

Co-editors

Volume 1: Starting Up - Edward Shorter

Volume 2: Neurophysiology - Max Fink

Volume 3: Neuropharmacology - Fridolin Sulser

Volume 4: Psychopharmacology - Jerome Levine

Volume 5: Neuropsychopharmacology - Samuel Gershon

Volume 6: Addiction - Herbert D. Kleber

Volume 7: Special Areas - Barry Blackwell

Volume 8: Diverse Topics - Carl Salzman

Volume 9: Update - Barry Blackwell

Volume 10: History of the ACNP - Martin M. Katz

VOLUME 2

NEUROPHYSIOLOGY

ACNP
2011

VOLUME 2

Max Fink

NEUROPHYSIOLOGY

Preface
Thomas A. Ban

PREFACE
Thomas A. Ban

In Volume 1 of this series, 22 clinicians and basic scientists reflected on their contributions to the "starting up" of neuropsychopharmacology (NPP). The central theme was the adoption of a behavioral methodology for the detection of psychotropic properties of drugs (see Brady, Cook, Dews and Stein, Volume 1). In Volume 2, the emphasis shifts to the detection of the action of drugs on the functional activity of the brain. There are two complementary approaches, with corresponding methodologies for neurophysiological research in NPP. One is focused on the electrical activity of the brain, using electroencephalography (EEG), and the other on cerebral blood flow (CBF) and metabolism, using brain imaging.

The bridge between neurophysiological and behavioral (psychiatric) research is the conditioned reflex (CR). The origin of the idea that the conditioned reflex is at the core of mental activity is in Wilhelm Griesinger's adoption of "reflex activity," as the basis of all brain activity, and his introduction of the concept of "psychic reflex," in the mid-1840s.[1, 2] His notion that mental activity is reflex activity became a feasible proposition by the end of the 19th century after the delineation of the structural underpinning of reflex activity in the brain by Camillo Golgi's description of "multi-polar cells" in the cerebral cortex,[3] Ramón y Cajal's recognition of the "neuron," as a structural and functional unit of the nervous system,[4, 5] and Charles Sherrington's postulation that the "synapse" is the functional site of transmission from one neuron to another.[6, 7, 8]

The concept of "psychic reflex" became accessible to scientific study in the early 20th century through Ivan Petrovich Pavlov's discovery of the CR.[9] His findings that verbal signals could replace sensory signals in CR formation opened a path for research in which mental activity is perceived as CR activity in the second (verbal) signal system and studied with conditioning methods (see Ban, Volumes 4 and 9). Pavlov's postulation that CR formation is based on the opening of formerly non-operating paths in the brain[10, 11, 12] became demonstrable by the 1990s[13] (see Kandel, Volume 3). Between the mid-1930s and late 1950s, a series of centrally acting substances, including alcohol,[14] amphetamine,[15] adrenaline and acetylcholine,[16] mescaline,[17] chlorpromazine and reserpine,[18] was studied on CR activity in animals[19, 20, 21] by Horsley Gantt and his associates in the United States.

In the 1960s interest shifted from the study of the effect of psychotropic drugs on the CR in animals to the effect of these drugs on the human electroencephalogram. Recognition that electrical activity is a natural property of the living brain dates back to Emil Du Bois-Reymond's detection of electric currents (action potentials), from the peripheral nerves and brain of frogs with a galvanometer in the late 1840s.[22, 23] His discovery that living brain generates electricity was substantiated independently in the mid-1870s by Richard Caton and Vasilij Jakovlevich Danilevskii, who recorded electrical currents and the fluctuations of these currents from the cerebral hemispheres of rabbits, monkeys,[24] and dogs.[25]

It was Hans Berger, in the 1920s, who first recorded electrical activity from the human brain through the intact skull. He introduced EEG, a technique for recording the electrical activity of the brain,[26] and showed that the spontaneous waking EEG was "sensitive to" hypoxia, hypocapnia, barbiturates, bromides, caffeine, cocaine, chloroform, morphine, scopolamine, and insulin coma.[27, 28] By the time the new psychotropic drugs were introduced in the 1950s, research on the electrical activity of the brain also included "sleep EEG,"[29] with the recognition of rapid eye movement (REM) sleep,[30, 31] "topography,"[32] "functional EEG,"[33, 34] and the study of "evoked (event related) potentials" (ERP).[35, 36, 37, 38]

In the 1980s research was extended to the study of brain metabolism, as measured by cerebral blood flow. The roots of this research lie in the assumption frequently held in the 1920s, that deficient oxidative processes play an important role in the pathogenesis of mental syndromes and especially of schizophrenia.[39] To stimulate oxygen consumption, carbon dioxide inhalation was tried in "catatonic" patients,[40, 41] and nitrous oxide inhalation in "psychoses,"[42] with equivocal results.[43] Juda Quastel's report in 1939 that oxygen uptake in the brain is much greater in vivo than in vitro,[44] and the introduction of the first quantitative in vivo measurement of CBF by Dumke and Schmidt in 1943,[45] led in the 1970s to the introduction of brain imaging techniques, suitable for the study of structure-activity relationships in the brain. Prior to their introduction, information on the living human brain was limited to structural changes revealed by pneumoencephalography[46] and carotid angiography,[47] and the only relatively consistent finding relevant to psychiatry was enlarged cerebral ventricles in schizophrenia first reported by Jacobi and Winkler in 1921.[48, 49]

Early studies on structure-function relationships, as for example the linking of "motor aphasia" to a lesion of the posterior part of the frontal lobe by Paul Broca in 1861,[50] and of "sensory aphasia" to the posterior part of the temporal lobe by Carl Wernicke in 1874,[51] were based on pathological anatomical findings, mainly in stroke patients.[52]

Research from the morgue moved to the study of the living brain of animals with the introduction of electrical stimulation by Fritch and Hitzig in 1870.[53]

Electrical stimulation was adopted in the study of the structure-function relationship in patients undergoing brain surgery by Wilder Penfield in the early 1950s.[54] His findings, that electrical stimulation of certain parts of the temporal lobe (TL) evoked déjà vu experiences and old memories, contributed to the recognition of the role of the TL in memory storage.[55]

Introduction of the chronic implanted electrode technique in animals by Walter Rudolf Hess in 1932, and his studies of the diencephalon, thalamus and hypothalamus,[56] extended the scope of the use of electrical stimulation in the study of structure-function relationships in the brain. In 1954, James Olds and Peter Milner found that rats with metal electrodes implanted in their nucleus accumbens, repeatedly pressed a lever controlling the delivery of an electric current, as if they were seeking pleasure by electrical activation of the region.[57] The discovery of "a pleasure center," involved in the "reinforcement" of behavior by "reward," provided the key for the identification of the cerebral structures involved in "operant (instrumental) conditioning," a form of learning, in which a motivational (emotional) factor, i.e., pleasure or punishment, is involved in the acquisition of CR.[58]

In 1939 James Papez suggested that emotions are processed through a reverberating circuit in the brain – which consists of the cingulate gyrus, hippo-campus, amygdala, mammillary bodies, hypothalamus and anterior thalamus – before becoming subjectively-experienced feelings in the cerebral cortex.[59, 60] The "Papez circuit" is also referred to as "limbic lobe," because its site corresponds with Paul Broca's "great limbic lobe,"[61] and "visceral brain," because of its numerous connections with the autonomic nervous system.[62]

The subjective experience of feelings depends on the state of arousal of the cerebral cortex regulated by brain stem structures. In 1949 Moruzzi and Magoun reported that electrical stimulation of the ascending reticular formation in the brain stem of animals produced a generalized activation and desynchronization of the EEG with increased cortical activity, whereas depression of the same structures produced the opposite effect.[63] They suggested that the reticular activating system (RAS) is the structure involved in the regulation of the states of arousal, consciousness, wakefulness and sleep.[64]

In 1949, the same year that Moruzzi and Magoun's report was published, Herbert Jasper demonstrated that stimulation of the thalamic reticular formation has a similar effect as stimulation of the brain stem reticular formation but with the activation restricted to the region that corresponds with the stimulation.[65] Combining Moruzzi and Magoun's findings with Herbert Jasper's, Henri Gastaut in the late 1950s formulated a hypothesis about the brain mechanisms involved in acquiring a CR.[66, 67]

This was the state of art in neurophysiology as relevant to NPP in the 1950s, at the time that the first set of psychotropic drugs was introduced. The findings reviewed in the first part of this Preface provide the background to the research conducted by the interviewees whose transcripts are included in Volume 2.

Interviewees & Interviewers

The twelwe transcripts in this volume, as in the first volume, are based on videotaped interviews with 21 interviewees. From the group, twelve are trained psychiatrists (Aghajanian, Andreasen, Bloom, Callaway, Feinberg, Fink, Gillin, Hartmann, Itil, Kaim, Sugerman and Weinberger); two of them (Aghajanian and Bloom) involved exclusively in basic research. From the remaining nine interviewees, one (Kessler) is a radiologist, four (Delgado, Kety, Longo and Sokoloff,) are MDs, and four (Bradley, Holzman, E. Killam and K.Killam) are PhDs, all involved in different areas of research in neurophysiology related to NPP. All but two interviewees (Bradley and Longo) are ACNP members; six (Callaway, Delgado, Fink, Kety, E. Killam and K. Killam) were founders, and two (E. Killam and K. Killam,) were presidents of the College.

All interviews were conducted in a period from 1993 to 2007, and with the exception of two, they were done at the annual meetings of the College. From the two interviews done between annual meetings, one (Kaim's) was conducted in Washington DC, and the other (Bradley's) in London, England.

The 21 interviewees were interviewed by twelve interviewers. Nine of these (Joel Braslow, William Bunney, Jonathan Cole, Leonard Cook, Eva Killam, Keith Killam, Irwin Kopin, David Kupfer and Steven Potkin) conducted one interview apiece. Of the remaining three, one (Andrea Tone) conducted two interviews; another (Leo Hollister) conducted three, and the third (Thomas Ban) conducted seven. In one instance, instead of an external interviewer, two interviewees (Keith Killam and Eva King Killam, husband and wife,) interviewed each other Ten of the interviewers are peers of the interviewees, and two (Braslow and Tone) are historians. One of the latter (Braslow) is also a trained psychiatrist.

By the time the editing of Volume Two was completed, seven of the interviewees (Philip Bradley, Christian Gillin, Philip Holzman, Seymour Kety, Eva Killam, Keith Killam and Arthur Sugerman), and four of the interviewers (Jonathan Cole, Leo Hollister, Eva Killam and Keith Killam), had passed away.

Contributions of Interviewees

In the following section some of the contributions of interviewees to the development of neuropsychopharmacology are reviewed.

Five interviewees (Fink, Callaway, Itil, Kaim and Sugerman) were engaged in studying the effects of psychotropic drugs with the employment of the **EEG in humans**. In the 1950s, *Samuel Kaim* studied the effect of new drugs on the seizure threshold in epileptics with Metrazol (pentylenetetrazol).[68] He also employed the EEG for monitoring drug effects.[69] Kaim was among the first to note that chlordiazepoxide in alcohol withdrawal could prevent seizures in delirium tremens.[70, 71]

Enoch Callaway introduced in the 1960s the "two-tone method" for studying ERPs in schizophrenia.[72, 73] He found significantly lower two-tone correlations in schizophrenia than in normal controls or in hospitalized psychiatric patients with another diagnosis. Callaway also revealed that two-tone correlations increased with clinical improvement, approaching normal values with effective phenothiazine treatment[74, 75, 76, 77] (*see also* Heninger, Volume 8.)

Max Fink was one of the first (in 1958) to report on the effects of chlorpromazine (CPZ) on the human EEG.[78] Fink introduced electronic frequency analysis in the evaluation of the electroencephalogram[79] and in the early 1960s set up the first EEG laboratory employing digital computer technology to study the effect of psychotropic drugs.[80, 81]

Turan Itil also reported in 1958 on the EEG effects of chlorpromazine,[82] and spearheaded research during the 1950s on the effects of antipsychotic and antidepressant drugs on the human EEG.[83, 84] In the 1960s Itil and Fink in collaboration developed "the quantitative pharmaco-EEG"[85, 86] for screening and classifying psychotropic drugs, monitoring changes in the course of treatment, and predicting treatment outcomes in individual patients.[87]

In the 1960s, *Arthur Sugerman* was among the first to employ quantitative EEG in the screening and evaluation of new psychotropic drugs.[88, 89] Sugerman was also one of the first researchers to show that treatment with antipsychotics by increasing the amplitude variability of brain waves corrected the reduced amplitude variability in schizophrenia.[90, 91]

Three of the interviewees (Hartmann, Feinberg and Gillin) were engaged in studying the effects of psychotropic drugs on the **sleep EEG.** *Ernest Hartmann* discovered in the 1960s that drugs which increased norepinephrine (NE) levels in the brain decreased D-sleep.[92, 93] He also noted that L-DOPA could increase nightmares and induce vivid dreams.[94, 95]

Irwin Feinberg revealed during the 1960s that the relative excess of fast β activity in the EEG seen in schizophrenia is associated with an increased number of awakening periods and decreased amount of time spent in deep-sleep stages.[96, 97] Feinberg divided hypnotics into GABAergic modulators (e.g., barbiturates, benzodiazepines), which decrease, or even eliminate, deep Stage 4 sleep, and glutamate antagonists, which increase deep sleep.[98] He also demonstrated that GABAergic modulators increased only "subjective sleeping time" whereas glutamate antagonists also increased the duration of sleep.[99, 100]

J. Christian Gillin demonstrated in the 1980s that REM induction is mediated by muscarinic M_2 receptors.[101, 102] He also showed that selective serotonin reuptake inhibitors lose their REM-suppressing effect with tryptophan depletion.[103, 104, 105] Gillin was a member of the team which studied the effect of sleep deprivation on brain metabolism.[106, 107]

Five interviewees (Kety, Sokoloff, Kessler, Andreasen and Weinberger) were engaged in studying the effects of psychotropic drugs on CBF and **brain metabolism**. *Seymour Kety* developed, in collaboration with Carl Schmidt, the first method for measuring overall cerebral blood flow (CBF) and metabolism in man in the mid-1940s.[108] The Kety-Schmidt nitrous oxide method was sensitive to the effects of barbiturates, insulin coma and electroshock.[109] In the mid-1950s, Kety with his collaborators also developed the first method for studying regional cerebral blood flow (rCBF) and metabolism with the use of trifluoriodomethane (TFDM).[110]

In the late 1970s *Louis Sokoloff*, a disciple of Kety, replaced oxygen consumption with glucose utilization, and developed an autoradiographic method with deoxyglucose for measuring rCBF and metabolism in man.[111] Subsequently, by replacing deoxyglucose (DG) with fluorodeoxyglucose (FDG), Sokoloff rendered the method suitable for use with a scanner[112] and opened the path for the introduction of positron emission tomography (PET).[113, 114]

Robert Kessler was a member of the team which introduced cerebral glucography into psychiatric research with PET in the early 1980s.[115] The team showed that the "anteroposterior gradient" of glucose use ("hypofrontality") was decreased statistically not only in schizophrenia, as shown by SPECT imaging,[116] but also in affective illness.[117]

Nancy Andreasen introduced magnetic resonance imaging (MRI) in the study of schizophrenia in the mid-1980s. She revealed thalamic abnormalities[118] and smaller frontal lobes in schizophrenia [119] than in the normal population. In the mid-1990s Andreasen postulated that a dysfunctional prefrontal-thalamic-cerebellar circuitry was the culprit for the cognitive dysfunction in schizophrenia.[120]

Daniel Weinberger introduced, in the mid-1980s, topographical imaging with the use of radioactive xenon in the study of schizophrenia.[121] He found that administration of the Wisconsin Card Sorting Test (WCST) did not produce an increase in CBF in the dorsolateral prefrontal cortex of this population.[122] Weinberger was among the first to combine molecular genetic research with functional brain imaging in the study of schizophrenia.[123, 124]

One of the interviewees, *Philip Holzman*, discovered in the mid-1970s that an abnormality of the smooth pursuit eye movement (SPEM),[125] a discrete neurological deficit, was present in 80 percent of patients with schizophrenia and in 40 percent of the first degree relatives of patients.[126, , 127] He perceived the population with an abnormality of SPEM as an **alternative phenotype** of the schizophrenic population and determined that a single gene could account for the tracking dysfunction.[128] The gene was located by Arolt and his associates on the short arm of chromosome 6p in the mid-1990s.[129]

Four interviewees (Longo, E. Killam, K. Killam and Bradley) were engaged in research studying the effect of psychotropic drugs on the **activity of the brain in animal models**. *Vincenzo Longo* was first to report, in 1954, on the "synchronizing" effect of chlorpromazine (CPZ) on the EEG of rabbits.[130] He suggested that the action of CPZ was on midbrain reticular formation structures and classified CPZ as a "ganglioplégique central."[131, 132] In the early 1960s Longo presented his findings in neurophysiological research with centrally acting drugs in rabbits in an "electroencephalographic atlas for pharmacological research."[133]

The Killams, Eva and Keith, were among the first (in the 1950s) to study the effects of the new psychotropic drugs on the brains of animals by using electrophysiological measures.[134, 135, 136] *Eva King Killam* was first to report on the effect of mephenesin on the brain stem reticular formation[137, 138] and to demonstrate the differential effect of anesthetics and interneuronal blocking agents on EEG arousal and recruitment responses evoked from the brain stem.[139, 140] *Keith F. Killam* studied the effects of psychotropic drugs on evoked electrical activity of the brain.[141] He was the first to report on the effect of psychotropic drugs on pathways of the reticular formation,[142] and on the reticular formation in general.[143] The Killams developed a screening test in baboons for anticonvulsants.[144, 145]

In the early 1950s *Philip B. Bradley* introduced chronic implanted electrodes in studying the effects of psychotropic drugs on the electrical activity of the brain in conscious cats.[146, 147, 148] In the late 1950s he suggested that central depressants and stimulants, such as barbiturates and amphetamines, act directly on arousal mechanisms in the brain stem, whereas antipsychotics and psychotomimetics like CPZ and LSD act indirectly, via afferent collaterals on arousal mechanisms.[149, 150] Bradley was among the first to study the effects of centrally acting drugs on the electrical activity of single neurons.[151, 152, 153]

One of the interviewees, *José Manuel Rodriguez Delgado*, was first to employ **chronic implanted electrodes** in humans to study the effects of electrical and chemical stimulation of specific brain areas.[154, 155, 156] He also explored the use of chronic implanted electrodes in the treatment of schizophrenia, epilepsy and depression.[157]

Two interviewees (Aghajanian and Bloom), were engaged in research on the study of the **neurophysiology of neurotransmitters.** By studying the firing rate of single neurons, *George K. Aghajanian* revealed during the 1970s some of the essential properties of serotonergic,[158, 159] noradrenergic[160] and dopaminergic neurons.[161] In collaboration with Steve Bunney, Aghajanian showed that antipsychotics and amphetamines affect single cell activity of dopaminergic neurons in the opposite direction.[162] He also demonstrated that serotonergic neurons continuously release 5-HT in slow tonic firing [163] whereas the tonic firing of noradrenergic neurons is reactive to sensory stimulation.[164]

During the 1960s and 1970s *Floyd E Bloom* characterized the neuroanatomy and neurophysiology of the NE system by employing microiontophoresis and electron microscopy combined with fluorescence histochemistry.[165, 166, 167] In the 1980s and 1990s Bloom contributed to the characterization of neuropeptides and "other mediators."[168, 169, 170]

The contributions of Aghajanian and Bloom provide a bridge between neuro-physiology and neuropharmacology, covered in Volume 3 of this series.

Interviewees included in Volume 2 entered the field at different stages in the development of NPP. Hence, the transcripts cover fifty years of history during which various neurophysiological methods were in the forefront at the different periods for studying the action of psychotropic drugs in the brain.

By the 1970s the emphasis on neuronal processing at the site of the synapse had shifted from electrical to chemical transmission, and with this shift, the conceptual framework of the operation of the brain changed. While the EEG has remained a most useful guide for clinicians in the use of psychotropic drugs, the information generated with the employment of brain imaging techniques about the differential effect of drugs on signal transduction and regional brain metabolism in clinically distinct psychiatric populations was to provide more specific cues than the EEG for research in NPP.

Max Fink, the editor of this volume, is a clinical psychiatrist (*see* Fink, in this Volume and in Volume 9.) He was one of the leaders in moving American psychiatry, embedded in psychoanalysis, into the neuropsychopharmacological era. Fink was also instrumental in rendering the EEG a suitable instrument for clinical research in the pharmacotherapy of psychiatric disorders. His Introduction and Dramatis Personae complements the information in the transcripts.

REFERENCES

1   Griesinger W. Über psychische Reflexactionen. Arch f Physiol Heilk 1843; 2: 76–81.
2   Griesinger W. Die Pathologie und Therapie der Psychiatrischen Krankheiten. Stuttgart: Krabbe; 1845.
3   Golgi C. Sulla fine struttura dei bulbi olfattorii. Riv Sper Freniatr Med Leg Alienazioni Ment 1874; 1: 405–25.
4   Cajal SR. La fine 'structure` des centres nerveux. Proc R Soc London 1894; 55: 444–67.
5   Cajal SR. Histologie du Système Nerveux de L'Homme et des Vertébrés. Paris: Maloine; 1909.
6   Foster M, Sherington CS.Textbook of Physiology. London: Mcmillan; 1897.
7   Garrison FH. History of Medicine. Philadelphia/London: WB Saunders Company; 1960.
8   Sherrington CS.The Integrative Action of the Nervous System. London: Scribner; 1906.
9   Pavlov IP. The scientific investigation of the psychical faculties or processes of higher animals. Science 1906; 24: 613-9.
10   Pavlov IP. Conditioned Reflexes. Translated by GV Anrep. Oxford: Oxford University Press; 1928.

11   Pavlov IP. Conditioned Reflexes and Psychiatry. Translated by WH Horsley Gantt. Chicago: International Publishers; 1941.

12   Ban TA. Conditioning and Psychiatry. Chicago: Aldine; 1954.

13   Kandel ER. In Search of Memory. The Emergence of a New Science of Mind. New York: W.W. Norton & Company; 2006. p.165–318.

14   Gantt WH. Effect of alcohol on cortical and subcortical activity measured by the conditioned reflex method. Bull Johns Hopkins Hosp 1935; 56: 61–83.

15   Alpern R, Finkelstein N, Gantt WH. Effect of amphetamine (Benzedrine) sulphate upon higher nervous activity. Bull Johns Hopkins Hosp 1943; 73: 287–99.

16   Freile M, Gantt WH. Effect of adrenalin and acetylcholine on excitation, inhibition and neuroses. Trans Am Neurol Assoc 1944; 70: 180–1.

17   Bridger WH, Gantt WH. Effect of mescaline on differentiated conditional reflexes. Am J Psychiatry 1956; 113: 352–60.

18   Gliedman L, Gantt WH. The effect of reserpine, chlorpromazine, morphine on the orienting response. In: Gantt WH, editor. Physiological Basis of Psychiatry. Springfield: Charles C. Thomas; 1958. p. 196–206.

19   Stoff DM, Bridger WH, Gantt WH. The first American psychopharmacologist. In: McGuigan FJ, Ban TA, editors. Critical Issues in Psychology, Psychiatry and Physiology. A Memorial to W. Horsley Gantt. New York/London: Gordon and Breach Science Publishers; 1987. p. 177–87.

20   McGuigan FJ, Ban TA, editors. Critical Issues in Psychology, Psychiatry and Physiology. A Memorial to W. Horsley Gantt. New York/London: Gordon and Breach Science Publishers; 1987.

21   Ban TA. Conditioning Behavior and Psychiatry. New York/London: Aldine; 2008.

22   DuBois-Reymond EH. Untersuchungen bei Tierische Elektrizität. Berlin: G. Remmer; 1848.

23   Horányi B. Ideggyogyászat. Budapest: Medicina; 1962.

24   Caton R. The electric currents of the brain. Brit Med J 1875; 2: 278–9.

25   Danilevskii VY. Research on the Physiology of the Brain. Moscow: Thesis; 1875.

26   Berger H. Über das elektroencephalogramm des menschen. Arch Psychiatr Nervenkr 1929; 87: 527–70.

27   Gloor P. The work of Hans Berger and the discovery of the electroencephalogram Electroencephalogr Clin Neurophysiol 1969; 28 (Suppl): S1–S36.

28   Fink M. Psychoactive drugs and the waking EEG. 1966–1976. In: Lipton MA, DiMascio A, Killam KF, editors.. Psychopharmacology: A Generation of Progress. New York: Raven Pess; 1978. p.691–8.

29   Loomis AL, Harvey EN, Hobart GA. Cerebral states during sleep as studied by human brain potentials. J Exp Psychol 1937; 21: 127–44.

30   Aserinsky E, Kleitman N. Regularly occurring periods of eye motility and concomitant phenomena during sleep. Science 1953; 118: 273–4.

31   Shorter E. A Historical Dictionary of Psychiatry. New York: Oxford University Press; 2005.

32   Walter W. The Living Brain. New York: W.W. Norton; 1963.

33   Lieberson WT. Functional electroencephalography in mental disorders. Dis Nerv Syst 1945; 5: 1–2.

34   Itil TM. Invited discusson of Dr. M. Fink's paper (Human psychoharmacology and functional electro-encephalography.) In: Efron DH, Cole JO, Levine J, Wittenborn JR, editors. Psychopharmacology. A Review of Progress. 1957–1967. Washington: Public Health Service Publications No 1836. Superintendent of Documents Government Printing Office; 1968. p. 509–22.

35   Pravdich-Neminsky W. Ein Versuch der Registrierung der elektrischen Gehirnerscheinungen. Zbl Physiol 1913; 27: 951–60.

36   Dawson CD. Cerebral responses to electrical stimulation of peripheral nerve in man. J Neurol Neurosurg Psychiat 1947; 10: 134–40.

37   Shagass Ch. Pharmacology of evoked potentials in man. In: Efron DH, Cole JO, Levine J, Wittenborn JR, editors. Psychopharmacology A Review of Progress. 1957–1967. Washington: Public Health Service Publications No 1836. Superintendent of Documents. Government Printing Office; 1968. p. 483–92.

38   Shagass C, Straumanis JJ. Drugs in human sensory evoked potentials. In: Lipton MA, DiMascio A, Killam KF, editors. Psychopharmacology: A Generation of Progress. New York: Raven Pess; 1978. p. 699–710.

39   Freeman W. Psychochemistry: Some physicochemical factors in mental disorders. JAMA 1931; 97: 293–6.

40   Loevenhart AS, Lorenz W, Waters RM. Cerebral stimulation. JAMA 1929; 92: 880–3.

41   Hinsie LE, Barach AI, Harris MM, Brand E, McFarland RA. The treatment of dementia praecox by continuous oxygen administration in chambers and oxygen and carbon dioxide inhalations. Psychiatry 1934; 8: 334–71.

42   Alexander FA, Himwich HE. Nitrogen inhalation therapy for schizophrenia. Preliminary report on technique. Am J Psychiatry 1939; 96: 643–55.

43   Lehmann HE. Before they called it psychopharmacology Neuropsychopharmacology 1993; 8: 291–303.

44   Quastel JH. Metabolism of brain and nerve. Ann Rev Biochem 1939; 8: 435–62.

45   Dumke PR, Schmidt CF. Quantitative measurement of cerebral blood flow in the macacque monkey. Am J Physiology 1938; 138: 421–31.

46   Dandy W. Ventriculopgraphy following injection of air into the ventricles. Ann Surgery 1918; 68: 5–11.

47   Moniz E. Injections intracarotidiennes et substances opaques. Presse méd 1927; 35: 969–71.

48   Jacobi W, Winkler H. Encephalograhische studien am chronische schizophrenen. Arch Psychiatr Nervenkr 1927; 81: 299–332.

49   Huber G. Pneumoencephalographische und psychopathologische Bilder bei endogenen Psychosen. Berlin: Springer; 1957.

50   Broca PP. Perte de la parole ramolissement chronique et destruction partielle du lobe antérior gauche du cerveau. Bull Soc Anthropologique 1861; 2: 235–8.

51   Wernicke C. Der Aphasische Symptomencomplex. Bresalu: Cohn & Weigert; 1874.

52   Pichot P. A Century of Pychiatry. Paris: Roger Dacosta; 1983.

53   Fritsch GT, Hitzig E. Über die elektrische Erregbarkeit des Grosshirns. Arch Anat Physiol Wissentchaftliche Med Leipzig 1870; 37: 300–32.

54   Andreasen NC. Brave New Brain. Conquering Mental Illness in the Era of the Genome. New York: Oxford University Press; 2001.

55   Penfield W, Jaspers H.Temporal Lobe Epilepsy and the Functional Anatomy of the Brain. NewYork: Little, Brown and Company; 1953.

56   Hess WR. Hypothalamus and Thalamus. Stuttgart: Thieme; 1956.

57   Olds J, Millner P. Positive reinforcement produced by electrical stimulation of the septal area and other regions of rat brain. J Compr Physiol Psychiatry 1954; 47: 419–27.

58   Iversen SD, Iversen LL. Behavioral Pharmacology. Oxford: Oxford University Press; 1975.

59   Papez W. A proposed mechanism of emotions. Arch Neurol Psychiatry 1937; 38: 725–43.

60   Kaplan HI, Saddock BJ. Synopsis of Psychiatry, Behavioral Sciences, Clinical Psychatry. Fifth ed. Baltimore: Williams & Wilkins; 1988.

61   Broca P. Anatomie comparée des circonvolutions cérebralés; le grand lobe limbique. Rev Anthropol 1878; 1: 385–498.

62   MacLean PD. Psychosomatic disease and the "visceral brain." Recent developments bearing on the Papez Theory of Emotions. Psychosom Med 1949; 11: 338–53.

63   Moruzzi G, Magoun HW. Brainstem reticular formation and the activation of the EEG. Electroencephalogr Clin Neurophysiol 1949; 1: 455–73.

64   Lehmann HE, Ban TA. Psychiatric research in America. In: Oldham JM, Riba MB, editors. Review of Psychiatry. Volume 13. Washington/London: American Psychiatric Press; 1994. p. 27-54.

65   Jasper HH. Diffuse projection system: the integrative action of the thalamic reticular system. Electroencephalogr Clin Neurophysiol 1949; 1: 405–19.

66   Gastaut H. Etat actuel des connaisances sur l'electroencephalographie du conditionement. Electroencephalogr Clin Neurophysiol 1957; 6 (Suppl): S133–S138.

67   Gastaut H. Some aspects of the neurophysiological basis of conditioned reflexes and behavior. In: Wolstenholme GE, O'Connor, editors. Neurophysiological Basis of Behavior. London: Churchill; 1958.

68   Kaim SC, Rosenstein IN. Anticonvulsant properties of a new psychotherapeutic drug. Dis Nerv Syst 1960; 21 (Suppl): S46–S52.

69   Hollister LE, Bennett JL, Kaim SC, Kimball I. Drug-induced EEG abnormalities as predictors of clinical response to thiopropazate. Am J Psychiatry 1963; 119: 887–8.

70   Kaim SC, Klett CJ, Rothfeld B. Treatment of the acute alcohol withdrawal state: a comparison of four drugs. Am J Psychiatry 1969; 125: 1640–6.

71   Kaim SC, Klett CJ. Treatment of delirium tremens. A comparative evaluation of four drugs. Quart J Stud Alcohol 1972; 33: 1065–72.

72   Callaway E, Jones RT, Layne RS. Evoked response and segmental set of schizophrenia. Arch Gen Psychiatry 1965; 12: 83–9.

73   Malerstein AJ, Callaway F. Two-tone average evoked response in Korsakoff patients. J Psychiatric Res 1969; 6: 253–60.

74   Callaway E. Invited discussant of Dr. Shagass' paper on Pharmacology of evoked potentials in man. In: Efron DH, editor. Psychopharmacology A Review of Progress 1957–67. Washington: Public Health Service Publication No`1836; 1968. p. 493–5.

75   Callaway E. Historical development of psychopharmacology. In: Ban TA, Healy D, Shorter E, editors. Reflections on Twentieth-Century Psychopharmacology. Budapest: Animula; 2004. p. 169–73.

76   Callaway E. Asylum. A Mid-Century Madhouse and Its Lessons about Our Mentally Ill Today. Westport: Praeger; 2007.

77   Callaway E. Brain Electrical Potential and Individual Psychological Differences. New York: Grune and Stratton; 1975.

78   Fink M. EEG and behavioral effects of psychopharmacological agents. In: Bradley PB, Deniker P, Radouco-Thomas C, editors. Neuropsychopharmacology. Proceedings of the First Intarnational Congress of Neuropsychopharmacology. Amsterdam/London: Elsevier Publishing Company; 1959. p. 442–6.

79   Fink M. Itil T, Shapiro DM. Digital computer analysis of the human EEG in psychiatric research. Compr Psychiatry 1967; 8: 521–38.

80   Fink M. EEG and human psychopharmacology. Ann Rev Pharmacol 1969; 9: 241–58.

81   Fink M. Pharmaco-electroencephalography. A Selective History of the Study of Brain Responses to Psychoactive Drugs. In: Ban TA, Healy D, Shorter E, editors. Reflections on Twentieth-Century Psychopharmacology. Budapest: Animula; 2004. p. 661–72.

82   Bente D, Itil TM. A comparison of various phenothiazine compounds on the human EEG. In: Bradley PB, Deniker P, Radouco-Thomas C, editors. Neuropsychopharmacology. Proceedings of the First International Congress of Neuropharmacology. Amsterdam/London: Elsevier Publishing Company; 1959. p. 496–8.

83   Itil, TM. The first use of placebo. In: Ban TA, Healy D, Shorter E, editors. The Rise of Psychopharmacology and the Story of CINP. Budapest: Animula; 1998.p. 157–60.

84   Itil T. Elektroenzephalographische Befunde zur Klassifikation neuro- und thymoleptischer Medikamente. Med Exp 1961; 5: 347–63.

85   Itil M, Shapiro DM, Fink M. Differentiation of psychotropic drugs: quantitative EEG analysis. Aggressologie 1968; 9: 267–80.

86   Itil T, Fink M. Anticholinergic drug-induced delirium: experimental modification, quantitative EEG and behavioral correlations. J Nerv Ment Dis 1966; 143: 492–507.

87   Fink M, Shapiro D, Hickman C, Itil T. Quantitative analyis of the electroencephalogram by digital computer methods. III: Applications to psychopharmacology. In: Kline NS, Laska E, editors. Computers and Electronic Devices in Psychiaatry. New York: Grune & Stratton; 1968. p. 108–23.

88   Sugerman AA. A pilot study of fluoropipemide (Dipiperone). Dis Nerv Syst 1964; 25: 355–8.

89   Sugerman AA, Herrman J. Molindone. An indole derivative with antipsychotic activity. Clin Pharmacol Ther 1967; 8: 261–5.

90   Goldstein L, Sugerman AA, EEG correlates of psychopathology. In: Zubin J, Shagass C, editors. Neurobiological Aspects of Psychopathology. New York: Grune & Stratton; 1969. p. 1–19.

91   Sugerman AA. Remembrance of drugs past. In: Ban TA, Healy D, Shorter E, editors. The Triumph of Psychopharmacology and the Story of CINP. Budapest: Animula; 2000. p. 78–81.

92   Hartmann E. Effects of psychotropic drugs on sleep: The catecholamines and sleep. In: Lipton MA, DiMascio A, Killam KF, editors. Psychopharmacology: A Generation of Progress. New York: Raven Pess; 1978. p. 711–28.

93   Hartmann E. The biochemistry and pharmacology of the D-state (dreaming sleep). Exp Med Surg 1969; 27: 105–20.

94   Hartmann E, Russ D, Oldfield M, et al. Dream content effect of L-DOPA. Sleep Res 1980; 9: 153–4.

95   Hartmann E. On the pharmacology of dreams and sleep (the D-state). J Nerv Ment Dis 1968; 146: 165–73.

96   Feinberg, I, Braun M, Koresko RL, Gottlieb F. Stage 4 sleep in schizophrenia. Arch Gen Psychiatry 1969; 21: 262–6.

97   Feinberg I, Koresko RL, Gottlieb G. Further observations on electrophysiological sleep patterns in schizophrenia. Compr Psychiatry 1965; 6: 21–4.

98   Feinberg I, Maloney T, Campbell G. Effects of hypnotics on the sleep EEG of healthy young adults: new data and psychopharmacologic implications. J Psychiatr Res 2000; 34: 423–8.

99   Feinberg I, Walker J, Price J, Price L, Floyd T, March J. Flurazepam effects on slow wave sleep: Stage 4 suppressed but number of Δ waves constant. Science 1977; 198: 847–9.

100   Feinberg I, Campbell IG, Schoepp DD, Anderson K. The selective group of GLu2/3 receptor agonist LY 379268 suppresses REM sleep and fast EEG in rat. Pharmacol, Biochem Behav 2002; 73: 467–74.

101   Velazquez-Moctezuma J, Gillin JC, Shiromani PJ. Effects of specific M1, M2 muscarinic receptor agonists on REM sleep generation. Brain Res 1989; 503: 128–31.

102   Gillin JC, Sutton L, Ruiz C, Golshan S, Hirsch S, Warmann C, Shiromani PJ. Dose dependent inhibition of REM sleep in normal volunteers by biperiden, a muscarinic antagonist. Biol Psychiatry 1991; 30: 151–6.

103   Moore P, Gillin JC, De Modena A, Seifritz E, Clark C, Stahl S, Rapaport M, Kelsoe J. Rapid tryptophan depletion, sleep electroencephalogram and mood in men with remitted depression on serotonergic reuptake inhibitors. Arch Gen Psychiatry 1998; 58: 201–2.

104   Landott H-P, Kelsoe JR, Rapaport MH, Gillin MJC. Rapid tryptophan depletion reverses phenelzine-induced suppression of REM sleep. J Sleep Res 2003; 12: 13–8.

105   Evans L, Kelsoe J, Rapaport H, Resovsky K, Sutton L, Gillin JC. Effect of rapid tryptophan depletion on sleep electroencephalogram and mood in subjects with partially remitted depression on bupropion. Neuropsychopharmacology 2002; 27: 1016–26.

106   Wu JC, Gillin JC, Buchsbaum MS, Hershey T, Johnston JC, Bunney WE. Effect of sleep deprivation on brain metabolism in depressed patients. Am J Psychiatry 1992; 149: 538–43.

107   Wu JC, Gillin JC Schachat C, Darnell LA, Fallon JH, Bunney WE. Sleep deprivation PET correlations of Hamilton symptom improvement ratings with changes in reactive glucose metabolism in patients with depression. J Affect Disord 2008; 107: 181–5.

108   Kety SS, Schmidt C. The nitrous oxide method for quantitative determination of cerebral blood flow in man: theory, procedure and normal values. J Clin Invest 1948; 27: 475–83.

109   Kety SS, Woodford RB, Harmel MH, Freyhan F, Appel K, Schmidt C. Cerebral blood flow and metabolism in schizophrenia.The effects of barbiturates, semi-narcosis, insulin coma and electroshock. Am J Psychiatry 1948; 104: 765–70.

110   Landau WM, Freygang WH, Rowland LP, Sokoloff L, Kety SS. The local circulation of the living brain: values in the unanesthetized cat. Trans Amer Neurol Assoc 1955; 80: 125–9.

111   Sokolov L, Reivich M, Kennedy C, Des Rosiers MH et al. The [^{14}C] deoxyglucose method for the measurement of local cerebral glcose utilization. Theory, procedure, and normal values in the conscious and anesthetized albino rat. J Neurochem 1977; 2: 897–916,

112   Reivich M, Kuhl D, Wolf A, Greenberg J, Phelps M, et al, Measurement of local cerebral glucose metabolism in man with 18 F-2-fluoro-2-deoxy-d-glucose. Acta Neurol Scand 1977; 56 (Suppl 64).

113   Phelps MF, Huang SC, Hoffman EJ, Selin C, Sokoloff L, Kuhl DE. Tomographic measurement of local cerebral glucose metabolic rate in human with [^{18}F] 2-fluoro-2-deoxy-d-glucose: validation of method. Ann Neurol 1979; 6: 371–88.

114   Sokoloff L. Per aspera ad astra. The road to metabolic mapping and imaging of local functional activity in the nervous system. In: Ban TA, Healy D, Shorter E, editors. Reflections on Twentieth-Century Psychopharmacology. Budapest: Animula; 2004. p.277–89.

115   Buchsbaum M, Ingvar DH, Kessler R, Waters RN, et al. Cerebral glucography with positron tomography. Arch Gen Psychiatry 1982; 39: 251–9.

116   Ingvar DH, Franzen G. Abnormalities of cerebral blood flow distribution in patients with chronic schizophrenia. Acta Psych Scandinavica 1974; 50: 426–62.

117   Buchsbaum MS, DeLisi LE, Holcomb HH, Kessler RM. Anterioposterior gradient in cerebral glucose use in schizophrenia and affective disorders. Arch Gen Psychiatry 1984; 41: 1259–66.

118   Andreasen NC, Arndt S, Swayze W. Cizadlo T, et al. Thalamic abnormalities in schizophrenia visualized through magnetic resonance image averaging. Science 1994; 266: 294–8.

119   Andreasen NC, Nasrallah HA, Dunn V, Olson S, et al. Structural abnormalities in the frontal sytem in schizophrenia. A magnetic resonance imaging study. Arch Gen Psychiatry 1986; 43: 136–44. 492–507.

120   Andreasen NC, O'Leary DS, Cizadlo T, Arndt S, et al. Schizophrenia and cognitive dysmetria: A positron-emission tomography study of dysfunctional prefrontal-thalamic-cerebellar circuitry. Proc Nat Acad Sci USA 1996; 93: 9985–90.

121   Weinberger DR, Berman KE, Zec RF. Physiological dysfunction of dorsolateral prefrontal cortex in schizophrenia I. Regional cereral blood flow (rCBF) evidence . Arch Gen Psychiatry 1984; 43: 114–24.

122   Goldberg TE, Weinberger DR, Berman KF, Pliskin NH, Poss MH. Further evidence for dementia of the prefrontal type of schizophrenia. Arch Gen Psychiatry 1987; 44: 1008–14.

123   Weinberger DR, Egan MF, Bertolino A, Callicott JH, Mattay VS, Lioska BK, Berman I. Neurons and the genetics of schizophrena. Biol Psychiatry 2001; 50: 825–44.

124   Wonodi I, Mitchell BD, Stein OC, Elliott LE, et al. Lack of association between COMT gene and deficit schizophrenia. Behav Brain Functions 2006; 2: 42–50.

125   Holzman PS, Proctor LR, Hughes DW. Eye tracking pattern in schizophrenia. Science 1973; 181: 179–91.

126   Holzman PS, Levy DL, Proctor LR. Smooth pursuit eye movements, attention and schizophrenia.. Arch Gen Psychiatry 1976; 45: 641–7.

127   Ban TA. Neuropsychopharmacology: the interface between genes and psychiatric nosology. In: Lerer B, editor. Pharmacogenetics of Psychotropic Drugs. New York: Cambridge University Press; 2002. p. 36–56.

128   Hartman PS, Kringlen E, Mathysse SW, Flanagan A, et al. A single dominant gene can account for eye tracking dysfunction and schizophrenia in offspring of discordant twins. Arch Gen Psychiatry 1988;45: 641–7.

129   Arolt V, Lencer R, Nolte A, Pinnow M, Schwinger E. Eye tracking dysfunction is a putative phenotype susceptibility marker of schizophrenia and maps to locus on chromosome 6p in families with multiple occurrence of the disease.. Am J Med Genetics 1996; 67: 564–579.

130   Longo VG, Von Berger GP, Bovet D. Action of nicotine and of the "gangliopleqique centraux" on the electrical activity of the brain. J Pharmacol 1954; 111: 349–59.

131   Bovet D, Longo VG. Pharmacologie de substance reticule du tonic cerebral. In: Proceedings of the 20th International Congress of Physiology 1956; 1; 306–29.

132   Longo VG. Experimental electroencephalography and its impact on neuropsychopharmacology. In: Ban TA, Healy D, Shorter E, editors. The Triumph of Psychopharmacology and the Story of CINP. Budapest: Animula; 2000. p. 33–7.

133   Longo V. Electroencephalographic Atlas for Pharmacological Research. In: Longo VG. Rabbit Brain Research. Volume 2. Amsterdam:Elsevier; 1962.

134   Killam KF. Studies of LSD and chlorpromazine. Psychiat Res Rep 1956; 6: 35–45.

135   Killam EK, Killam KF. The effects of psychotherapeutic compounds on central afferent and limbic pathways. Ann NY Acad Sci 1957; 66: 784–805.

136   Killam EK,Killam KF. Phenothiazine: pharmacologic studies. Proc Res Nerv Ment Dis 1959; 37: 245–65.

137   King ER, Unna KR. The action of mephenesin and other interneuron depressants on the brain stem. J Pharmacol 1954; 111: 293–301.

138   Killam EK. Pharmacology of the reticular formation. In: Efron DH, Cole JO, Levine J, Wittenborn JR, editors. Psychopharmacology. A Review of Progress 1957–1967. Washington: Public Health Service Publications No 1836; 1968. p. 411–45.

139   King EE. Differential action of anesthetics and interneuron depressants upon EEG arousal and recruitment responses. J Pharmacol Exp Ther 1956; 116: 404–17.

140   King EE. Differential action of anesthetic and multineuronal blocking agents on EEG arousal and recruitment responses evoked from the brain stem. Fed Proc 1954; 13: 375–6.

141   Killam KF. Pharmacological influences upon evoked electrical activity in the brain. In: Garattini S, Ghatti V, editors. Psychotropic Drugs. Amsterdam: Elsevier; 1957. p. 244–51.

142   Killam KF, Killam EK. Drug action on pathways involving the reticular formation. In: Jasper HH, Proctor LD, Knighton RS, Noshay WC, Costello RT, editors. Reticular Formation of the Brain. Boston: Little Brown & Company; 1958. p. 111–22.

143   Killam KF. Drug action on the brain stem reticular formation. Pharmacol Rev 1962; 14: 175–223.

144   Killam KF, Naquet R, Bert J. Paroxysmal responses to intermittent light-stimulation in a population of baboons (papio papa). Epilepsia 1966; 7: 215–9.

145   Weinberger SB, Killam EK. Alterations in learning performance in the seizure prone baboon. Effects of elicited seizures in chronic treatment with diazepam and phenobarbital. Epilepsia 1978; 10: 301–16.

146   Bradley PB, Elkes J. The action of atropine, hyoscyamine, physostigmine, and neostigmine on the electrical activity of the conscious cat. J Physiol (London) 1953; 120: 14–5.

147   Bradley PB, Elkes J. The action of amphetamine and D-lysergic acid diethylamide (LSD 25) on the electrical activity of the brain of the conscious cat. J Physiol (London) 1953; 120: 13–4.

148   Bradley PB, Elkes J. The effects of some drugs on the electrical activity of the brain. Brain 1954; 80: 77; 117–20.

149   Bradley PB. The central action of certain drugs in relation to the reticular formation of the brain. In Jasper HH, Proctor LD, Knighton RS, Noshay WC, Costello RT, editors. Reticular Formation of the Brain. Boston: Little Brown & Company; 1958. p. 123–49.
150   Bradley PB, Key BJ. The effect of drugs on arousal responses` produced by electrical stimulation of the reticular formation of the brain. Electroencephalog Clin Neurophysiol 1958; 10: 97–110.
151   Bradley PB. Methods and analysis of drug-induced behavior in animals. In: Bradley PB, Deniker P, Radouco-Thomas C, editors. Neuropsychopharmacology. Proceedings of the First Intarnational Congress of Neuropharmacology. Amsterdam/London: Elsevier Publishing Company, 1959, 11–19.
152   Bradley PB. A personal reminiscence of the birth of psychopharmacology. In: Ban TA, Healy D, Shorter, editors. The Triumph of Psychopharmacology and the Story of CINP. Budapest: Animula; 2000. p. 25–32. 153 Bradley PB, Mollica A. The effect of adrenaline and acetylcholine on single unit activiy in the reticular formation of the decerebrate cat. Arch Ital Biol 1958; 96: 168–86.
154   Delgado JMR, Hamlin H, Chapman P. Technique of intracranial electrode implacement for recording and stimulation, and its possible value in psychiatric patients. Conf Neurol. 1952; 12: 315–9.
155   Delgado JMR. Permanent implantation of multi-lead electrodes in the brain. Yale J Biol Med 1952; 24: 351–8.
156   Delgado JMR. Evaluation of permanent implantation of electrodes within the brain. Electroencephalogr and Clinical Neurophysiology 1955; 7: 637–44.
157   Delgado JMR. Physical Control of the Mind. Towards a Psychosocialized Society. New York: Harper & Row; 1977.
158   Aghajanian GK, Warren EF, Sheard MH. Lysergic acid diethylamide sensitive neuronal units in the midbrain raphe. Science 1968; 161: 706–8.
159   Aghajanian GK, Asher IM. Histochemical fluorescence of raphe neurons. Selective enhancement by tryptophan. Science 1971; 172: 1159–61.
160   Aghajanian GK, Cederbaum JM, Wang RY. Evidence for norepinephrine-mediated collateral inhibition of locus ceruleus neurons. Brain Res 1977; 136: 570–7.
161   Bunney BS, Aghajanian GW. Mesolimbic and mesocortical dopaminergic systems: physiology and pharmacology. In: Lipton MA, DiMascio A, Killam KF, editors. Psychopharmacology: A Generation of Progress. New York: Raven Press; 1978. p.159–70.
162   Bunney BS, Walters JR, Robert RH, Aghajanian GK. Dopaminergic neurons: effect of antipsychotic drugs and amphetamine on single cell activity. J Pharmacol 1973; 185: 560–71.
163   Aghajanian GW, Wang RY. Physiology and pharmacology of central serotonergic neurons. In: Lipton MA, DiMascio A, Killam KF, editors. Psychopharmacology: A Generation of Progress. New York: Raven Press; 1978. p. 171–84.
164   Bunney BS, Aghajanian GK. Dopamine and norepinephrine innervated cells in the rat prefrontal cortex: pharmacological differentiation using microiontophoresis techniques. Life Sci 1976; 19: 1983–9.
165   Bloom FE. Electrophysiological pharmacology of the single nerve cell. In: Efron DH, Cole JO, Levine J, Wittenborn JR, editors. Psychopharmacology. A Review of Progress. 1957–1967. Washington: Public Health Service Publications No 1836; 1968. p.355–74.
166   Bloom FE. Central noradrenergic system: physiology and pharmacology. In: Lipton MA, DiMascio A, Killam KF, editors. Psychopharmacology: A Generation of Progress. New York: Raven Press; 1978. p. 133–42.
167   Moore RY, Bloom FK. Central catecholamine neuron system: anatomy, physiology of the norepineph-rine and epinephrine system. Ann Rev Neurosci 1979; 2: 113–68.
168   Koob GF, Bloom FE. Behavioral effects of neuropeptides: Endorphins and vasopressin. Ann Rev Physiol 1982; 44:571–82.
169   Bloom FE. Neuropeptides and other mediators in the central nervous system. J Immunol 1985; 135: 743–5.
170   Hokfelt T, Bartfai T, Bloom FE. Neuropeptides. Lancet Neurology 2003; 2: 463–72.

CONTENTS

ABBREVIATIONS

A	adenosine
AchE	acetylcholinesterase
ACNP	American College of Neurpsychopharmacology
ACTH	adrenocorticotropic hormone
ADP	adenosine diphosphate
AIDS	acquired immunodeficiency syndrome
AMP	adenosine monophosphate
AP	Associated Press
APA	American Psychiatric Association
ApoE4	apolipoprotein E
APPA	American Psychopathological Association
ASPET	American Society for Pharmacology and Experimental Therapeutics
ASTP	army specialized training program
ATP	adenosinetriphosphate
AV	arterio-venous
AZT	zidovudine (azidothymidine)
BA	Bachelor of Arts
BAP	British Association for Psychopharmacology
BDNF	brain derived neurotrophic factor
BMA	British Medical Association
BP	behavioral pharmacology
BPRS	Brief Psychiatric Rating Scale
BP	British Pharmacological Society
BZ series	3-quinuclidinyl benzilate series
C	cervical
^{14}C	radioactive isotope of carbon
CBF	cerebral blood flow
CSF	cerebrospinal fluid
CINP	Collegium Internationale Neuro-Psychopharmacologicum
CNS	central nervous system
CO_2	carbon dioxide
COMT	catechol-O-methyl transferase
CPZ	chlorpromazine
CR	conditioned reflex
CS	conditional stimulus
CSF	cerebrospinal fluid
CT	computerized tomography

Cyclic AMP	cyclic adenosine monophosphate
D	dopamine receptor
D-sleep	dreaming state (REM) in sleep
D-state	dreaming state
DEA	Drug Enforcement Agency
DFO	diisopropylfluorophosphate
DNA	deoxyribonucleic acid
DND	discrete neurological deficit
DOPA	dihydroxyphenylalanine
DSM	Diagnostic and Statistical Manual series (of the American Psychiatric Association)
DSc	Doctor of Science
DST	dexamethasone suppression test
DT	delirium tremens
ECDEU	Early Clinical Drug Evaluation Unit
ECT	electroconvulsive therapy (electrically-induced seizures)
EEG	electroencephalography
EM	electron microscope
EMI	Electrical and Music Industries
ERP	event related potential
FASEB	Federation of American Societies for Experimental Biology
FDA	Food and Drug Administration
FDG	fluorodeoxyglucose
fMRI	functional magnetic resonance imaging
FSS	first signal system
GABA	γ-aminobutyric acid
GB-94	mianserin
GI Bill	Servicemen's Readjustment Act
G protein	guanine nucleotide binding protein
HLA	human leukocyte antigen
5-HT	5-hydroxytryptamine (serotonin)
5-HTP	5-hydroxytryptophan
HIV	human immunodeficiency virus
IBM	International Business Machines
ICI	Imperial Chemical Industries
ICT	insulin coma therapy
IMI	imipramine
IND	investigational new drug
IPEG	International Pharmaco-EEG Group
IRB	Institutional Review Board
IRP	Intramural Research Program

IUPHAR	International Union of Pharmacologists
JECT	Journal of ECT
K	potassium
LAAM	levo-α-acetylmethadol
L-DOPA	levodopa
LINC	Laboratory Instrument Computer
LSD	lysergic acid diethylamide
LY354740	eglumegad
M	muscarinic receptor
M 100907	[R-(+)-alpha-(2,3-dimethoxyphenyl)-1-[2-(4-fluorophenyl]-4-piperidinemethanol
MA	Master of Arts
MAO	monoamine oxidase
MAOI	monoamine oxidase inhibitor
Mass	Massachusetts
MCAT	Medical College Admission Test
MD	Medical Doctor
MDL 100907	M100907; ritanserin ($5HT_{2a}$ antagonist)
MDMA	3,4-methoxylenedioxymethamphetamine
MIT	Massachusetts Institute of Technology
MRC	Medical Research Council
MRI	magnetic resonance imaging
MS	Master of Science
MZ	monozygotic twins
Na	sodium
NAMI	National Alliance on Mental Illness (originally known as National Alliance for the Mentally Ill)
NARSAD	National Alliance for Research in Schizophrenia and Depression
NAS	National Academy of Sciences
NASA	National Aeronautics and Space Administration
NCDEU	New Clinical Drug Evaluation Unit
NE	norepinephrine
NHS	National Health Service
NIDA	National Institute on Drug Abuse
NIH	National Institutes of Health
NIMH	National Institute of Mental Health
NINDB	National Institute of Neurological Diseases and Blindness
NJ	New Jersey
NMDA	N-methy-D-aspartic acid
NMS	neuroleptic malignant syndrome

N_2O	nitrous oxide
NOSIE	Nurses' Observation Scale for Inpatient Evaluation
NPP	neuropsychopharmacology
NRC	National Research Council
NREM	non-REM (sleep)
NY	New York
NYU	New York University
PCP	phencyclidine (Sernyl)
PDR	Physicians' Desk Reference
PEG	pneumoelectroencephalography
Penn	University of Pensylvania
PET	positron emission tomography
PGH	Philadelphia General Hospital
PGO	ponto-geniculo-occipital
pharmaco-EEG	pharmaco-electroencephalography
PHS	Public Health Service
PNAS	Proceedings of the National Academy of Sciences
POMC	pro-opio-melanocortine
PR	Puerto Rico
PSC	Psychopharmacology Service Center
PTSD	post-traumatic stress disorder
RAF	Royal Air Force
RAS	reticular activating system
rCBF	regional cerebral blood flow
REM	rapid eye movement (sleep)
RNA	ribonucleic acid
RO5069	chlordiazepoxide
SBP	Society of Biological Psychiatry
SK&F	Smith, Kline & French
SKF-525A	ß-dimethylaminoethyl diphenylpropylacetate hydrochloride
SPECT	single photon emission tomography
SPEM	smooth pursuit eye movements
SSRI	selective serotonin reuptake inhibitor
SSS	second signal system
St.E	St. Elizabeths Hospital
TFDM	trifluoriodomethane
THC	tetrahydrocannabinol
TL	temporal lobe
TLC	Assessment of Thought, Language and Communication
TRH	thyrotropin-releasing hormone
TSH	thyroid-stimulating hormone

UC	University of California
UCLA	University of California Los Angeles
UCSF	University of California San Francisco
UK	United Kingdom
UMDNJ	University of Medicine and Dentistry of New Jersey
UP	University of Pennsylvania
UR	unconditional reflex
USD	University of San Diego
VA	Veterans' Administration
VMA	vanyllylmandelic acid
WAW	William Allanson White Institute
WCST	Wisconsin Card Sorting Test
WHO	World Health Organization

INTRODUCTION & DRAMATIS PERSONAE
Max Fink

The discovery of electricity in the mid-18th century was an exciting novelty that quickly led to its trials in medicine. By 1804 Giovanni Aldini and Benjamin Franklin had safely applied electric currents in melancholic patients, with seeming success.[1] The motor cortex was electrically stimulated and mapped by Edouard Hitzig and Gustav Theodor Fritsch in 1870.[2] Electric currents were observed from the surgically exposed brain of dogs in 1874 by English scientist Richard Caton.[3] A half century later, in 1929, the German psychiatrist Hans Berger reported electric rhythms from the intact head of humans.[4]

That electric rhythms permeated the brain brought brain structure and function front and center in the study of psychiatric illness. Mental and physical paradigms evoked passionate (although less bloody) arguments, similar to those that embroiled the wars of Catholics and Protestants. The conflicts between the somatic therapists and the psychoanalysts were deflected by a sudden enthusiasm for pharmacology that quickly dominated psychiatric practice and research. This science nurtured another compelling conflict, between those who believed that any animal regardless of its position in Nature's developmental tree was an appropriate model for man, and those who saw human pharmacology as *sui generis*.

Berger modified the electrocardiograph to amplify brain signals, renamed it the electroencephalograph, and gave neuropsychiatrist-clinicians reliable measures of brain functions in the living human. Studies of brain waves replaced neuropathology of the cadaver, the major tool of neuroscience in the 19th century. The EEG was first applied in seizure disorders and to the newly introduced treatments of electroshock, insulin coma, and leucotomy. When psychoactive agents arrived in the clinics, the proven science was immediately applied to studies of the new drugs. The clinicians who developed this science took two tracks: those who studied intact humans using scalp electrodes and those who implanted electrodes in animals to record cellular electrical activity.

Berger recorded oscillating currents from the scalp of patients, reporting changes with vigilance, drugs, seizures, sleep and age. His 1929 publication *Über das Elektroenkephalogramm des Menschen* was followed by 12 additional reports, the last in April 1938. Tragically, Nazi laws forced his discharge from his hospital position with the loss of his laboratory. His successful suicide followed soon thereafter.

The EEG is markedly altered during and after induced seizures (ECT) and insulin-induced comas (ICT). The changes are progressive and persist for weeks after the last treatment. Recordings are painless, can be repeated without risk, and are sensitive to moment-to-moment changes in brain physiology. In the 1950s, the EEG effects of ECT were reported by ACNP members *Herman Denber*, *Joel Elkes*, *Max Fink*, *Sidney Merlis*, and *George Ulett*, and it was relatively easy to apply the same instruments and methods to study the new psychoactive agents as they were introduced.

Presentations at international conferences in Paris in 1957 and the CINP meeting in Rome in 1958 introduced clinicians to the new science. In a memorable session in Rome, *Turan Itil* and *Dieter Bente* described their experience with chlorpromazine (CPZ) and imipramine (IMI) from their Erlangen laboratory. Each medication had distinguishable effects on EEG frequencies and amplitudes. CPZ elicited seizure activity, while IMI did not. After their presentation, *Max Fink* from New York City's Hillside Hospital described the same findings for the same medications. This immediate independent replication established a science of pharmaco-electroencephalography (pharmaco-EEG) that flourished for three decades.[5]

Human Pharmaco-EEG Studies

EEG laboratories were established in the asylums in the 1940s. The effects of amobarbital and amphetamines, the seizures of ECT, and the comas of ICT were already well described when LSD, then chlorpromazine, meprobamate and imipramine startled the clinicians with their effects in the severely ill.

Psychoactive agents – substances that cross the brain's blood-brain barrier and alter the fluids bathing brain cells – influence the frequencies, amplitudes, and patterns of waveforms in the resting EEG of alert subjects. The effects of chronic treatment and acute intravenous administration were catalogued in patients, and then in normal adult volunteers.[6] At first, these changes in electric patterns were considered specific for individual chemicals, but as more substances were studied, class-specific patterns emerged. The EEG effects of substances clinically identified as "antipsychotic" differed from those considered "antidepressant" or "psychostimulant." The EEG signatures of hallucinogens, deliriants, and anxiolytics added to the identifiable patterns. The chemicals that failed to influence brain electrical activity were found to be clinically inert, no more effective than placebos.[7, 8, 9, 10]

The first studies scanned paper records by page turning, seeking identifiable patterns and estimating the changes in frequencies and amplitudes using clinical guidelines. To assure quantitative measurements, electronic analyzers and then digital computer analyzer systems were developed and applied. *Max Fink* and *Turan Itil* used successively improving digital computer analyzers to measure changes in frequency and electric power and to measure drug effects across the spectrum of psychoactive drugs. Amplitude analysis was applied by *Arthur Sugerman* working with *David Engelhardt*, *Carl Pfeiffer* and *Leonide Goldstein*. *Sam Kaim* examined the effects of addicting substances, the minor tranquillizers, alcohol, opioids, and opioid antagonists. *Herman Denber*, *Sidney Merlis* and *Sidney Malitz* characterized different compounds in their clinical studies of new drugs in asylum populations.

Itil's laboratories in St. Louis and New York became the principal training center for the pharmaco-EEG leaders, with Werner Herrmann in Berlin, Bernd Saletu in Vienna, Masami Saito in Japan, Sevket Akpinar in Turkey, and Jovan Simeon in Ottawa as graduates. Their assays defined many new active drugs developed in their countries' laboratories.

The sleep EEG was the focus of interest of *Irwin Feinberg*, *Ernest Hartmann*, *Chris Gillin*, *Enoch Callaway* and *Turan Itil*. As a science of evoked electrical potentials developed, Callaway and Itil described the effects of psychoactive drugs on this measure of brain electrical activity.

The Association-Dissociation Controversy.

Did the EEG reflect differences in clinical changes with psychoactive drugs, or were the measured changes epiphenomena of limited clinical significance? Human studies reported different EEG patterns for antidepressant, antipsychotic and anxiolytic drugs. These observations were formulated in a hypothesis of the *association of EEG and behavior*. Pharmacologists working with animals reported no such relationship and formulated a dictum of *dissociation between the EEG and behavior*[11] Since much of industry support for pharmacology was based on the assumption that the studies could predict human effects, the clinicians' challenge required defense.

In the mid-1960s these different experiences were presented at meetings of the ACNP, CINP, and SBP. The pharmacologists described anticholinergic drugs as eliciting "sleep EEG" records with high voltage burst activity in dogs, cats, rabbits and monkeys when the animals were restless with running motor movements. Examined closely, these animals were not "sleeping" but were delirious. They were neither able to carry out normal commands nor to make their usual responses to sensory cues. Their EEG showed a preponderance of fast frequencies and a lack of patterned sleep stages. The *dissociation* reported by pharmacologists resulted from their limited range of observations – limiting measures of behavior to motor functions only, and limiting the EEG to visual measures of the superficial similarity between the EEG of normal sleep to that occurring in delirium.

The assumption of a direct predictive relationship between findings in animals and humans ignores species differences in brain chemistry developed during evolution. The brain is well shielded from external injury by the skull and meninges, and internally by a physiologic blood-brain barrier that excludes foreign substances from impacting brain cells. Each animal species is unique in what it allows through these barriers, a resultant of the millennia of differences in feeding patterns and exposures to toxic agents. Evolution influences the responsivity and tolerance of species to potential chemical toxins. A well-known example of species specificity is the opioid induction of excitement in felines but sedation in bovines and man. The ability of animal breeders to develop genetic lines that are either seizure-prone or seizure-tolerant to noise and light is a classic example that is commonly used in selecting animals for study. I observed the differential tolerance of beagles and setters to anticholinergic deliriants.[12] Species differences challenge the accepted pharmacology fallacy that animals are automatic surrogates for man. Species dissociations in psychopharmacology are a warning that predictions for humans from observations in animals are at the scientist's and society's hazard.

Laboratory Neurophysiology

By mid-century technological advances had made possible the recording of electrical oscillations from the brain surface, then clusters of cells, then from individual cells. Chemicals were first applied by massive dosing through oral and parenteral routes and then by localized administration to single or a few contiguous cells. After working with *Joel Elkes* at St. Elizabeths Hospital, *Floyd Bloom* developed microiontophoresis techniques to study drug effects in cats and rabbits. The metabolism of the cyclic AMP and noradrenaline systems, and the effects of endorphins, opioid peptides, alcohol, and almost all psychoactive chemicals were catalogued. His neuropharmacology texts describing these technical achievements became standard college teaching vehicles.

Extensive single neuron cell recordings by *George Aghajanian* at Yale, *Philip Bradley* in the UK, *Vincenzo Longo* in Italy, and *Eva* and *Keith Killam* at various sites in California extended the knowledge of the impact of various substances on the electrical firing rates of neurons. The effects of marketed psychoactive drugs on the multiplicity of neurotransmitterswere elegantly described, offering a confusing catalog of drug effects. The transmitter hypothesis of CNS active drug effects is elaborate but so far has been poorly related to human behavior.

The contributions of *Philip Bradley* are illustrative. After studying the human EEG with Grey Walter at Burden Neurological Institute, and describing the effects of LSD in man, Bradley turned to single cell recordings in animals. His examination of atropine and physostigmine led him to support the dissociation hypothesis of *Abraham Wikler* that the behavioral consequences of these drugs were not related to their EEG effects. He was the principal protagonist in the controversy that is defined in the conference proceedings published in 1968 cited earlier.

In addition to depth recordings, the Killams developed a baboon model of epilepsy, following the work of Robert Naquet of Marseilles. Keith Killam was active in computer analysis early in the era, building a LINC computer. Later he developed telemetry systems to monitor free-ranging animals. Studying flicker-evoked seizures, the Killams studied the relative potencies of anticonvulsants.

Brain Structure Imaging.

Soon after the discovery of X-ray, recordings pictured the skull and its defects. With air injected into the spinal canal as a contrast substance, shadows of the ventricles were seen (pneumoencephalography). Egas Moniz received the Nobel Prize in Medicine in 1949 for his introduction of lobotomy and of carotid angiography, a technique which illustrated the brain's vascular circulation. Both techniques were painfully invasive and risky. Computed tomography (CT), magnetic resonance imaging (MRI), and positron emission tomography (PET) offered less invasive images of brain activity. *Nancy Andreasen, José Delgado, Philip Holzman* and *Robert Kessler* applied these imaging systems to studies of patients.

Nancy Andreasen examined the relationship between symptom patterns of schizophrenic patients – the positive and negative symptoms – and brain structure. Her studies defined loss of brain structure as a marker for chronic psychosis.

Abnormalities in eye movements are found in the severe mentally ill. *Philip Holzman* reported abnormalities in pursuit eye movements and diminished vestibular nystagmus as a marker in psychotic patients and in their first-degree relatives. *José Delgado* began with animal studies of lobotomy and implanted electrodes demonstrating that stimulation of specific loci has identifiable effects on the animal's movement and attack behavior. His dramatic demonstration of control of a charging bull in a bullfight arena startled the public.

Prologue or Epilogue?

After more than eighty years of studies of the impact of chemical agents on the electrical rhythms in man what have we learned? The blood-brain barrier is selectively permeable to many chemical substances that alter the electrical and chemical activity of brain cells, thereby altering behaviors. These are the "psychoactive" substances. Chemicals that do not breach this barrier are inert in their influence on behavior.

Do the changes in electrical rhythms relate to the interpersonal behaviors that challenge clinicians? Apparently yes; some chemicals alter brain rhythms, motor behavior and vigilance in predictable fashions. In man, we associate the EEG changes with changes in mood, orientation, and thought, and we have achieved success in predicting clinical drug effects. Agents that affect the human brain are identified, and the variations in EEG rhythms are associated with specific behaviors. Agents that elicit hallucinations and delusions with clear orientation are distinguished from deliriants that affect thought as well as orientation, and from those that minimize or inhibit such thoughts. Some agents alter mood; some increase motor activity while others inhibit and sedate. For each behavior, the change in EEG pattern bears a predictive relationship.

Electrically-induced seizures produce slow frequencies and increase amplitudes of resting EEG rhythms. These changes are necessary accompaniments to assure behavioral change. Patients who do not show systematic EEG change do not change their behavior.[13, 14] Is the same true for antidepressants, anxiolytics or antipsychotics? We believe so, but we have lost both clinical and research interest in documenting this relationship.

Alas, the effects of drugs on brain rhythms are species sensitive. Explanations based on neurotransmitter measures, especially when these are recorded in animals, have not been helpful. Similarly, the connections between single cell recordings and human behavior have been elusive. The present brain imaging methods are too gross to define the subtle changes in behavior that interest psychiatrists and neurologists. Of these technologies – brain imaging, single cell recordings, EEG recordings in animals and in humans – we are left with the thought that the scalp recorded EEG is still the most promising instrument. Recordings using scalp electrodes are not invasive, are sensitive to moment-to-moment chemical and behavior changes, and may be repeated as often and for as long as the researcher wishes. The stories embedded in these interviews teach readers that more detailed studies are warranted. Sadly, pharmaco-EEG methods involving alert and sleeping patients are no longer active areas of inquiry.

Role of Government Research Support

The impetus for the rapid spurt in pharmaco-EEGstudies in the period of 1955 to 1985 came from extensive support from the National Institute of Mental Health (NIMH). The Federal government established the National Institute (later Institutes) of Health (NIH) in 1930 with a special program for mental health research added in 1946. The Clinical Center opened in 1953. Reports of dramatic effects with the new psychoactive drugs encouraged Congress to establish the Psychopharmacology Service Center (PSC), with Jonathan O. Cole as its first Director, in 1956. A PSC Clinical Committee supported clinical trials through an Early Clinical Drug Evaluation Unit (ECDEU) program begun in 1959.[15] The first awards went to recently established research units in the asylums. Generous funding encouraged more accurate assessments of behavior by multi-item symptom rating scales for clinicians and for patients, replacing global ratings of "improvement." The PSC was the first scientific unit at NIH to use digital computer technology to analyze their data. The first multivariate statistical analyses at NIMH examined behavior rating scales from the ECDEU unit at Hillside Hospital. ECDEU funding supported clinical studies of putative psychoactive substances.

NIMH funding targeted to psychopharmacology attracted a host of academic laboratory scientists like bees to pollen-laden plants. The laboratories in academia and industry were distant from patient populations so their interest necessarily shifted to animal models. The laboratory scientists extolled their sciences as royal roads to understanding brain functions and abnormal behavior. Animal behavior, physiology, and pharmacology were equated to that of humans. An enthusiasm for neuroscience encouraged more imaginative hypotheses and more grandiose promises attracting more and more research funding. Leaders of NIMH were drawn from the academy and the laboratory, not from the clinic. Attracted by imaginative and fanciful theories based on animal studies, research funding was directed to the laboratory neurosciences and clinical trials were starved for independent support By the mid-1980s the clinical ECDEU program disappeared. Industry marketing managers and the academic leaders of NIMH, many of whom had no active clinical experience beyond their student years, directed funds to multi-site collaborative studies with study design, data analysis, and reports managed from within the industry. These studies were designed to collect the minimal data needed to convince official government agencies to approve marketing of drugs. Tragically, no novel medication for the effective relief of a psychiatric illness has been developed in the past three decades.

In the 1970s, as new agents were tested, European clinicians described "golden placebos" – drugs with minimal effects on behavior and minimal risk of unpleasant effects. These included many of the SSRIs, atypical neuroleptics, and mood stabilizers. EEG studies of these substances failed to find more than minimal brain effects in patients or in volunteers at the recommended dosages and yet the marketing proceeded enthusiastically. The failure of pharmaco-EEG studies to define EEG and behavior profiles for these compounds was considered a black mark against the science. Sadly, the predictions that the drugs had minimal clinical effects proved accurate as the recent large government-sponsored multi-site studies of newly marketed agents find minimal differences compared to placebo.

Clinical research in the asylums was further inhibited by anger engendered by the medical experiments in Nazi Germany and Soviet Russia. Laboratories established in prisons for volunteer participation in medical trials were shut down. The few clinical research centers that sought to continue their studies found new barriers in Institutional Review Board (IRB) requirements. By the end of the 20th Century the freedom of exploration by individual clinicians that marked early psychopharmacology had ended.

These interviews reflect the excitement of the investigators as they explored the impact of CNS active substances on behavior. Neuroscience technology has moved on to awesome bio-engineering methods, seeking individual genetic variations in the response to psychoactive agents. Single cell and scalp recorded EEG are now historical footnotes, similar to the experiences with leeches and maggots. One can hope that the move away from clinical studies will reveal more of nature's secrets, although the history of how little has been learned from animals and imaging methods is not promising.

Dramatis Personae

The following pages introduce the Dramatis Personae of this volume in enough detail to give a framework for understanding their contributions.

Clinical Research

Max Fink graduated from New York University in 1945, and obtained residency training in neurology and psychiatry at Montefiore and Bellevue Hospitals in New York. A final year of residency at Hillside Hospital, a private sanitarium for the mentally ill in New York, was followed by a fellowship in clinical EEG. In 1954 he established the hospital's EEG Laboratory. When psychoactive drugs came to the hospital in 1954, he recorded the acute and chronic effects in patients. In 1959 he replaced hand measurements with the outputs of an electronic frequency analyzer. In mid-1962 he established the Missouri Institute of Psychiatry in St. Louis, creating a new laboratory for EEG analysis using digital computer methodology. An IBM 1710 system was programmed with the multivariate statistical analyses done at the mainframe computers at Washington University. Turan M. Itil came to St. Louis in 1964 and together they explored many psychoactive substances. Fink returned to New York in 1966 to develop a new pharmaco-EEG laboratory at the New York Medical College, using the state-of-the-art IBM 1800 system. Joined by Donald Shapiro they catalogued the effects of known and putative psychoactive substances. Interest in opioids, opioid antagonists, cannabis and cannabinoids broadened the known drug profiles. In 1972 he moved the pharmaco-EEG laboratory to the State

University of New York at Stony Brook, continuing his studies until 1985. In the late 1960s Fink revived his interest in ECT studies. In the 1970s he was a member of the APA Task Force on ECT, writing his textbook *Convulsive Therapy: Theory and Practice* in 1979. In 1985 he established the journal *Convulsive Therapy*, now *Journal of ECT* (JECT). In the last decade he has published detailed texts on the clinical syndromes of catatonia in 2003, and melancholia in 2006, in collaboration with Michael Alan Taylor. He also wrote a treatise on ethics in electroconvulsive therapy with the Swedish ECT expert and ethicist Jan-Otto Ottosson in 2004.

Enoch Callaway received his BA and MD from Columbia University in 1947, with residency training in Worcester State Hospital and the University of Maryland. His research career began with studies at the University of Maryland. He moved to the Langley Porter Institute at the University of California at San Francisco in 1958, where he continued his studies until retiring as Professor Emeritus. In 1975 he published *Brain Electrical Potentials and Individual Psychological Differences*, and in 1978 and 1979 he edited volumes of studies of human evoked potentials. Noch wrote about his own work as follows:

"I started out interested in neuroendocrinology and wrote my first paper on cortisol response to ECT. But I soon fell under the spell of Hudson Hoagland and electrophysiology. Charles Shagass got me intrigued by event-related potentials (ERP), and most of my research had to do with that. Unfortunately "what we thought would be a window on the mind turned out to be a peephole into a hall of mirrors." The work on ERPs and intelligence, however, has an offspring in Alan Gevins' and SAM Technology Inc. (a company that develops neurological tests of mental functions), while the work on schizophrenia goes on with David Braff and colleagues in San Diego. But I have been easily distracted, and unrelated topics including ethnobotany, parallel distributed processing networks, vitamins in autism, eye movement desensitization and reintegration, prevented me from single-minded pursuit of my main line of research! And then I have always loved seeing patients, which has taken its share of my energy. But all told, I have had fun, and I hope done more good than harm."

In 2007 he published a refreshing memoir of his experiences at the Worcester State Hospital in *Asylum: A Mid-Century Madhouse and its Lessons about Our Mentally Ill Today*. The hospital was the center of his endocrine and electrophysiology research with Hudson Hoagland as his mentor.

Turan M. Itil received an MS and MD from Istanbul University, moving to the University of Tübingen in Germany for residency training. In 1953 he joined the faculty at the University of Erlangen. With Dieter Bente and Fritz Flügel he explored the EEG effects of new psychoactive substances. He described the changes induced by chlorpromazine in 1954, reserpine in 1956, and sleep changes with these drugs in 1957. In 1958 he met Max Fink at the CINP meeting in Rome and they began an active collaboration. Itil moved to St. Louis in 1964 to set up the EEG Laboratory at the Missouri Institute of Psychiatry. Using digital computer methods in collaboration with Donald Shapiro, and studying acute effects in human volunteers, Itil developed a quantitative methodology to predict the clinical class of putative substances. The first studies on anticholinergic drugs in patients elicited differences from animal studies; he was a principal proponent of the hypothesis of an association of EEG and behavior. In 1972 he identified the antidepressant profile of GB-94, a new agent developed by Organon scientists in Oss, Holland. His description conflicted with predictions made by the pharmacologists. The research director at Organon, Jack Vossenaar, gambled on clinical trials and, after their success, mianserin was released for clinical use. The model of pharmaco-EEG prediction was verified. An interest in sleep EEG led Itil to study methods of automatic scoring of sleep EEG using digital computer methods. In 1974 he moved to New York Medical College and established the HZI Research Center Laboratory in Tarrytown. He continued to study and predict the application and dosage ranges of putative compounds, identifying active and inactive agents among natural and synthetic hormones, psychostimulants, and cognitive enhancers. He also established outpatient clinics assessing dementia by EEG and neuropsychologic methods. In addition to establishing the science of pharmaco-EEG, Itil was mentor for many leading pharmaco-EEG scientists: Werner Herrmann in Berlin, Bernd Saletu in Vienna, Masami Saito in Osaka, and Sevket Akpinar in Ankara. Itil retired in 1993.

Samuel C. Kaim graduated in medicine in Zurich, Switzerland. His interest in psychiatry was stimulated by the lectures of Hans Maier, successor to Eugen Bleuler. He continued in psychiatry at the Burghölzli in 1937–1938, in charge of ECT and ICT, and in 1938 he earned his passage to the United States, transferring a violent psychotic patient to New York. He developed skills in EEG beginning in 1950 at the VA Hospital in Coral Gables. His first studies were in Metrazol (pentylenetetrazol) activation to assess epilepsy and his first psychoactive drug study was a clinical and EEG trial of chlordiazepoxide (RO5069) in alcoholism, epilepsy, and status epilepticus. After presenting his work at the VA Central Office he was invited to assume the position of Chief of Psychiatric Research at the VA in Washington in 1960. During the Vietnam War he successfully lobbied the White House and Pentagon to recognize the extent and severity of substance abuse in returning veterans. He managed the VA cooperative studies of l-α-acetyl-methadole (LAAM) and after 21 years succeeded in getting it marketed. He next monitored the NAS studies of naltrexone in opiate dependence.

A. Arthur Sugerman graduated from Trinity College Medical School, Dublin, in 1952. He began his psychiatric education in Newcastle with Sir Martin Roth, migrated to the United States in 1959, and joined Carl Pfeiffer, Leonide Goldstein and Henry Murphree at the New Jersey Neuro-Psychiatric Institute in 1961. An early member of the NIMH ECDEU program, he established a pharmaco-EEG unit to assay new psychoactive drugs. His pharmaco-EEG reports began in 1963 with studies of deanol, phenothiazines, synthetic TRH, and numerous newly introduced substances during the next two decades. The principal tool of amplitude analysis was developed and applied to these studies. Later in Sugerman's career an interest in alcoholism research led to a position as Medical Director of the Carrier Clinic, and teaching at the UMDNJ-Robert Wood Johnson Medical School. In the last decades of his life he enthusiastically wrote book reviews.

After completing his BA at City College and MA at Swarthmore, *Irwin Feinberg* received his MD at New York University in 1955. His postgraduate work, in Boston, at NIMH and St. Elizabeths, was punctuated by a year in Paris with Prof. Jean Piaget. Since 1989, he has been Professor of Psychiatry at UC-Davis. His research career began with studies of critical flicker fusion, the Funkenstein Test, and disturbances in oxygen metabolism in dementia – this latter work in the NIMH laboratory of Louis Sokoloff. Feinberg soon found his interest in EEG and sleep EEG recording. He described the characteristics of the sleep EEG and relations to eye movements and memory. He catalogued the effects of amphetamines, barbiturates and benzodiazepines on the sleep EEG. He developed an effective automatic sleep EEG scoring system. Puzzled over the significance of sleep in behavior, he demonstrated the beneficial effects of sleep on immediate memory. In the 1980s his interest in the sleep of adolescents led to a hypothesis of the failure of maturation and loss of synaptic changes in young people as the basis for the symptoms of schizophrenia.

J. Christian Gillin, a leader in sleep research, graduated from Harvard College and received his MD from Case Western Reserve in Cleveland, Ohio, in 1966. After residency training at Stanford University, he developed an interest in the physiology of sleep at NIMH (1971–1982), moving on to the VA Medical Center at San Diego in 1982. His first research interest was in the transmethylation hypothesis of schizophrenia but his major contributions were in sleep studies, following his experiences with William Dement at Stanford. At NIMH Gillin's group replicated the finding of short REM latency as a marker of severe depression. They examined the cholinergic hypothesis for REM sleep developing the Cholinergic REM Induction Test using arecoline and physostigmine, and applied Delgado's Tryptophan Depletion Test for serotonin deficiency. Studying the effects of psychotropic drugs on sleep parameters, he reported the suppression of REM sleep by MAO inhibitors.

He was a leader in sleep societies and the founding editor of the ACNP journal *Neuropsychopharmacology* in 1987.

A dedicated researcher in the physiology of sleep, *Ernest Hartmann* obtained his undergraduate degree at the University of Chicago, MD at Yale University, and postgraduate studies at the Albert Einstein College in the Bronx, Massachusetts Mental Health Center in Boston, and the National Institute of Mental Health. He completed training at the Boston Psychoanalytic Institute. Since the early 1970s, Ernest has been on the faculty of Tufts University. He developed an interest in sleep early and has focused his studies on the mechanism of dreaming – its relation to EEG measures, physiology (as in relation to menstruation), effects of a wide range of psychoactive compounds, diet (as in the effects of l-tryptophan), and the behavioral changes following REM deprivation. Combining his experience in psychoanalysis and sleep, he became interested in what might underlie primary process thinking and defense mechanisms of psychotic illnesses. The first of his nine books was *The Biology of Dreaming* in 1967, followed by *The Functions of Sleep* in 1973, *The Sleeping Pill* in 1978, and *The Sleep Book* in 1987. A popularizer of sleep concepts, Ernest wrote *Boundaries of the Mind: A New Psychology of Personality* in 1991 and *Dreams and Nightmares* in 1998, as well as many chapters on sleep in various multi-author volumes on psychotropic drugs and compendia of physiology.

Growing up in New York City, *Philip Holzman* completed undergraduate work at City College, and then performed his military service between 1943 and 1946. Intrigued by Freudian philosophy, he returned to City College, and on the recommendation of Gardner Murphy, a leading psychologist, he went to the Menninger Foundation for psychoanalytic training. He received his PhD in experimental psychology at the University of Kansas in 1952, and became a training analyst, writing books on psychoanalytic technique and the Rorschach test. In 1968 he was attracted to Chicago by Daniel Freedman. He has spent a good part of his research career in studying vestibular nystagmus in schizophrenia, describing diminished nystagmus in catatonia, cataloguing smooth pursuit eye movements in schizophrenia, and finding no effect on it of psychoactive drugs.

Laboratory Research

Philip Bradley served in the British army for six years and went on to pharmacologic training. He studied nerve potentials in insects and then worked with Joel Elkes obtaining training in EEG recording with W. Grey Walter in Bristol. In various positions he studied the pharmacology of anticholinergic drugs in animals, the sedation threshold and effects of LSD; in man, and changes in EEG following lobotomy. He recorded the changes in EEG with psychoactive drugs but most of his laboratory work was in micro-recording of changes in single neurons, the technique of microiontophoresis. With other pharmacologists, notably Abraham Wikler, he concluded that the EEG effects of drugs were not associated with the observed behaviors. In 1966 he participated in a symposium on anticholinergic drugs in animals and man, edited the proceedings with Max Fink. It was published as *Anticholinergic Drugs*, volume 28 of *Progress in Brain Research*. Philip Bradley was a founder of the CINP, an active leader in the British Pharmacological Society, and Editor of *Neuropharmacology*.

Keith and *Eva Killam* worked together at various sites in California on electrophysiology in animals. Keith received a degree in engineering at Tufts University and after working in the Philadelphia laboratories of Smith, Kline & French (SK&F) he received his PhD in pharmacology at the University of Illinois, returning to SK&F to assay new pharmacologic agents. His major work was done at UCLA with Horace Magoun. He next moved to Stanford and in 1968 became chairman in pharmacology at UC-Davis Medical School. Eva King graduated from Sarah Lawrence College and obtained her PhD from Illinois, where she met Keith. They married in 1958, and collaborated in all their studies. Much of their work was in the EEG of seizure disorders, working on the relation to cognition with James Olds and E. Roy John. With Robert Naquet of Marseilles they developed the baboon model of inducing seizures by flickering light. They bred animals for ever-lower seizure thresholds, ending with animals that seized spontaneously. Keith was a grantee of the early computer analysis programs, first working with a home-built LINC computer. When ever-smaller recorders became available, he developed telemetry devices to study free roaming animals with digital computer processing of the EEG signals. In pharmacology, they studied the role of various drugs on GABA, seeking more effective anticonvulsants.

Vincenzo G. Longo obtained his MD in 1948. He was mentored by the Nobelist Daniel Bovet and for most of his professional life Longo has been at the Laboratory for Therapeutic Chemistry at the Istituto Superiore de Sanità in Rome. A classical pharmacologist, he studied the EEG effects of a wide range of psychoactive drugs, publishing an atlas of the effects of drugs on the EEG of the rabbit and a text in 1972, *Neuropharmacology and Behavior*. One early study showed that the tremors induced by nicotine were indistinguishable from those in Parkinson's disease. Longo describes his laboratory as tackling many problems at once, seeking to benefit from "evoked serendipity." Since 1985, as an officer of Italy's major research institute, he describes his work as mainly administrative.

After receiving his MD in 1958, *George K. Aghajanian* remained at Yale for his career and since 1974 as Professor of Psychiatry and Pharmacology. Working with Dan Freedman and Floyd Bloom early in his career and with

William Bunney later, he studied the effects of psychoactive drugs on brain metabolism, focusing early on serotonin metabolism. When he was called to military duty he was assigned to the Edgewood Chemical Laboratory studying anticholinergic compounds. His major contributions have been in recording electrophysiologic properties of monoaminergic neurons, first serotonin and then dopamine. He has described the role of serotonin metabolism in atypical antipsychotics and developed the concepts of metabotropic receptors. He is the winner of many awards.

Floyd E. Bloom received his MD from Washington University, St. Louis in 1960. Further training at Yale University in histochemistry and electron micros-copy led to his developing a Cytochemical Pharmacology Laboratory at St. Elizabeths Hospital. In 1975 he moved to the Salk Institute as head of the Center for Behavioral Neurology. In 1989 he again moved a short distance to become Chairman of the Scripps Research Institute. His early studies focused on microiontophoresis recordings from the locus coeruleus and raphé nuclei mapping the serotonin and norepinephrine systems. He next mapped neuro-peptide systems in the brain with interest in ß-endorphin and opioid peptides. Floyd is best known for his mentoring many neuroscientists, his textbooks and popular books on neurochemistry, and lately as the Editor of *Science*.

José Manuel Rodriguez Delgado received his MD in Madrid in 1942. As a medical student, Delgado was doing brain research in monkeys with Juan Negrin, an eminent physiologist and political leader, who had to leave Spain when Franco became Head of State. After the Civil War in the early 1940s, Delgado continued his brain research, implanting electrodes, recording electri-cal currents, doing ablation experiments in chimpanzees in Madrid. Seeking better laboratory conditions, Delgado came to Yale University to work with John Fulton. He stimulated animals by electricity, electromagnetic waves, and chemicals, carefully identifying functions of different brain nuclei. Delgado also worked with patients. He is best known for his control of animal behavior by remote stimulation of implanted electrodes. In 1971 he was invited back to Spain to start the Physiology Department at Autonoma University Medical School. In the past two decades, during the 1980s and 1990s he has become more philosophical, interested in the meaning of brain function, mind, and ethics. In 1969 he published a classic summary of brain research in *Physical Control of the Mind: Toward a Psychocivilized Society*.

Brain Imaging

Seymour Kety received his MD in 1940 from the University of Pennsylvania. In 1943 he joined the Department of Pharmacology of the University where he developed the method that was to become known as the Kety-Schmidt N_2O

method for measurement of cerebral blood flow and metabolism in unaesthesized humans. In 1948 Kety was appointed Professor of Clinical Physiology in the Graduate School of Medicine at the University of Pennsylvania. In 1951 Kety left UP to become Scientific Director of both the National Institute of Mental Health and the National Institute of Neurological Diseases and Blindness (later National Institute of Neurological Disorders and Stroke) of the National Institutes of Health. In 1957, he resigned from his post and in the years that followed he held various positions, e.g., Henry Phipps Professor and Chairman, Department of Psychiatry, Johns Hopkins University; Professor of Psychiatry, Harvard University; and Director, Laboratories for Psychiatric Research, Mailman Research Center, McLean Hospital. In 1983 he retired from Harvard and returned to the NIMH from which he retired in 1996. In 1972, with Max Fink and James McGaugh, he organized the Dorado Beach international symposium on the mechanisms of electroconvulsive therapy, published as the *Psychobiology of Convulsive Therapy* in 1974. Kety's research was instrumental in opening up the field of cerebral circulation and metabolism. Together with several collaborators he developed a functional method for measuring local blood flow that was to be developed further into functional brain imaging. Kety's research also contributed to providing evidence of a major genetic component in the etiology of schizophrenia.

Louis Sokoloff received his MD in 1946 from the University of Pennsylvania. In 1949, after a year of internship at the Philadelphia General Hospital, and two years of service in the army as Chief of Neuropsychiatry at a station hospital in Camp Hill, Virginia, Sokoloff joined Seymour Kety to study cerebral blood flow and brain metabolism in the Department of Physiology and Pharmacology at the University of Pennsylvania. In 1954, he moved to the National Institute of Mental Health and stayed as Chief of the Laboratory of Cerebral Metabolism until his retirement in 2004. Sokoloff is recognized for his research in the development of a methodology for the metabolic mapping and imaging of local functional activity of the nervous system in animals and humans.

Beginning as a scholar of English literature, *Nancy Andreasen* obtained a PhD in 1963 at the University of Nebraska and then an MD at the University of Iowa in 1970. Her postgraduate work has been at the University of Iowa. Early on she became interested in schizophrenia and when Iowa obtained a CT scanner and later an MRI, she identified the loss of tissue in chronically ill psychotic patients. Referring to her findings, she says:

"What I think this is telling us is that schizophrenia is not located in a specific part of the brain. The essence of schizophrenia is that it's a disease that affects many different parts of the brain that normally have to work together, that aren't working together well, are not communicating with each other. So, it's a disease of disconnections."

In recording the psychopathology of psychotic patients she developed scales to separately identify positive and negative symptoms. She has been often honored for her work, and has published more than a dozen books, including the popular volumes *The Broken Brain* (1984) and the *Brave New Brain* (2001). In the past decade she has been Editor of the *American Journal of Psychiatry*.

A graduate of Yale College and Medical School, *Robert Kessler's* postgraduate studies were in Ann Arbor and Boston and then at the NIH Clinical Center where he developed skills in brain imaging using positron emission tomography with various ligands. He moved to Vanderbilt University as Professor of Radiology in 1984. His extensive bibliography of studies in animals, patients and volunteer subjects reflects his efforts to identify brain lesions that are the basis for abnormal behavior. In his interview, speaking of his studies in mice, Bob noted:

"At some point, what we learn in animals has to be translated into humans and it's not going to be very straightforward; and if you just look, closely, at the anatomy of rats and mice and look at the anatomy of the human brain, that's a pretty long leap. Now, genetically, it may not be so long, but in terms of the actual circuitry, it may be bigger than people think. And, so, I began thinking at some point, we're going to have to examine the human condition to validate what we know in animals to make sure that it really applies."

Daniel Weinberger received his MD in 1976 from the University of Pennsylvania and completed his residency in psychiatry in 1977 at the Massachusetts Mental Health Center in Boston. He joined, in the same year, the Adult Psychiatry Branch of the Intramural Research Program of NIMH as Research Ward Director, and rose to become chief of the Clinical Brain Disorders Branch of the Program in 1986. In 2004, he was appointed director of the IRP's newly established Genes, Cognition and Psychosis Program. Weinberger is recognized for his research bridging neuroimaging and molecular genetics with cognition. He is the recipient of numerous honors and awards for his contributions, including the A.E. Bennett Foundation Award for Clinical Sciences of the Society of Biological Psychiatry in 1981, the Morton Prince Award of the American Psychopathological Association in 1984, ACNPs Joel Elkes Award in 1989, and the American Psychiatric Association's Foundations Fund Prize for Research in 1991.

REFERENCES

1   Bolwig T, Fink M. Electrotherapy of melancholia: The pioneering contributions of Benjamin Franklin and Giovanni Aldini. JECT 2009; 25: 15–8.

2   Shorter E. A Historical Dictionary of Psychiatry. New York: Oxford University Press; 2005.
3   Brazier MAB. A History of Neurophysiology in the 19th Century. New York: Raven Press; 1988.
4   Gloor P. Hans Berger on the Electroencephalogram of Man. Electroenceph Clin Neurophysiol 1969; 28 (Suppl): 1–350.
5   Fink M. Pharmaco-electroencephalography: A note on its history. Neuropsychobiology 1985; 12: 173–8.
6   Fink M. A Selected Bibliography of EEG in Human Psychopharmacology 1951–1962. Electroenceph Clin Neurophysiol 1964; 23 (Suppl.)
7   Fink M. EEG and human psychopharmacology. Ann Rev Pharmacol 1969; 9: 241–58.
8   Fink M. EEG classification of psychoactive compounds in man: Review and theory of behavioral associations. In: Efron D, editor. Psychopharmacology A Review of Progress 1957–1967. The Proceeding of the Sixth Annual Meeting of the American College of Neuropsychopharmacology. Washington: Public Health Service Publications No. 1836 Superintendent of Documents. US Government Printing Office; 1968. p. 497–507.
9   Fink M, Itil T. Neurophysiology of the phantastica: EEG and behavioral relations in man. In: Efron D, editor. Psychopharmacology A Review of Progress 1957–1967. The Proceedings of the Sixth Annual Meeting of the American College of Neuropsychopharmacology. Washington: Public Health Service Publications No. 1836. Superintendent of Documents. US Government Printing Office; 1968. p. 1231–40.
10 Fink M and Itil T. EEG and human psychopharmacology: IV: Clinical antidepressants. In: Efron D, editor. Psychopharmacology A Review of Progress 1957–1967. The Proceedings of the Sixth Annual Meeting of the American College of Neuropsychopharmacology. Washington: Public Health Service Publications No. 1836. Superintendent of Documents. US Government Printing Office; 1968. p. 671–82.
11 Bradley P, Fink M, editors. Anticholinergic Drugs and Brain Functions in Animals and Man. Amsterdam: Elseview; 1968.
12 Fink M. Pharmaco-electroencephalography. A`selective history of the study of brain responses to psychoactive drugs. In: Ban TA, Healy, D, Shorter E, editors. Reflections on Twentieth-Century Psychopharmacology. Budapest: Animula; 2004. p. 661–72.
13 Fink M. Convulsive Therapy: Theory and Practice. New York:Raven Press; 1979.
14 Fink M. Electroconvulsive Therapy. A Guide for Professionals & Their Patients. New York: Oxford University Press; 2009.
15 Fink M. A clinician-researcher and ECDEU: 1959–1980. In: Ban TA, Healy D, Shorter E, editors. The Triumph of Psychopharmacology and the Story of the CINP. Budapest: Animula; 2000. p. 82–92.

INTERVIEWEES & INTERVIEWERS

PART ONE

Electrophysiology and Neuropsychopharmacology

Clinical Research

MAX FINK

Interviewed by Jonathan O. Cole
San Juan, Puerto Rico, December 11, 1995

JC: I am Dr. Jonathan Cole. I'm a past president of the ACNP, and a founding member. I'm interviewing Dr. Max Fink* on behalf of the History Task Force. I was the subject of such an interview myself; though, it was so long ago that I forget exactly what happened. An outline was provided and I'm going to converse with Dr. Fink around issues raised in the outline. Dr. Fink is currently, I believe, a Professor of Psychiatry at the State University of New York at Stony Brook. Why don't you tell how you got into psychopharmacology and what happened thereafter?

MF: I finished medical school in 1945, and my recollection from my days at Bellevue was that I was already a psychopharmacologist as a student, mainly because we were involved in a number of projects, one of which was to treat catatonic patients with barbiturates. One professor treated some catatonic patients with amphetamine, and as a student I got involved. When I finished medical school, I decided to go into neurology and spent a couple of years training at Montefiore Hospital in the Bronx; then I decided to become a psychiatrist as well, and continued training at Bellevue. I then went to Hillside Hospital in January 1952. During that time, as it was the fashion in those days – this was 1947 to 1953 – I went to the William Alanson White Institute of Psychoanalysis. I became Board Certified in neurology in 1952, psychoanalysis in 1953 and psychiatry in 1954.

JC: Wow! Were there more double boarded people then than now?

MF: Most of the young people in my class who went into neurology took psychiatry as well, because neuropsychiatry was the discipline; the split between neurology and psychiatry occurred, I think, sometime in the nineteen fifties. So, many of my co-workers were neurology-boarded, and then boarded in psychiatry. It was customary. Psychoanalysis was the unique part. There were few of us who were willing to do that, mainly because my mentor at that time, Morris Bender, who was professor of neurology, would have asked me to leave. It was a very, very strong point of contention. Psychoanalysis was considered a "no no" for neurologists. So, I kept it a secret until I finished.

JC: Despite the fact that Freud was a neurologist before becoming a psychiatrist; although I guess, he never became a psychiatrist in one sense.

MF: Besides Morris Bender I had a lot of fine neurology teachers. Joseph Gerstmann of Vienna was one of the teachers at Bellevue, and a family

---

* Max Fink was born in Vienna, Austria in 1923.

friend. Bernard Dattner also of Vienna was another teacher, and also a family friend. At Bellevue, I had both Wortises, S. Bernard and Joseph, as teachers. One of the finest neurologists I ever met was Edward Weinstein. He was a psychoanalyst as well as a neurologist. In the William Alanson White (WAW) the leading figure was David McKenzie Rioch, the neuropsychiatrist.

JC: I knew David Rioch in Washington, sometime after.

MF: He was one of the teachers who ran a course at the WAW Institute. That was a strange situation; he taught in Washington, DC, and we used to go down Fridays and spend all day Saturday with him, every other week for about eight weeks, even though we trained in New York. At the same time I was taught by his wife, Margaret Rioch, and that was fun.

JC: Interesting. What did you do after all that training?

MF: I think that's important. In 1952, at Hillside, I was going into practice. That's what everybody did. Hillside had taught me how to administer ECT and insulin coma, and as I was finishing my year and completing my Neurology Boards, they asked whether I would work half time and run the insulin coma and ECT suites. So when I went into practice in late 1953, I worked at Hillside half time. But in 1953, as I was about to go into practice, there was an announcement that the National Foundation for Infantile Paralysis offered a Fellowship. I applied and was awarded it for twelve months. I spent my time learning EEG at Mount Sinai. I like to tell the story that I earned one hundred and fifty dollars a month as a Fellow. My rent in Manhattan was one hundred and fifteen dollars a month. So, my wife, my son, and I had to live on, literally, thirty-five dollars a month, plus the benevolence of my mother-in-law and my parents. When I finished in 1953, I began a practice and was in practice from 1953 to 1958. And then, NIMH stepped in.

After I learned EEG I went back to Hillside in 1953. They had no EEG device and I went to the head of the hospital, Israel Strauss, and said, "Would you like to have an EEG Service?" His response was, "How much does it cost?" I replied, "Five thousand dollars." And a few days later, I received a phone call that the Dazian Foundation had given me a grant for five thousand dollars for an EEG device. So we started to do EEGs at Hillside in 1954. At that point, NIMH announced a program for grant awards. I wrote a grant application to study the EEG during ECT, and also insulin coma. The number was M-927, among the first thousand applications, and that's how I began a research career.

Once I had the grant, Hillside Hospital set up a research program, and appointed me director. They were going to call me "Director of Research." I didn't like that. In those days, a term for people like myself was "Experimental Psychiatrist," because we administered the drugs or ECT or whatever. And, that's how it happened that my research career started. The grant was awarded and it was, at that time, in 1954, that Henry Brill held a meeting at Creedmoor State Hospital to present the first data on chlorpromazine from studies throughout the State of New York. He had set up studies in Marcy State Hospital, Buffalo; Manhattan State; Central Islip, and each of the local research directors, who became founders of the ACNP, presented. Joe Miller, the medical director of Hillside Hospital, sent me to the meeting. I listened to the presentations and was amazed at what I heard. When I came back, I called the Smith, Kline & French representative and said, "I want some Thorazine." I got it and we introduced chlorpromazine at Hillside. Within a short period, we had Thorazine, ECT and insulin coma studies. And, that's the way the Hillside program started. The next big step was LSD. Actually, LSD came just before chlorpromazine. We had LSD at Hillside. In those days, you may remember, some people thought that having an LSD experience would make you a better psychiatrist.

JC: Yes, indeed.

MF: So, I introduced LSD to Hillside and offered every resident an LSD experience, in the EEG laboratory – the whole routine. Then, when Thorazine became available, we were able to show that the EEG effects of LSD could be blocked by Thorazine. And that was one of the first papers of a drug interaction monitored by EEG. When, a few years later, imipramine became available, we were puzzled. We did the EEG of chlorpromazine; we did the EEG of imipramine and they were different. By that time, Don Klein had joined me; Max Pollock, Robert L. Kahn, and Nat Siegel were psychologists on the team, all of whom were being paid from M-927 or subsequent grants.

The next big step was your invitation to join the PSC Clinical Committee. In 1958, I was torn, because I was working every afternoon and evening as a practitioner, and couldn't do that, the research work and manage the ECT and insulin coma units. One day, Joe Miller asked, what would it take, to bring me on full-time? In those days, I was paid $12,500 annually from Hillside. I said, "Just double it and I'll give up my private practice." He agreed and my starting salary as Director of the Department of Experimental Psychiatry was $25,000 a year. For that, we could live very nicely in those days with no problem at all. And I've been a full time academic ever since. I've not gone back to private practice at any time.

The next big step came from you, which is why I've always said I'm very grateful. You invited me to be part of the PSC Clinical Committee, and it was there that I learned a great deal about clinical research. I met the people who were developing rating scales. It was a very exciting, interesting time. I remember being a site visitor and learning how people were doing things. I remember the meetings that started the NCDEU, held at different centers; two were held at Hillside over the first few years.

JC: At what point did you get into EEG?

MF: As I said, I learned EEG in 1953 at Mount Sinai Hospital in New York with Hans Strauss, and got my first grant to do EEG and ECT research in 1954. Then we did the EEG with chlorpromazine followed by all the interaction studies. In 1958, I met George Ulett who had built a device in St. Louis, which was an analog analyzer. For ten thousand dollars he'd build one for me. I went to you at NIMH, and you added ten thousand dollars, as a supplement to my grant. I got this analyzer and we began to do quantitative EEG in 1959. When I moved to Missouri in 1962, which is another story, George Ulett made money available for digital analysis and that's how we moved from the analog to digital computer analyses. That experience in quantitative EEG, went on from 1959 to 1985, when I stopped.

JC: But Turan Itil continued?

MF: Right. I met Turan in 1958. We were at the CINP meeting in Rome and that was an unusual experience, because he and I were on the program one after the other. We did not know each other, and it was just Max Fink, Turan Itil, EEG and chlorpromazine. I like to tell the story that I presented my slides and he got up and presented his slides and we could have presented the same talk, exchanging the slides, because we had the same findings. We've been very good friends ever since. When I moved to Missouri, I invited Turan to join us from Erlangen, Germany. He came in 1963.

JC: He continues to use quantitative EEG to work up new drugs.

MF: Well, he is one of the world leaders in quantitative EEG.

JC: Quantitative EEG had its run, and then sort of dropped out.

MF: That's an unfortunate story. Quantitative EEG is one of the best imaging methods that we have. You can tell whether a drug has a central effect, whether that central effect is of a certain type or not. For example, we learned to classify drugs and how to predict what a psychotropic drug would do. We learned that if you have a patient, for example, whose reaction to a psychoactive substance is unusual, that person is not having the same brain effects due to the drug that others have. Turan has used this methodology to explain what is known as therapy-resistant psychosis and therapy-resistant depression. There are people to whom you give large doses of the drug, and they don't have any EEG effect, and therefore, they don't have the behavioral effect. Actually, if you want to talk about EEG quantification, the big issue in the 1950s was whether or not there was a relationship between the brain changes and the EEG changes and behavior. You remember Abraham Wikler?

JC: Yes

MF: Abe had published a paper in 1952, in which he said, quite clearly, that there was dissociation between the EEG and behavior. Now, this was work done in dogs. Soon thereafter, in the next four or five years, there was a series of papers in pharmacology journals, each of which argued that the EEG and behavior are dissociated. However, by 1961, I, Turan Itil, George Ulett, Joyce Small and Charles Shagass, were convinced that, in man, the EEG and behavioral response to psychoactive drugs were correlated. You could predict what the behavioral consequences were of a substance or of a treatment like ECT, if you examined the EEG measures. By 1966, we had conferences on EEG association or EEG dissociation. The 1966 conference was published by Elsevier in 1968 in *Anticholinergic Drugs and Brain Functions in Animals and Man*. That was one of my first books, which I edited with Philip Bradley.

JC: How did you get oriented toward ECT?

MF: I did ECT as a medical student.

JC: You are known, at least in some quarters, as an expert on ECT around the world.

MF: Actually, in my lifetime, I was the first in the research world who was both a psychopharmacologist and an electroencephalographer. In 1966, I became a drug abuse specialist but went back to ECT in 1967. Anyhow, ECT was an experience I had in medical school, but paid no attention to. On January 2, 1952, however, when I arrived at Hillside as a psychiatric resident, the medical director picked me and said, "Come with me." We went to the ECT suite and he showed me how to give ECT, and after he treated three or four patients, he walked out and left the rest for me to do. From that time on, I was the resident in charge of ECT at Hillside.

JC: Well, in the medical model, you "See one, do one, teach one."

MF: That's exactly what happened to me. At the same time I didn't realize ECT was in one corner of the suite while down the hall was the twenty-two bed insulin coma unit. A few days later the medical director said, "Now, you're in charge of insulin coma, as well." One of the first things we did in 1954 was set up a random assignment study of patients to receive insulin coma or chlorpromazine; thirty patients in each cell. In 1958, we published a report that Thorazine did as well as insulin coma, was safer, less expensive, and easier to use. Safety was the most important issue, because insulin coma has a death rate of about 2% of patients treated; so we replaced insulin coma with chlorpromazine. Also, in one of the most important early studies at Hillside, supported by NIMH, we studied

EEG and ECT; we measured neuropsychological test performance, language behavior and the effect of Amytal (amobarbital) on the EEG and speech. All of that was published, between 1955 and 1960. By the late 1950s, early 1960s, it became obvious that imipramine, chlorpromazine and all the other drugs essentially replaced ECT.

When I moved to Missouri in 1962, I stopped doing ECT. The only reason I went back to it in 1967, was because a young man came to me one day, who was a resident at New York Medical College, which is where I went after my Missouri experience. He wanted to do a study of unilateral-bilateral ECT. That young man was Richard Abrams and together we did a unilateral-bilateral study. We also did a multiple monitored ECT study in 1970–71.

The thing that intrigued me was how does ECT work? I went to NIMH and said I wanted to run a meeting on the mechanism of action of ECT. They suggested that I should have Seymour Kety as co-director of that meeting. Seymour and I met and he said that we should also have a third director; and they invited Jim McGaugh from UC Irvine. The three of us met with NIMH in Washington in 1971 and set up the meeting, held in 1972, on the Mechanism of Action of Convulsive Therapy. The presentations of the conference, held in Puerto Rico at the Dorado Beach Hotel, were published in 1974 in *Psychobiology of Convulsive Therapy*. That really started me to thinking about mechanisms of action. In the middle seventies, you may remember in 1975, 1976 and 1977, we suddenly got interested in neuroendocrines, mainly because of the TSH response to TRH and the dexamethasone suppression test. In 1978, I set up a set of studies at the VA in Northport on ECT and TSH response to TRH and DST, published that material in 1979, and wrote a paper on the "Neuroendocrine Theory of ECT" with Jan-Otto Ottosson of Sweden.

By that time something else had also happened. In 1975, the APA asked me to be a member of the APA Task Force on ECT and I spent three years, from 1975 to 1978 on that. Suddenly, I was one of the nation's experts on ECT. I didn't start that way. It was because I spent three years learning the stuff. In 1978, we published the Task Force report, and then in 1979, I had learned enough to write a textbook. My textbook on ECT appeared in 1979. It was very well received. As a matter of fact, in 1980, it received the Anna Monika Award, and that was a shot in the arm so I've continued my interest in ECT ever since.

By 1985, we were aware that we needed some better education about ECT. After a plenary lecture at the CINP congress in Florence, Italy, the publisher of Raven Press, Alan Edelson, asked me to edit an ECT journal for his company. I created the journal *Convulsive Therapy* and ran that quarterly for nine years. I stepped down as editor two years ago and turned it over to Charles Kellner. In 1987, the APA set up a second Task Force on ECT and invited me to be a member. And so, I've been active in, and written extensively on ECT; I treat patients with ECT, and I'm best known by most people for being an ECT expert. But it's the fourth or fifth of my lives; I've done other things.

JC: You've done a lot.

MF: The only thing I'm sorry about is that I've failed to convince the psycho-pharmacology world that ECT is a reliable, effective, and useful way to change brain function and behavior. It is the brain function and behavior relationship that is, in my mind, the central part of psychopharmacology. Every one of the psychotropic drugs that are effective is because they change brain function, and whether you get involved with the neurohumors, the receptors or the neuroendocrines, it is the totality of brain function that's changed. I've been very much disappointed, that societies like the ACNP and the Society of Biological Psychiatry, have turned their backs on ECT and don't see it as a very effective central mechanism for changing brain function in a therapeutic way. Indeed, it has an efficacy which is often better than the drugs available for certain illnesses.

JC: ECT, certainly, I think, is coming back in frequency of use. I don't know whether there's any good data on it, but . . .

MF: Oh, there is.

JC: The hospitals I'm familiar with in Boston, anyway, used to give three or four people ECT on a Monday, Wednesday and Friday morning and they're now giving between twelve and twenty ECTs. Sometimes they're overflowing and giving it also on Tuesdays and Thursdays. It might be due partly to managed care, but I think more people are realizing that there are patients who like it better than other treatments and are using it because it does work.

MF: It's also a wonderful theoretical model, because the actual measurement of what happens to the brain is quantitative. You give one seizure, two, four or whatever you wish, and don't have to worry about administering drugs, wondering what percentage gets to the brain. You don't have to worry about the first pass effect and how much is destroyed in the liver or conjugated and put out in the urine. And you do not have to worry about compliance. You know exactly what you've done. You know when you've done it, you have time relations that are superb, and you have the EEG which traces every effect during the seizure and, then, during the course of the illness, measures the inter-seizure EEG. The EEG is a very wonderful tool.

JC: One of the thing I've wanted to be able to do and nobody, I think, including Turan, has done, is to get EEGs on people before and after they start to go on medication and see what happens. I kept thinking that a forty-eight hour EEG might well predict who's going to get better and who isn't. My timing may be wrong.

MF: No, actually, I think Turan has done that. He has a set of experiments in which he gave an IV dose of a drug, an IV dose of a second drug, and by measuring the EEG he showed that those who have the major EEG change have the better therapeutic effects.

JC: Those are the ones in whom the drug is going to work.

MF: And his data are very compelling. It's a sad thing that this and other societies have put aside the EEG.

JC: Once in a blue moon they will have a study group or a special day, but it's not a core event in the program.

MF: It used to be. In the first decade of the ACNP we had sessions on EEG as a regular feature. It was an important part of the work, just like we had neuropsychology sessions.

JC: I think you need people to keep pushing, which is part of the problem. I'm no longer organizing sessions here. I've enough projects without trying to establish groups to do this. How did Taylor and Abrams come to do the work with you at New York Medical College?

MF: Taylor and Abrams were my residents. They were the two most brilliant residents I've ever had. Taylor, as a resident, replicated the Pitts and McClure experiment, the IV administration of lactate to stimulate a panic attack. And then he applied to NIMH, received the grant, but the Navy called him. The grant was put in abeyance but when he got back, he no longer went back to that research. He and Abrams did superb studies in mania and catatonia. They showed the signs of catatonia to be more prevalent in mania than in schizophrenia and more prevalent in depression than in schizophrenia. They published that work in 1976 and 1977. Abrams had started doing ECT research with me in 1967. Eventually, he's become the author of a dominant ECT textbook. His book has replaced mine, since I wrote mine in 1979 and have never rewritten it. Taylor and Abrams are still active.

JC: One of the byproducts of your insulin coma and Thorazine study was that I worked for about seven years trying to get somebody to fund an insulin coma research award to see whether failures on standard antipsychotics would benefit from insulin coma.

MF: Those of us who've done insulin coma work are chagrined by the fact that this wonderful technique, offering an opportunity to study glucose metabolism, brain function, and a whole host of variables, was replaced prematurely. Insulin coma has never had a chance again. It's really a very dangerous procedure. In the Hillside experience, on average, we lost by death two patients a year and that's a bit much.

JC: I heard that glucagon would prevent that. I'm not sure that's true.

MF: Oh, there were many things that we tried, and it was an interesting experience in those days. The way people died was that they went into prolonged coma that was eventually fatal in some. One or two deaths we had at Hillside were thought to be cardiovascular.

JC: It's probably just as well that I couldn't get it funded and resurrected. I think we've covered a lot of the things. I know you were giving courses on ECT, because we talked about that recently. I'm sure a lot of psychiatrists get through their residency without seeing ECT or, at best, seeing three or four treatments. So my question is what credentials you should have to take over an ECT service?

MF: I'm asked a great deal about ECT training and give a lot of lectures. I travel around the country. I've recently helped re-establish ECT in Uruguay, in Holland and in France. It's been a lot of fun! I would say the most important things that I've done, that I'm proudest of, is that I have been a clinician who spent most of my time treating people, and I've applied quantitative methods and good methodology in studies, first of EEG and psychopharmacology, then narcotics, opioids, and narcotic antagonists.

We didn't talk about my marijuana/hashish experience in Greece. For a couple of years I had a contract from NIMH, before NIDA, to do a study of cannabis. We took US marijuana and US THC-Δ-9 to Athens and brought Greek hashish to New York. We compared the effects of hashish, THC-Δ-9 and marijuana on EEG, on behavior, psychological tests and language. It was a fascinating experience, and demonstrated quite clearly, that marijuana does change brain function acutely and chronically. Tolerance develops and withdrawal does occur. In many ways, it is another central nervous system drug to which one develops tolerance and changes in behavior.

JC: Do you have any feeling about claims that marijuana does things to at least some people with AIDS that is not done by THC?

MF: Not at all. It's obvious that marijuana and hashish have many more substances in them than THC-Δ-9, a single purified extract. There are other active ingredients in marijuana, and if some people say that marijuana is broader in its effect than THC-Δ-9, they are probably right. The problem is we don't have the kind of experience to justify that conclusion.

JC: In the kind of things you measured marijuana was markedly different from hashish?

MF: Well, hashish differs in the sense that intravenous THC-Δ-9 did not actually replace the effects of smoked hashish. It was a different experience, but the EEG effects were the same; they were in the same direction, but quantitatively they were much less with THC. We could not relate exactly the THC-Δ-9 content to the amount in the hashish, but you would never do that exactly.

JC: You also worked with heroin. Would you like to say anything about that?

MF: It's important to tell people that there was a time in the United States, when it was legal for physicians and researchers to get heroin and administer it to patients. We administered heroin and measured the EEG effects. We did blockade studies with cyclazocine, a narcotic antagonist. When naloxone was first introduced by a company in Long Island, one of the first samples was given to us at New York Medical College because we were known for doing research in that area. We administered naloxone to our volunteers and then to each of us, and found that by itself it did not do anything. But it was a direct opioid antagonist. That was an interesting experience. We did work with l-α-acetyl-methadole (LAAM), and also with methadone. That was another piece of psychopharmacology that isn't ordinarily included in today's psychopharmacology culture. People no longer talk about the narcotics. They put that aside. It's another field, just like EEG is another field.

JC: Parenthetically, I'm currently undergoing my first malpractice suit for giving buprenorphine to a patient for depression. The drug certainly worked. This lady I gave it to spent a year and a half in bed; then after I started treating her wih buprenorphine she got a job within two weeks. But she also immediately became obsessed about being physically dependent on the buprenorphine. I thought it was better that she was working, whether she was or wasn't dependent. Anyway, sooner or later she signed herself in somewhere and did not have any withdrawal symptoms when taken off buprenorphine. Then she started snorting heroin after discharge. I was no longer taking care of her at the time. Who knows, I may end up in court yet.

MF: The buprenorphine EEG profile is that of a narcotic antagonist, even though it has agonist properties. It is primarily an antagonist that has the profile of tricyclic antidepressants, and therefore, your use of buprenorphine as an antidepressant is justified by the EEG model as a predictor of treatment effects.

JC: Actually, I got the idea of using it from a German study.

MF: In the past twenty years I have been defending doctors in cases in which patients have developed tardive dyskinesia. Let me tell you something else I've done lately. A clinician experimentalist has unique opportunities to use his skills. When we treat patients and see something unusual that is an opportunity. That was how Roland Kuhn discovered imipramine. In 1987, I was called to see a patient who was in a manic delirium, and at the same time, she was suffering from lupus erythematosus. I took one look at her and suggested the way to stop her delirium was to give her a few ECT. Of course, the internist said, "No"; the family said, "No." Everybody objected, but five weeks later, on a Friday afternoon, they called me and said, "Now, you can treat her." We gave her ECT and she recovered. At the time she was catatonic, rigid, mute, withdrawn and had to be tube and IV fed. Since that time, we've begun studying catatonia, and identified that catatonia is present, as Taylor and Abrams had described, in patients with affective illness, more often than in patients with schizophrenia. In 1990, I wrote an article with Mickey Taylor, arguing that catatonia should be treated as a separate entity in DSM-IV. We sent it to the DSM-IV committee. They actually changed DSM-IV by adding a new category 293.89 as "catatonia secondary to a medical condition."

JC: Now there's a category for it?

MF: There is now a category for "catatonia, secondary to a medical condition." What is important is that catatonia is very responsive to ECT. Indeed, the first patient in whom seizures were induced pharmacologically, on January 23, 1934, was a catatonic patient. He had been mute and required tube feeding for four years. The first one getting ECT in Rome in 1938 was a catatonic patient. And so catatonia is a different entity than schizophrenia, which doesn't ordinarily respond well to ECT. We've just written a few papers on catatonia, and I'm very excited. This is a whole new life for me. It is beyond the EEG and even beyond conventional ECT.

JC: Do you think there are catatonics now showing up, or are we just recognizing them better? I think I've seen more catatonics in the past five years than I have seen previously.

MF: I think what we're recognizing is that catatonia is a syndrome; it's a motor syndrome in psychiatry. As soon as a patient comes in with psychosis, they're given neuroleptics and that tends to squelch the syndrome. In some patients, it makes it much worse and we call that syndrome the Neuroleptic Malignant Syndrome (NMS). The NMS Syndrome is a malignant form of catatonia and it should be treated as such. That's something that will appear in the next issue of *Biological Psychiatry*.

JC: Which I finally subscribed to, after forty years. Good. I think that's about all I've got. Anything else you would like to say for the record? I think we've covered most you've done.

MF: What I would like to say as a historical note is that starting off as a clini-
      cian and doing experimental work has been quite rewarding. I am rather
      pleased about the kind of life I've had. One of the questions is, am I happy
      the way things turned out? I am. Actually, I've refused to quit work, even
      though I'm going to be seventy-three in January. I feel that teaching and
      doing clinical work is important. I think that the experimental approach to
      clinical work has been a marked and added advantage. I have asked a
      number of questions of a theoretical nature, and I think we have learned
      a great deal about EEG and drugs. We are now involved with develop-
      ing a GABAergic theory for catatonia. I'm not sure where that's going to
      go, as we're still trying to collect some data. But the application of clini-
      cal experience, experimental paradigms, quantification, which I think is
      terribly important, and measurement; each of these are very satisfying. I
      think if somebody listens to this, it will be important to note that the stu-
      dents we've had, have been very important to me. And the fact was also
      important that people like yourself are willing to support the nutty things
      that we wanted to do. It's critical that society recognizes young investiga-
      tors. One of the main reasons why I got into a research career was that
      I presented a paper at the Society of Biological Psychiatry in 1958, and
      received the first A.E. Bennett Award.

JC: Oh, my goodness.

MF: As a result of that, the people at Hillside thought, well, this is great.

JC: Gee, you must be doing something great. . . .

MF: I must be doing something great. The NIMH support, the Grant, M-927, I
      received to study EEG effects of ECT in 1954 was very important for me,
      it had an important effect on my life.

JC: Good. You may be pleased to know that my son is an attending at
      St. Elizabeths, and he covers the ECT service when the ECT guys are on
      vacation.

MF: There is one other question that they want you to ask me and that is, what
      do I see as happening in the next five years?

JC: Oh, dear. At the past presidents' lunch, they raised the question that Fuller
      Torrey is claiming that he's analyzed the grant program of the NIMH and
      decided that eighty percent of the grants fall outside the mission of the
      Institute and should be farmed out to the National Science Foundation
      and Neurology Institute or some place. Who knows where that will
      end up?

MF: Without trying to be critical, the reality is that somewhere in the 1970s,
      American psychiatry adopted this neuroscience approach. The Society
      for Neuroscience was very successful in the late 1960s, when it was cre-
      ated. Molecular neuroscience has dominated our field during the past

decades, and not only in this society, but also the Society of Biological Psychiatry and the American Psychiatric Association; they've all been contaminated by it. What I see, at the present time, is that we have missed, in this society, what we were originally brought together for. The original group consisted of psychiatrists, psychologists and laboratory scientists. And, if I remember correctly, Jon, it was one-third, one-third and one-third in the original group.

JC: Yes.

MF: I'm not sure how long ago but the meetings and the intent of this group to study the effect of chemicals on the human mind has changed. Somewhere chemicals in the animal took over. We have, literally, lost the human being in this society. It sounds like sour grapes. It's not; it is merely as I see it.

JC: I think it's true; there is usually, in any half a day, one session I have some interest in. There used to be a choice of three or four and I'd have to decide which one I wanted to go to. From George Zubenko's talk yesterday in my honor I didn't understand a word he was talking about, and I wasn't sure whether I wanted to or not. I mean, it was gene expression and what not.

MF: Well, I think your session yesterday was in the old style. The only problem was that they didn't give me and others a chance to raise some questions. But I would say, in the next five years, this society will either be changing direction or become a molecular science society that is going to lose all the clinicians.

JC: They're going to go to Don Klein's and they're going to Paul Wender's.

MF: The neuroscientists are rather glib about schizophrenia, about all the terms that we use in clinical psychiatry, and that's unfortunate. Schizophrenia is a complex disorder and it's not easy to diagnose it, and it's not easy to follow its course, and it's not very stable. It's hard to know the difference between manic-depressive insanity, or a bipolar disorder and schizophrenia. And, what's going to happen in the next few years? If the clinicians bring themselves together, and maybe with Fuller Torrey, urge that clinical rather than laboratory work is the core issue be supported, then we might come back. If not, I think we will have to have a new explosion, a new interest somewhere, but it will not be here.

JC: You may well be right. Schatzberg and I are rewriting our *Handbook on Clinical Psychopharmacology* with a new guy named Chuck DeBattista. He is doing about a third of the work and getting some money for it. I was both amused and horrified when I was reading what must be his section, on Mood Stabilizing Drugs; he's got about four pages on all we don't know about how lithium works. I'm not sure it's worth putting four pages into second messengers and calcium channels when we really don't know how they work. It's unclear how to apply the fantasies, the sort of metapsychopharmacology that he's propounding. By trying to be more scientific than we can be, it's causing confusion.

MF: There is a very popular book published right now. Gates, the multi-billionaire, the head of Microsoft, has written a book. He tells a story about the difference between hardware and software. He recognized that hardware had a future, which expanded and expanded, but that software was the future where things really mattered, in terms of developing the computer revolution. The chemistry of the brain is clearly the hardware. The things that psychiatrists used to deal with and still deal with, are broader than the hardware. We can go and do all the hardware stuff that the scientists are telling us, but ultimately, it's the human mind. It might sounds negative, but it's the human mind and it's the human expression that really matters in psychiatry, and is the basis for psychopharmacology and the place where we should look. I will stop there. Thank you very much, Jon.

JC: I read another book that fascinated me. It was a lovely description of a bipolar patient's way through life, all the shenanigans she and her psychiatrist went through, trying to get her to take lithium. He was trying to give her too high a dose or one thing or another, but the issue, she devoted thirty pages to, was the fact that lithium worked. For a good old fashioned manic, having lithium work was a problem. When you're used to dancing through the rings of Saturn and somebody tells you, "My God, you look normal today," it sounds like an insult.

MF: It's a good book. Unfortunately, she is too defensive. Anyway, thanks very much, Jon.

JC: Thank you.

ENOCH CALLAWAY III

Interviewed by Thomas A. Ban
Acapulco, Mexico December 13, 1999

TB: This will be an interview with Dr. Enoch Callaway* for the International Archives in Neuopsychopharmacology of the ACNP. It is December 1999. We are at the annual meeting of the College. I'm Thomas Ban. You have been involved in neuropsychopharmacology since the field was born. Could we start with your recollections about the introduction of chlorpromazine in the United States?

EC: Right after it became available in the US, Smith, Kline & French invited a lot of us to dinner at Trader Vic's. I still remember those thick lamb chops. That was the first time I enjoyed a meal paid for with drug house money.

TB: When and where did you first hear about chlorpromazine?

EC: I think that was at the APA meeting in 1955 or 1956. People were very much divided about it. There were those people who said, "Oh, this drug is terrible. It's going to cover over symptoms, and the patients will never recover. The only way you truly recover from anything is to work it through with psychoanalysis." And there were other people who hailed it as a miracle drug.

TB: What got you interested in psychopharmacology?

EC: I'll tell you a story buried in the archives of dead people's heads. Worcester was the birthplace of the contraceptive pill, and the people there were at the forefront of endocrinological research in psychiatry. I was resident and research fellow and we had done some studies with schizophrenics measuring cortisol in their urine. That was largely because we could measure cortisol and not many other people could. So we would collect 24-hour urine samples. Our assays were not very sensitive, but you could extract enough cortisol from a 24-hour sample for an assay. The schizophrenics had low cortisols. Later that turned out to be due to the fact that we studied them in the wintertime when they had scurvy.

We knew that cortisol didn't cure schizophrenia. In fact, it could produce a psychosis. But Armour had extracted and purified ACTH, so Hoagland and Pincus decided that maybe ACTH would cure schizophrenia. Those first doses cost about a half a million dollars, because they were made from camel pituitaries. It was my job to line up four matched schizophrenics. I thought that from three thousand patients, matching four would be a snap. Well, I learned something about combinational mathematics. It took me more than a month to do it, but I ended up with four schizophrenic males pretty well matched on all the important

---

* Enoch Callaway III was born in La Grange, Georgia in 1924.

variables. They looked so much alike you might have thought they were quadruplets. And so, we started our study. Every day I would rate the patients using the Malamud-Sands Rating Scale. I don't know whether you remember Harry Freeman? He was a very taciturn gentleman, and he would come in every morning with four syringes with peanut oil, two with placebos and two with ACTH. He would inject the four patients and leave. He wouldn't speak to anybody to make certain he was keeping the study blind. Little by little, two of the patients started to improve. They began to comb their hair. They stopped talking about their delusions. They began to look like they were about ready for discharge.

Then one morning the nurse said to me, "Noch, I think that you should look at Bill and John. They're developing acne and humps on their back." Bill was one that we thought was a drug patient, and John was one we thought was a placebo patient. Both were developing Cushing's disease from the ACTH. It took us about another four days to finish up the planned trial, but by that point our two recovering schizophrenics had regressed rapidly. Almost the whole ward was sitting around in mourning. When the study was done, I remember, I was sitting at my desk writing up the report and feeling terribly let down. Harry Freeman came in and said, "Cheer up Noch. Suppose by chance it had come out the other way. We could have spent millions of dollars on an ineffective treatment." So, I learned there's something to be said for failures in drug trials.

TB: So, you had been involved in psychopharmacological research since you were a resident in Boston?

EC: Not Boston. There's a saying in Boston, "What do you think of Worcester? As a hole?" I was attracted to Worcester because I was interested in neuroendocrinology and I did a few neuroendocrinologic studies, but Hudson Hoagland and neurophysiology seduced me away. I can remember Hoagland's first lecture on the EEG, and it seemed to me that this was more likely to tell us what's going on in the mind than measuring steroids in the urine. Before I knew it Hoagland had inveigled me into becoming the de facto electroencephalographer at Worcester. When I finished my work at Worcester, Jake Feinsinger asked me to come down with him to start the new department at the University of Maryland. I went to work with him because there were two very good psychoanalytic institutes in Baltimore and I intended to start my psychoanalytic training.

TB: Was this in the early 1950s?

EC: This was in 1950–51. Jake was very interested in having his young people do research, which pleased me. But just before I left Worcester, Sid Sands the clinical research director was replaced by a young man named Nate Kline. I overlapped with Nate by about three months, but Nate was an experience, and I still think he was one of psychiatry's outstanding people. God knows he had faults. There was no problem identifying those, but if his critics had done as much good as Nate did, the world would be a better place.

TB: So you moved from Worcester to Baltimore in Maryland.

EC: I moved to Baltimore.

TB: And it was in Baltimore where you set up your first EEG laboratory?

EC: I didn't do much EEG work there because I hadn't been at Baltimore very long before the Korean War started. The army quickly ran out of medical officers in Korea, and they called up the Navy medical officers and assigned them to the army to become battalion surgeons, which was not a very pleasant prospect. At that time, Jake Feinsinger had a contract with the Army Chemical Center to study effects of anticholinesterase nerve gases. That was supposed to be top secret. I arrived at Edgewood, and Harold Himwich said, "Your work will be secret, but here's *Life Magazine* and if you read this article, you'll figure out what we're doing and where you fit in." When I finished my training at Fort Sam Houston, they began assigning people to different army battalions at the front in Korea. When I went in for my assignment, there were red stamps all over my papers. This army colonel said, "Well, Dr. Callaway, I see you're cleared for top secret." I said, "Yes, sir." He said, "And you know something about chemical warfare." "Yes, sir." For a bleak moment I could see myself as a chemical warfare officer in Korea. Then the Colonel said, "Well, we're sending you back to the Army Chemical Center." So I spent much of the Korean War at the Army Chemical Center, which was a rather unexpected benefit from my interest in research.

TB: So you worked with Himwich in Edgewood and not in Illinois?

EC: I worked with him when he was at Edgewood, before he went to Galesburg. Harold was the director of research for the Army Chemical Center, and one of the more delightful human beings that it has been my pleasure to know. He and Wilhelmina provided a sort of a constant enthusiastic spirit to our research group. While I was in the military I noticed some very curious things about the effects of nerve gas on attention. The first job I was given was to measure the nervousness that nerve gas was supposed to produce. Charlie Shagass had developed a method for measuring that, which involved the administering of loud sounds. How much one jumped seemed to be related to nervousness. So I replicated Charlie's set-up and used his method on people exposed to nerve gas and controls. And lo and behold, the people exposed to nerve gas seemed much calmer and startled less than the controls.

TB: Did you use any electrophysiological measure?

EC: We did electromyograms. We had the person try to hold their arms still, but in a somewhat tense position. Then we blasted 95 db sounds in their ears. Subjects jumped less when they had been exposed to nerve gas.

TB: What did you do after the war ended?

EC: Well, after the war, I went back to the University of Maryland and tried to follow up the observations I had made in the army. At that time I worked with Bob Grinnell. I didn't get back to EEG for a while because I had a career award in research. I think Danny Freedman, I and another gentleman whose name I don't remember, were the first to get those awards.

TB: What were you studying in your research?

EC: As I said before I was following up the observations I made in the army and I was also trying to identify drugs that affected startle responses in people. We were looking at drugs like amphetamine, atropine and scopolamine.

TB What did you find?

EC: We found that amphetamine did not make people startle more. Now today that would not surprise anybody, but then that's what we were giving it for, to increase startle. In the meantime, the University of California was building a new research wing at Langley Porter Institute. This was just about the time in the mid-1950s when I went to the APA meetings in San Francisco and first heard of chlorpromazine. My wife, being from Oklahoma, had always wanted to move to California. I had no interest in California myself, but being a good husband, we went to the meeting. At my wife's suggestion I called Alex Simon and asked him about job possibilities in California. Alex said, "We are building a new research wing. During the APA, come out and I'll take you around and show it to you. We've already offered John Lilly the job of chief of research. You know John don't you?" I said, "Sure." Alex said, "I'll be showing John around and we'd love to have you come along." So I went out to California. Alex showed me around with John. They were building this beautiful, spanking new research wing, and they were going to have four research positions. I said, "John, you're so lucky." He replied, "Yeah, isn't it wonderful?" We parted, and I went back home to Baltimore.

After a couple of days the phone rang. It was Alex Simon, and he said, "Noch, can you take that job I offered to John Lilly?" I said, "What happened?" He said, "Well, John ran off with the wife of a psychoanalyst from Oakland, and he's gone to the Caribbean to talk to dolphins." I said, "Well, let me come out and talk to you about it." And of course my wife was jumping up and down in the chair saying, "Yes, yes!" And so that's how I got to Langley Porter. My interest in electronics had developed in the course of measuring electromyograms. At Edgewood, they gave me an EEG machine and a Gray Walter analyzer. But it seemed that each time I got the analyzer tuned it was time to quit work, and I don't think I ever got an experiment run with it. It was a very dicey piece of instrumentation. When I got to California, Charlie Shagass was just beginning to publish his stuff on evoked potentials. I had decided at this point that, while brain waves didn't seem to be windows on the mind, evoked potentials might be. And so the Office of Naval Research, the University of California and the State of California all pitched in and got me started on evoked potentials.

TB: What was your first project with evoked potentials?

EC: The first project was a fairly simple one. When we first got the computers, just being able to see evoked potentials was fascinating, and the early meetings in which we discussed evoked potentials were very much like third grade show and tell sessions, where people say, "Look what I've found," and, "Oh, I've seen something like that before." And nobody knew what any of what we saw meant. But clearly you could do all sorts of things to the stimulus or to the subject and change the pattern of evoked potentials. And so I thought schizophrenics, if anything, are more variable than normal subjects, so the differences between their evoked responses to repeated tones should be greater than those of normal people. We did a lot of work on that and published a number of papers on it. I collaborated with Manuel Donchin whose fame rests in his work on the P300 wave.

TB: Are we still in the 1950s?

EC: We are now in the early 1960s.

TB: After Worcester did you get any further training in EEG?

EC: No. After my residency I had psychoanalytic training, and also took math at Johns Hopkins through differential equations; two things that haven't had much value in my work. But, they were sure fun and interesting.

TB: Were your activities restricted to research in your laboratory, or were you also involved in clinical work?

EC: No, my activities were not restricted to lab research. I've always seen patients. I somehow feel my identity as a psychiatrist depends on seeing patients, but I probably have never spent more than half time seeing patients, and sometimes a lot less.

TB: So, at Langley Porter you were seeing patients and doing research.

EC: I was also teaching.

TB: What proportion of your time did you spend seeing patients?

EC: I suppose in those years when grants were easy to come by, I would see patients two nights a week, and when grants got tighter, I would see more. Actually, as director of research I was not supposed to have clinical duties in the department of psychiatry, but was allowed to see patients in the evening. So I saw patients in the evening and did my work in the daytime.

TB: But your responsibilities included teaching?

EC: Yes, and I was involved with both undergraduates and postgraduates. God knows how research would get done in the United States without graduate students and post-docs. With med students, I probably did mostly clinical teaching. The thing I particularly liked to teach was interview techniques for medical students and residents. They seem to think that they're born with a natural ability to interview patients. But they have to be taught.

TB: Where did your research support come from?

EC: From NIMH and the Office of Naval Research.

TB: Could you talk about some of the research projects you had been involved with at Langley Porter?

EC: One of the main themes that has gone through my work – and I am not so sure now that it was a good theme – was that neurotransmitters would be linked to cognitive processes. I thought there was some sense, some logic, in the way that acetylcholine seemed to modulate memory, and some sense, some logic in the way that dopamine seemed to modulate attention. As time passed I got more and more fascinated with that theme and was trying to design tasks that would pull apart acetylcholine and dopamine effects. I was also interested in designing tasks to detect the differences between the effects of drugs; for example the effects of the benzodiazepine clonazepam, and the ß-blocker propranolol. When I turned 65, NIH was getting harder and harder to deal with, and the Office of Naval Research said they wanted to fund younger people. They weren't funding anybody over 65. So I moved to the VA so I could get VA funds for my research. And for a while that worked out pretty well.

TB: Could we get back to your research with acetylcholine and dopamine?

EC: Well, at that time I thought that different neurotransmitters were associated with different kind of processes in the brain. I thought that there was a grand scheme of things that caused different neurotransmitters to be associated with different cognitive operations. It was only later that Crick, I think, wrote, "There is no grand scheme. God is simply a tinkerer." If I had read that 40 years earlier, I think I would have stuck to neuroendocrinology. But the EEG was very seductive for 'lumpers' like me. I thought we were going to see something that captured what's going on in the mind. I hope the functional MRI people will do lot better than we've done with EEGs. It's been a fascinating field, but I don't think it's very fruitful.

TB: You started to tell us before about your work with evoked potentials in schizophrenia. Could you tell us more about what you did and what you found?

EC: In our early studies we found that the P300 waves in schizophrenics were of lower amplitude and more variable than in normal subjects. And those were fairly durable findings. We worked with some pretty sophisticated signal detection methodology, but I don't think we got it to the point where it was of any practical use. One of my ex-UCSF colleagues, Alan Gevins, has developed some very sophisticated methods of de-blurring the EEG literally, making it an electronic lens that looks through the inter-vening tissues, and combining EEG data with behavioral data. That is very interesting. Don Jewett, who is the guy that discovered the far field evoked potentials, is incidentally another of my ex-colleagues. He is also one of those who quit academia to start their own companies. And Don has some stuff that looks very promising. But, if I had to wipe out a field of knowledge and do the minimum damage to psychopharmacology, I'm not sure that the EEG wouldn't be my first choice. I remember when Joe Wortis was giving Charlie Shagass' obituary. He said, "Charlie did all the right things in doing research. He just picked the wrong problems." And I think that may be the case here. But some of it seems to be potter-ing along. Not through me, but through people that were with me, as for example, the work in schizophrenia with Dave Freedman's recovery response, and Dave Braff's startle response. So there still seem to be fruit on branches of the tree, but they are pretty sparse.

TB: What would you consider your most important contribution?

EC: I suppose the students I've worked with. They are probably individually each one worth more than any contribution I made.

TB: Could you mention a few of your students by name?

EC: I was just talking about Dave Braff. I also had Reese Jones. Then there were lots of other people in the lab, such as Bob Freedman, David Servan-Schreiber, Kim Meador, and I don't know whether we should count Jack Mendelson. He was a medical student when I was a resident at the University of Maryland and I supervised him. But I really hate to do this because I'm going to forget to mention someone important. Oh yes, there was Monte Buchsbaum.

TB: Oh, he was your student?

EC: Medical student. Thinking of Monte reminds me of an interesting story. We had what, in those days, were considered outstanding computer facilities. I think we had a computer with 8000 bits of memory and punch-paper tape, really state of the art stuff. Monte was interested in fluctua-tion in reaction time. Later, I think that was popularized as the Rabbit

Effect. You make a mistake and slow down, and you don't immediately speed up again. It takes awhile for the effect of mistakes to wear off. I had been looking for relationships between human cycles such as diurnal cycles, cardiac cycles, breathing cycles, and variability in the EEG. So Monte learned Fourier analysis in a flash, like Monte learns things, and he asked, "Can I borrow your number for the Berkeley computer?" I said, "Sure," thinking that no medical student is going to run up a big bill on that mammoth Berkeley computer. But Monte disappeared for a week. It wasn't like him not to show up for work. Finally he came in, and he had six New York phone book sized batches of printout. He had looked at the sequence of reaction times a hundred different ways.

This reminds me that Adolph Pfefferbaum, Judy Ford, and Manny Donchin were also in my lab at some time. They were certainly pioneers in the P300 field.

TB: You had been involved in research with the new psychotropic drugs from the very beginning, starting with chlorpromazine. Would you like to talk about some of the drugs you were involved with?

EC: I was doing some research with LSD. We thought that serotonergic agents like LSD were involved in the pathogenesis of schizophrenia. So we did a study with LSD to see if benzyl antiserotonin would inhibit LSD psychosis. We did small studies in those days. We had three nurse graduate students who volunteered to be subjects: one got LSD alone; one got LSD and benzyl antiserotonin; and one got benzyl anti-serotonin alone. It was a double-blind study but we thought that it was immediately apparent who got what. One girl started to have florid hallucinations, one complained of headache, and the third didn't notice anything. So we said, "Well, the gal with the headache got the benzyl anti-serotonin; the gal with the florid hallucinations got the LSD; and the gal with nothing is the one who has had her psychosis blocked by the benzyl antiserotonin." Wonderful! I had someone stay with each one of them all night.

But the girl that didn't have any symptoms said to her monitor, "Look, I'm just very tired and I don't want you sitting around. Would you go and leave me?" And the lady, against all my instructions, left. That evening, I got a call at home from the head nurse. "You've driven one of my nurses crazy. She's sitting in front of the television set talking to it." I said, "Oh, shit. I'll get in the car and come in." I broke the blind, of course. The one that had the benzyl antiserotonin alone was the one that had the florid hallucinations in the lab; the one who had the headache had been given LSD; and the one hallucinating in front of the TV had LSD and benzyl antiserotonin. So, benzyl antiserotonin didn't do anything for LSD psychosis, but the power of the placebo effect was incredible.

I still hope that somebody will find there is some logic to psychophar-macology in terms of neurotransmitters. As a clinician, I have become less and less hopeful. Every so often I see a patient who has failed on three SSRIs, abysmally, and when I put him on a fourth he gets well beau-tifully. If all four drugs have similar neurotransmitter effects, that doesn't make much sense. In fact, I'm still convinced when I see a serious obses-sive patient who gets well on an SSRI that the old psychoanalytic theories of obsession made much more sense than the fact that they respond to a drug. You know, you could make such wonderful analytic interpretations about the content of the obsession.

TB: It looks like you are not very much impressed with SSRI antidepressants.

EC: Oh, I'm very impressed with them. But I'm not impressed with the theories.

TB: Do you remember your first publication?

EC: I think the very first thing I published was on cortisol output in the course of electric shock treatment.

TB: That was work done in Massachusetts?

EC: In Worcester.

TB: Where was it published?

EC: I think it was published in the *Journal of Nervous and Mental Disease*, which was a good journal in those days. Then I had a series of papers on schizophrenia with Monte Buchsbaum, Manny Donchin, Reese Jones, and Dave Braff. Toward the end of my research career I got very inter-ested in parallel distributed processing and neural network modeling, and I still think that something is going to come of that. One of the last papers I wrote was on neural network modeling to explain amphetamine effects. But then I think that the more recent work that Jonathon Cohen has done in the same area of research is much better and probably makes what I did quite obsolete.

TB: But it was your work that opened up the field of neural network modeling. Could you talk about your contributions in that area?

EC: Well, I don't want to take any credit for developing it at all. The credit should go to David Servan-Schreiber, who came to work in my laboratory. The idea I had was that each neurotransmitter has some unique global effect on cognitive processing. I was hoping one could design a network that would model changes in human behavior produced by changes in a particular neurotransmitter with changes in a particular parameter in the network. The neural networks are fairly simple arrangements of hypo-thetical modules placed in layers which interact with each other by either inhibition or excitation. You can take a very, very simple arrangement and model some amazing things, as Jonathon yesterday presented in his Stroop model, which I think has three layers and four neurons in each layer. It's very simple. Jonathon is not talking about norepinephrine, serotonin and other neurotransmitters. He's now talking about brain structures. And his notion that the frontal cingulate gyrus is a feedback loop that it's responding to conflict makes a lot of sense to me. As for which neurotransmitters are operating in the frontal cortex, there are GABA, glutamic acid, norepinephrine, serotonin and probably some others we don't even know yet. So, I think that looking for anatomical analogies to neural nets is going to be much more promising than looking at neurotransmitters. If I wasn't retired, I would get involved with people doing fMRI and neural net modeling to try and relate structures to functions.

TB: You are retired, but aren't you still involved in developing new drugs with a drug company?

EC: Are you referring to memantine?

TB: Yes. Could you elaborate on that?

EC: The drug company is called Neurobiological Technologies. Currently memantine is available in Europe. We are doing some work in neuropathic pain with it, and we shall soon break the double blind to see what happened. We have "very promising results" with it in Alzheimer's disease, and the company is making a big splash about that at the Alzheimer meeting in Stockholm. So that's been a lot of fun. We started out with Nancy Lee and Horace Lowe to work on dynorphin, but that has fallen by the wayside. I had a theory that turned out not to work. I thought that if you combined physostigmine and scopolamine you'd have sort of an imitation of nicotine effect that would help people stop smoking. But it did not work either. And every failed drug trial is about 10 million dollars down the tubes. But we may make it. We still have some work going on with the corticotropin-releasing hormone that seems to combat edema in a very curious way. It reduces peritumoral edema, it reduces post-surgical edema, and we're now looking at what else it does.

But my favorite hobby now is treating patients for the Family Service League, where I don't get paid and so I don't have to worry about managed care. Most of my patients are on welfare, so if I want to try a new drug all I have to do is deal with the pharmacist who oversees the program. He and I now have a cordial relationship, and I can almost get anything for my patients. So, it's fun.

TB: When did you first get involved in new drug development?

EC: I suppose when I was at Worcester. We did a study there giving methamphetamine to schizophrenics. There was a controversy whether methamphetamine would make them worse or better. And we found that it activated them, but it didn't necessarily make them sicker. They were just more active. Then as I mentioned before, I was interested in benzyl anti-serotonin. And later on I became very interested in what might be called nootropics. I was also working with MDMA before it became illegal, primarily to open people up for psychotherapy. It was an incredible agent.

TB: Do you think that MDMA is particularly suitable for opening up people for psychotherapy?

EC: Yes, and also some other amphetamine analogues.

TB: Are you still interested in psychotherapy?

EC: I guess what I'm interested in is the mind, and how you study it, regardless whether listening to a patient, or giving a drug, or looking at an evoked potential. One of my teachers once said that a lot of people are not interested in psychology and psychiatry because they are naturally intuitive and they know what is going on in people's minds. And there are others of us who are essentially psychologically tone-deaf, and we have to work to understand it. So for us, it isn't intuitively obvious what's going on. We are puzzled why it happens in one way and not in another. And I'm one of those people who are constantly puzzled by what is going on in somebody else's mind.

TB: And you would use any means to understand it.

EC: Yes.

TB: From all the different means you have tried which one would you trust the most?

EC: I think that what we are seeing now is a convergence of different methods, a combination of cognitive testing, drugs, fMRI, evoked potentials and others, and I feel kind of sorry for the new generation. They will need to be physicists, mathematicians, psychologists and pharmacologists all at the same time. We used to talk about interdisciplinary research, and the idea that there is some underlying general principle that brings all these disciplines together. We thought that by getting the mathematician, the physicist, the physiologist, and the psychoanalyst in the same room together, they would find the secret. One of the wonderful little phrases that came out of these brainstorming sessions was Carl Pribram's. He said, "Emotion is the ablative of motion. If you hit somebody, you don't experience the anger quite as much as if you sit still." But modern research is big business. Just look at the slides people present now. They say, "This is the team that worked with us," and there are four columns of names.

TB: What was actually your last publication?

EC: My last paper was published in the *California Fly Fisher* and was entitled "Two psychiatrists look at their obsession." I don't think it's going to be picked up by Medline. The last one before that was on the effect of cotinine, which is a metabolite of nicotine, on behavior.

TB: When was it published?

EC: About one and a half years ago.

TB: What are you doing these days? You have your clinical practice, and it seems that you are advising Neurobiological Technologies.

EC: And I do fly-fishing.

TB: And fly-fishing? When did you become a member of ACNP?

EC: I don't think I was there at the very first meeting but I think I was at the second one.

TB: So you became a member soon after it was founded, in the early 1960s?

EC: Yes.

TB: Were you ever an officer?

EC: I was on the Council.

TB: So you had been a councilor. Have you been actively involved with any other professional organization?

EC: Yes, I was involved with the Society of Biological Psychiatry. I was president of that organization at one point.

TB: So you were active in the Society of Biological Psychiatry.

EC: Yes. Joe Wortis was one of my favorite human beings. I was also president of the Society for Psychophysiological Research.

TB: Would it be correct to say that your primary area of research was psychophysiology?

EC: Yes.

TB: And you have been interested all through your career in new psychotropic drugs?

EC: Well, I'm trying to keep up with the new drugs for my small practice. As a matter of fact, a lot of people don't know that there is a listserv on the World Wide Web which is run by Ivan Goldberg in New York. There, one can find information that is usually not reported elsewhere. They describe difficult cases and their responses to drugs.

TB: So, you think that we are missing some important clinical feedback.

EC: Yes. There is a lot of what we could learn from uncontrolled research.

TB: You have been involved with psychopharmacology for almost 50 years. Do you think we have made major advances since the 1950s?

EC: Well, I have been interested lately more in history than before. I guess the older you get, the more interesting history becomes. During the past 50 years the other major event in psychiatry besides the introduction of psychotropic drugs was the community mental health movement. There are some interesting books on that. *Madness in the Streets* is one of them. It raises the issue that de-institutionalization started well before the introduction of the new psychotropic drugs. In fact, I remember that already at the time I left Worcester there were teams looking for patients to discharge. The idea that patients can be kept out of hospitals and treated at home is not new. But with the anti-psychiatry people it has led to the denial of mental illness with detrimental consequences, because if there is no mental illness there is no need to put up money to take care of psychiatric patients. So the state hospitals were closed or drastically reduced in size. And now in the United States – I don't know what Canada is like – but the state hospitals are being reopened as forensic institutes, because the only way that some people can get treated if they are seriously ill is to commit a felony. Unfortunately, long-term results of involuntary treatments aren't so good.

TB: In your evaluation, what was the contribution of new psychotropic drugs?

EC: Well, we don't see those chronic depressed patients and totally beat out obsessive-compulsives we used to see in the state hospitals. I think the big problem in depression is how to get primary care physicians to recognize anxiety and depressive disorders. Those disorders now are treatable; the problem is how to get physicians to recognize them. The other day, I saw a friend whose doctor had just said, "Well, you're 75 years old. Everybody is depressed when they're 75 years old." This is the opinion of a 45-year-old physician. Now, how do you educate these people?

TB: So we have made progress insofar as we don't see those chronic depressive and obsessive-compulsive patients. On this note we should conclude this interview with Dr Enoch Callaway. Thank you very much for sharing this information with us.

EC: Well, thank you. You are a very gentle interviewer.

TB: Thank you.

TURAN M. ITIL

Interviewed by Thomas A. Ban
San Juan, Puerto Rico, December 11, 2002

TB: This will be an interview with Dr. Turan Itil* for the Archives of the American College of Neuropsychopharmacology. I am Thomas Ban. We are at the Annual Meeting of the College in San Juan, Puerto Rico. It is December 11, 2002. Let's start from the very beginning. Where and when were you born? Tell us something about your education.

TI: I was born in Bursa, Turkey in 1924. Bursa is the old capital of the Ottoman Empire. My family moved to Eskisehir and then to Istanbul. I finished my high school at the Istanbul High School, and subsequently went to medical school and finished at the University of Istanbul, Medical School. And, after that, I went to military service for one year.

TB: Did you want to become a medical doctor all the time?

TI: Actually, I wanted to be an engineer, but I couldn't get into the engineering school. With my awards from the high school I was ultimately admitted to medical school. At that time, in Turkey, it was easier to get admitted to medical school than engineering. After I finished my military service, I went to Germany, where I was told that one of the most famous doctors alive was a professor at the University of Tübingen. His name was Ernst Kretschmer. Kretschmer, as you may know, wrote several books. He was one of the first biological psychiatrists of the century. I stayed at the Tübingen Clinic and finished my education in neurology and psychiatry there to become a neuropsychiatrist. When I joined the University in Tübingen, we were treating patients with phantom pain. These patients lost their arms or legs in the war and felt excruciating pain in their lost limb.

TB: Are we in the late 1940's?

TI: That is the beginning of the 1950s.

TB: When did you get to Tübingen?

TI: Just the beginning of the '50s. At that time, several of my professors told me that in a new article published by French people it was reported that promethazine, called Atosil, had a significant effect on relieving phantom pain. I was told to get the information and check out whether we should give it to our patients. So, I did that. According to the French publication Atosil was effective in phantom pain but not in all patients. So we started to give it to our patients. I found it unusual that some patients responded whereas others did not. So I asked my professors, "how can I predict which patient will show a response and which will not?" Several of them

---

* Turan M. Itil was born in Bursa, Turkey in 1924.

said, "There is no way to know in advance." Then another said, "why don't you read this publication from Dr. Berger? He claims that electroencephalography (EEG) would show the effects of the derivatives of opiates and barbiturates, as well as of mescaline, on the brain."

The next day I went to Fritz Flügel, and asked whether he thought I should learn EEG in order to see the effect of promethazine/Atosil on the brain. The obvious question was whether promethazine penetrates the blood-brain barrier in every patient. The EEG might show in which patient promethazine penetrated the blood-brain barrier and had an effect on the brain. He did not believe in Dr. Berger's findings and told me that I shouldn't bother to learn EEG. Then, I went to my neurology professor. His name was Ishman. I asked the same question, and he said, "That's not a bad idea. Why don't you go and learn it?" Over the next six months I started to learn about the EEG. It was at that time the first papers on the effectiveness of chlorpromazine in some psychotic patients were published by Deniker and Delay.

TB: Could you tell us something about Fritz Flügel?

TI: Flügel was a guest doctor like me, without pay, in Tübingen, and became chairman of one of the largest neuropsychiatry department in Germany, at Erlangen. Professor Flügel invited Bente first and then me to join him in his department, and one day he said to me, "We have a machine, but nobody's using it. Why don't you come and start to use it?" At the time, I was working with Dr. Dieter Bente who was one or two years older than me. He was also interested in EEG, but was always busy. It was just about that time that a meeting took place in Paris on chlorpromazine which Professor Flügel attended. When he returned from Paris, he was very enthusiastic and said that he wanted to talk to the Bayer people in Germany to get chlorpromazine. And indeed, a few weeks later, we got chlorpromazine and Professor Flügel said, "let us see whether chlorpromazine has any effect on the brain."

TB: Was this in 1955?

TI: The meeting took place in 1954, and we started to give chlorpromazine to all kinds of patients. To our surprise, we saw some effect. The findings became my first publication on a psychotropic drug. Our paper with Bente was published in 1954 with the title, "The Effect of Chlorpromazine on Human Brain."

TB: Was this the first publication on the effect of chlorpromazine on the human brain?

TI: Yes. There was an Italian publication before ours of the effect on the brains of animals; ours was the first publication on the human brain. We showed that chlorpromazine produced sleep-like effects. But the effects appeared to me more than just an effect that produces sleep. And after we published our paper, we also presented our findings at several meetings in Germany. There was no interest on the effect of the drug on the EEG; all people were interested in was that it induced sleep. To show that chlorpromazine-induced sleep was different from normal sleep we did a study in which we recorded sleep in a group of people after sleep deprivation and in another group after chlorpromazine administration. We found a significant difference between physiological and chlorpromazine-induced sleep. And, we published these findings as well. We also found that chlorpromazine had an effect in some people but not in others, something similar to what we saw with promethazine. We compared the effects of chlorpromazine and promethazine on the EEG, and found that even though both induced sleep, the brain sleep of patients was different with the two drugs. With chlorpromazine we saw slow-wave synchronized activities, and with promethazine, we saw fast activity.

TB: So, adding one methyl group to the side chain made a difference on the effect of the drug on the EEG.

TI: Exactly. In the meantime, there were important meetings taking place. First, the one in Milan, on Psychotropic Drugs, then the founding of the CINP in Zurich, and finally, the first CINP meeting in Rome.

TB: How did the psychiatric community respond to your findings?

TI: There was no response. At the time the German psychiatric society considered pharmacological treatment a gimmick of the drug companies. There were nineteen departmental chairmen in Germany, and only one, Professor Flügel, was involved with chemicals. They called him jokingly, the "chemical doctor," and he was not taken seriously. The first time that he was taken seriously was when he was invited to Switzerland to meet Professor Binswanger whose daughter had schizophrenia with hallucinations. She was treated unsuccessfully with psychotherapy, and he wanted to see whether the drug Flügel described to him would help his daughter. It did, and Binswanger was very impressed.

TB: So, Binswanger was impressed with the effects of chlorpromazine?

TI: He was very, very impressed. And of course, he was telling the other doctors and professors, so Professor Flügel started to have a reputation. Before that it was based on introducing occipital (cysternal) pneumoencephalography. Prior to that, pneumeoencephalography was always done by lumbar puncture. He used occipital puncture because prior to becoming a neuropsychiatrist he was a neurosurgeon.

TB: So, it was Flügel who introduced cysternal puncture. Was cysternal puncture, rather than lumbar puncture, used at the clinic?

TI: Yes, it was routine in our clinic, but not in every clinic in Germany. Lumbar puncture is still used a lot, because cysternal puncture has some dangers.

TB: It's very simple to do.

TI: Yes, and much less painful for the patient.

TB: There are much less after-effects.

TI: The after-effect is little because you need to inject much less air.

TB: Am I correct that you did your EEG studies with chlorpromazine in collaboration with Bente?

TI: Yes. In 1957 there was a meeting in Milan and Flügel took me along. It was the meeting where it was decided to found a society that was to become the CINP. It took place in a small room at the university.

TB: So you are one of the few people who attended the meeting at the Milan symposium that led to the founding of the CINP?

TI: There were no more than 20 people there.

TB: Can you recall the names of the people?

TI: No, I can't.

TB: I'm sure Trabucchi, who was president of the Milan symposium was there, and also that Garattini, who organized the symposium, was there.

TI: I remember that there was a long discussion about whether it should be a society of brain pharmacology, neuropharmacology, neuropsychiatry, or psychopharmacology. I think my boss and me were the only ones from Germany there, but I am not sure. The majority of the people were from Italy and Switzerland. There were also a couple of people from France and the United States. We really didn't understand what was going on. As a matter of fact, we were there accidentally. We were walking somewhere with my boss, when somebody said, "Oh, we have a meeting to form an organization." My boss shook his head and asked, "What organization?"

TB: This was in the spring of 1957.

TI: Yes. And then, we heard that in 1958, there would be a meeting in Rome. And the Rome meeting was probably one of the most important meetings in my life, because it was at that meeting that I presented on the differences in the effect of chlorpromazine and promethazine on the EEG. And just before I presented, Dr. Max Fink presented his findings. He described the effects of chlorpromazine on the brain, and that the effect of chlorpromazine is different from the effect of anticholinergic drugs. I presented my findings with chlorpromazine after him, and our findings were identical. We both got excited that the effects of chlorpromazine were different from both anticholinergic and antihistaminic drugs. We were also excited that we could almost use each other's slides to show the effects of chlorpromazine. So, we became the best of friends, and since we were the only people in the field of EEG in psychopharmacology, we began to correspond with each other to exchange information. As you know, at that time there was no e-mail or fax. As a result of my frustration in Germany, I started to have the idea of going to the United States to do my research in a more sophisticated setting.

In 1959 or 1960 I traveled around in Germany to show my slides to professors of physiology at universities; those famous professors looked at me, and said, "you might be right, but prove it." So I started to ask people, "How can I prove it?" And they replied, "you have to quantify your findings and apply statistics, to show that the effect is not by chance, but real. That's science." We never learned science in medical school, nor after medical school, and certainly not in our training in neuropsychiatry. In Erlangen, we were working very closely with Bayer. As a Turkish citizen in a German university, you could neither get an appointment nor be paid. So I was studying Bayer drugs at the University in Erlangen. At that time, everybody was looking for something better than chlorpromazine and for better methodology to study these drugs. We were, scientifically, absolutely like lay people. One of the scientists at Bayer, named Friedrich Hoffmeister, was a corresponding member of the American College of Neuropsychopharmacology; he was one of the top researchers at Bayer. He started to teach me about scientific methodology. At the time Bayer was interested in studying piperazine phenothazines.

TB: Could you tell us about the piperazine phenothiazines you worked with?

TI: One of them was Stelazine.

TB: We are in the late 1950s. Correct?

TI: Yes. At the time we thought that more effective drugs would have greater EEG effects. One of these drugs was called butaperazine; it had a greater EEG and behavioral effect. Clinically, it turned out to be a very effective compound.

TB: Butaperazine was studied but not introduced into clinical use in North America. I am wondering why?

TI: Butaperazine came to this country but not sold because, in the meantime, Stelazine was of interest. Butaperazine produced more extrapyramidal side effects than any of the other compounds, but as I said, at the time the idea was one would have better therapeutic effects with compounds which induced more extrapyramidal side effects. With that kind of belief we started to study the effects of reserpine. Reserpine was first introduced in Germany as an antidepressant, but Professor Flügel found it had therapeutic effect in psychotic patients.

TB: Reserpine was given for treating neurotic depression in some countries in those years. Right?

TI: Yes, I think it was given to patients with neurotic depression.

TB: At the same time, it was also reported that it caused depression when used in the treatment of hypertensive patients.

TI: We studied the effect of reserpine in psychotic patients, especially in schizophrenics, and we thought it was more effective than chlorpromazine. We had also seen more extrapyramidal side effects with it. Professor Flügel combined reserpine with chlorpromazine and found that the combination was better than either of the two drugs alone. But it also induced more Parkinsonian effects. We presented and published our findings, but then within six months, seven patients committed suicide while taking reserpine. At first, we couldn't link reserpine with the suicidal attempts, because many of those patients were receiving other drugs as well. But by giving only reserpine to some patients we observed that not only their suicidal thoughts increased, but also their energy level. So it was not a depressive affect alone, but together with an increase in anxiety and drive that led to suicide.

TB: Was it akathisia you saw with reserpine?

TI: Yes, patients had akathisia, anxiety and restlessness; they could not sit still.

TB: Were you the first to report it?

TI: Yes.

TB: This was in the late 1950s. How did it show up on the EEG?

TI: That was very interesting. When we did EEGs with the reserpine and chlorpromazine combination, what we saw was an increase in synchronization in the frontal area, the kind of effect seen in Parkinson's disease. In our model, that was supposed to be an indicator of better therapeutic effects. We thought the more we can change brain function, the better the therapeutic effects would be. And the changes we produced were in the direction that chlorpromazine alone had produced. It was about that time I started writing my thesis on the effect of drugs on the EEG as the prerequisite for being appointed as dozent. One area I was especially interested in was the identification of drugs with therapeutic effects using the EEG in schizophrenia. We started to call these drugs neuroleptics to differentiate them from sedative drugs. I completed and published my thesis and became a dozent at the University of Erlangen.

TB: What year was that?

TI: 1962. My thesis was published in the form of a book in Turkey and in Germany, but didn't have any impact. In the meantime, Max Fink invited me to the United States. When you become a dozent in Germany, you know that in five to six years you will become professor, even if you don't do anything, so I thought I should go to the United States to learn English and how to quantify the EEG. Max was working at the time with electronic frequency analyzers.

TB: Was Max Fink in St. Louis at the time?

TI: No, Max was in New York, in the Great Neck area. It was just about the time he got the wonderful offer from George Ulett to set up a research institute in St. Louis, Missouri. I was planning to visit Max Fink at Hillside Hospital, but about three months before my visit he told me that he was moving to St. Louis. He was planning to bring famous people, young people, from all around the world. I told him that I'm not so famous, but active, and he said I should come to St. Louis.

For me, of course, New York was a very attractive place; I didn't have any idea about St. Louis. One day I was sitting at the Rotary lunch in Nuremberg, and next to me was a young man whose father had the biggest brewery in the city. While I was talking to him, he said he had just come from Missouri, where he visited the Busch Company, the famous brewery in St. Louis. I said, "I am going to go to St. Louis. What kind of a city is it?" He shook his head, "It's terrible; cold with lots of snow in winter, and hot and humid in summer." I was shocked, but we had already planned our trip and were ready to leave.

I asked the University for a leave of absence for the year, and they approved my request. Then a very important thing happened. Bavaria did not have any rules that foreign citizens couldn't become dozents, so as soon you were appointed you automatically became a civil servant with pay. So as it turned out I became not only a dozent, but also an employee of the department and clinic. That was a big thing because I could go on sabbatical for a year. Now, sabbaticals are usually with pay, but because I was not a German citizen as yet they didn't want to pay me. In the meantime, Max Fink offered me $18,000 a year. I didn't know how much that was worth, so I wrote to my brother who was living in Toledo, Ohio, and asked him whether I could live on that money with my wife and my son. He wrote back saying, that's fantastic! He had been in the United States for thirteen or fourteen years and was making only $12,000 a year. So he told me that would be great money, and I should come immediately. So that's how I decided to come to the United States for one year.

But when I arrived to St. Louis I was shocked. In Erlangen we had 150 beds, and our EEG laboratories were working steadily. This was not the case at the Missouri Institute of Psychiatry. The name was great; the building was great and brand new, but there was nothing else. There were no patients and there were no machines. There was nothing. I said to Max, "What's going on?" He said, "Wait, I have lots of money. Just tell me what you need." I said to Max, an "EEG, of course." He replied, "No problem, just get the information about what kind of machine you want and we'll get it." Indeed, there was a lot of money from the state, a lot of space and plenty of patients, because the Missouri Institute of Psychiatry served nine state hospitals. Ulett was Commissioner of Mental Health for Missouri, and made Max Fink Director of the Institute so he could get patients from the state hospital system. Ulett was also professor at Washington University, and had Max appointed professor in the department. The plan was to create the necessary environment for research.

I was anxious thinking I had only twelve months and that might not be enough to set up a laboratory, learn English and how to quantify the EEG. While Max was recruiting Sam Gershon from Australia and young people from around the world he told me I should write an application for a new grant. I had no idea what a grant was or how to write one. But of course, he helped a lot with writing it. In Germany we had studied treatment-resistant schizophrenics and found that those with enlarged third ventricles and abnormal EEGs did not respond to butaperazine. We published our findings and Max and George Ulett read our reports.

TB: When did you publish those findings?

TI: 1958, 1959. Recently others found similar findings with MRI and CT scans.

TB: Similar to the findings you published in the late 1950s?

TI: After they read the German results they thought it was very interesting and suggested, "You should write a grant application to study schizophrenia and psychopharmacology." After I wrote the grant Jonathan Cole himself came with a group of people to review our request. It was approved for $70,000 annually, for five years. In addition Max had other grants. We had plenty of money. My time was up by then and I was supposed to go back to Erlangen. I had a very difficult decision to make; whether to go back to Germany or stay in the United States.

I returned to Germany with my wife and told Professor Flügel I was entertaining the thought of staying for one more year in St. Louis. I'll never forget his expression; he looked at me and said, "You are crazy. You worked like a slave for many years and now that you have become a dozent and will be a professor in two or three years, you want to leave for the United States. A professor in Germany is close to God; what do you want to do in the United States? Forget it." But his wife was much more understanding. She said, "People say to do research in the United States is much better than here." My wife who was critical of everything when we arrived in the States, by the end of our year in St.Louis, started to accept the American way of life and suddenly didn't like her native country.

That was crucial, and when we went back to St. Louis we started to look for a house. Our family was growing as were the laboratories at the Institute.

We started our psychopharmacology research in schizophrenia and that turned out to be a major project. Just recently, somebody became interested in writing my biography, and when he asked me what I would consider my greatest achievement I told him it was the quantification of the EEG. Max Fink was heavily involved with computers and we used them to analyze our data.

TN: What other important findings did you have?

TI: We discovered that all drugs that are effective on behavior have an effect on the brain and this effect can be demonstrated by using the quantified EEG. Probably even more important were our findings that drugs which have certain therapeutic effects show similar EEG changes. All antidepressants produce one type of effect; all neuroleptics produce another type of effect; all anxiolytic drugs produce yet another type, and all drugs we call cognitive activators or psychostimulants produce a fourth type of effect. So we published our findings which showed that drugs produce different effects on the quantitative EEG if they have different therapeutic properties.

TB: When did you publish these findings?

TI: In 1965–1966. About the same time, we accidentally discovered Tacrine that was to become the first anti-Alzheimer's drug. We were working with schizophrenic patients who had cognitive deficits, and were trying to figure out how to treat patients who seemed also to have – as indicated by their large ventricles and EEG changes – an organic state that interfered with the therapeutic effect of neuroleptics. We gave this kind of schizophrenic Ditran, a potent anticholinergic substance, to make them acutely psychotic and then treat them with neuroleptics. It didn't work, but when we gave them Tacrine, (tetrahydroacridane), a substance Sam Gershon brought from Australia, it controlled both their psychosis and confusion. It also reversed the EEG changes induced by Ditran. We published our findings is 1965. We wrote that Tacrine had a significant effect on human behavior, and reduced experimentally-induced confusion. We were not smart enough to relate experimentally-induced confusion to dementia. It was several years later that Bart Summers recognized the potential of Tacrine and pharmacologically similar drugs in the treatment of dementia. At the same time we found that schizophrenic patients have different EEG patterns from normal subjects. Then, we looked at psychotic, schizophrenic children and found similar differences between schizophrenic and normal children as we found in adults.

Finally, we took part in a WHO project in Copenhagen, with Sarnoff Mednick and Fini Shulsinger, and found that children at high risk for schizophrenia have significantly different EEG patterns than normal controls. They have more fast activity in their EEG. Since all neuroleptics decrease fast activity and increase α activity they correct these EEG changes in schizophrenia. Now, twenty-five years later, we recognized a similar pattern in patients with Alzheimer's disease where all cognitive enhancers that exist today, including memantine, increase α activity that is proportionately reduced with the severity of dementia. So, as in schizophrenia, in Alzheimer's demetia one can use EEG to measure therapeutic effects.

TB: How do you predict whether a drug will be therapeutic for a patient, using the EEG?

TI: Using a single test dose, you can predict whether a particular drug will produce the desired therapeutic effect in the central nervous system of a particular patient. You can see whether the drug modifies brain reactivity in the direction of normalizing the EEG. Based on this, we think that one can predict whether a particular drug will be effective in a particular patient. We call this method the test dose procedure of the quantitative pharmaco-EEG. We organized a society, the International Pharmaco-EEG Group (IPEG) and developed databases, like fingerprints, for antidepressants, antipsychotics, anxiolytics and cognitive activators.

TB: When and where did you move from St. Louis?

TI: In 1973 I moved to the New York Medical College, to Al Freedman's department because Max Fink had left the College and moved to Stony Brook University on Long Island. I set up laboratories at the College and at the VA and we established databases for findings with drugs on the quantitative EEG.

TB: How many drugs did you study and have in your database?

TI: We studied about 250 experimental drugs.

TB: Is your database accessible to everyone?

TI: Naturally. Many of the drug profiles are published.

TB: Would it be correct to say that clinical improvement is reflected in the EEG changes?

TI: That's right, and I thought the EEG was important in the detection of the psychotropic qualities of drugs. For example we examined hormones and found that mesterolone, a synthetic androgene preparation, in low dose shows an anti-anxiety pattern, and in high dose an antidepressant pattern on the EEG. The antidepressant effect of mianserin was discovered by this type of screening.

TB: We are running out of time. Is there anything important we left out you would like to add?

TI: When we published our findings all the drug companies wanted to have their drugs studied with quantitative EEG. We couldn't do this because studies with computerized EEG are very expensive. In the 1980s, the new computers completely changed the picture, and this was the time I moved into research and set up studies with Gingko Biloba in Alzheimer's disease, and also organized a multi-center trial with amitriptyline in a WHO program to show that its therapeutic effect can be predicted by EEG analyses. In the WHO study, we enrolled 450 patients. In the Alzheimer's study, we had 310 patients. I hope one day psychiatrists will be able to give a drug and be able to predict, with an automated EEG, whether a patient will respond to a psychotropic drug without waiting several weeks.

TB: Am I correct that you are still active in your research?

TI: I'm very active. I am very much concerned that drug therapy is given without checking the effect of drugs on the brain. So we are setting up memory centers where we can check with our EEG methodology the effect on the brain of the drugs given to patients.

TB: On this note we conclude this interview with Dr. Turan Itil. Thank you, Turan, for sharing this information with us.

TI: Thank you.

SAMUEL C. KAIM

Interviewed by Leo E. Hollister
Washington, DC, April 14, 1997

LH: It's Monday, April 14, 1997, and we're in Washington to continue video-taping the History of Psychopharmacology, sponsored by the ACNP. My name is Leo Hollister and I'm pleased to welcome today, my old friend and colleague, Sam Kaim.* Welcome, Sam.

SK: Thank you.

LH: I guess we've known each other for longer than we care to remember, what is it, 1960 to 1997?

SK: 1960 to 1997.

LH: Thirty-six years.

SK: Thirty-seven!

LH: That's a long time. Tell me, Sam, how did you get started in medicine and in psychiatry and, eventually, in psychopharmacology?

SK: I went to medical school in Zurich, Switzerland and the teacher who impressed me most was Hans Maier, the Chairman of Psychiatry at the Burghölzli. He was a dynamic man, had had five wives and many kids. He was a successor to Eugen Bleuler and I had occasion, during my stint there as a resident after graduation, to translate Bleuler's last paper into English for an American journal. That was a paper on "The Biological Memory of All Cells." This is way before anyone knew about DNA. Bleuler was really a wonderful, gifted man. He was a little fellow with a long beard with a lot of stories about him. After he retired and when Maier succeeded him, there's a story about Bleuler standing on a street corner in downtown Zurich and trying to get across the street. He'd put one foot down, then retreat, and did this for about thirty minutes. A policeman came over and said to him, "Old man, you look like I ought to take you to the Burghölzli," and Bleuler replied, "No, don't do that. I spent thirty years there. I've had enough of that place."

LH: Of course, he was the director for many years. He was the kind of charismatic teacher that got you interested in psychiatry. You eventually trained there, didn't you?

SK: I trained there after graduation and stayed for two years; it was during that period I got involved with psychopharmacology.

LH: We're talking about what date now?

SK: 1937 and 1938. I was in charge of the insulin shock and Metrazol convulsive therapies at the Burghölzli and used them in combination with other therapies, so they were the first two psychopharmacologic agents

---

* Samuel C. Kaim was born in New York, New York in 1911.

I worked with. Adolf Meyer used to visit periodically; I remember visiting the Phipps Clinic at Hopkins in Baltimore, and it was the mirror image of the Burghölzli. I felt like I'd stepped back in time to my own experience at the Burghölzli. The Burghölzli was quite a place and still is. Manfred Bleuler, Eugen's son, and I shared the podium at the University of Louisville on two occasions when they had their international psychopharmacology seminars.

LH: That was one of John Schwab's seminars?

SK: Schwab's, yes. One of our patients was Einstein's son, who had schizophrenia. I saw a piece in the paper recently; it was interesting that Einstein never visited him. He did send a hundred dollar check every month for his keep in our private wing. Imagine a hundred dollars a month at the Burghölzli, to have a private room and great therapists.

LH: You can't even get a glass of beer in a hospital these days for that.

SK: You could get a breakfast, maybe. Anyway, it was quite a place.

LH: Do you think that Einstein just couldn't deal with his son's mental illness?

SK: I don't know, I never met Einstein, but the son was interesting. Every time we gave him ground privileges, we'd have to revoke them. He had a habit of going behind the women patients and goosing them.

LH: Well, he wasn't totally crazy, was he?

SK: In 1938, after the Anschluss and the Nazis took over Austria, the New York Times correspondent in Berlin had his wife as a patient at the Burghölzli. She had broken down on the trip to Europe, When he decided Europe was getting too hot for his family, he asked me to accompany them on the boat from Paris back to the States.

LH: That must have been a nice assignment.

SK: Yes, except she was a violent, unpredictable patient who had a heart condition, so we couldn't sedate her very heavily. And she tried to jump overboard a couple of times. At one point, I was holding her ankles while she was trying to get through the porthole of the cabin! I earned five hundred dollars and our first class passage. That's how I got back to the States and out of Europe in time. In fact, Maier, who was half Jewish, told me how lucky I was to be an American.

LH: This was in 1938?

SK: Right. We brought her to the Hartford Retreat for treatment, which is now The Institute of Living.

LH: Who was in charge at The Institute of Living then?

SK: I think it was a man named Burlingame. I'm not sure. This goes back sixty years. Anyway, I spent four years in military service during World War II, and then I went into private practice in Illinois. After a short period, I went to the VA Hospital in Coral Gables.

LH: That would have been in 1950?

SK: Right. It was there I got involved with the EEG. I took training at the Medical College of Virginia in 1951, and subsequently a refresher course at the Boston VA. With the experience I had with Metrazol, I had a tool to use, the EEG activated by Metrazol, to assess the patient's threshold for convulsions.

LH: So you used a Metrazol activated EEG to predict how much shock to induce convulsion?

SK: I used the EEG, first, to assess the effect of various psychopharmacologic agents on patients who were restless, a little violent, and in some neurological cases. I was in charge of both psychiatry and neurology at the VA so I had sixty-eight patients under my care. I was usually the only psychiatrist. I used the drugs to quiet patients down, so I could do an EEG. Then, two men from Roche approached me, I think in 1958, with four numbered drugs.

LH: Hoffmann-La Roche?

SK: Yes. I found one of the drugs of interest. It was RO5069, which at the time was called methaminodiazepoxide, and later chlordiazepoxide, familiarly known as Librium. It was the first of the benzodiazepines brought over from Europe by Leo Sternbach, who had the drugs on his shelf for a long time. After he immigrated to the States, he got a job at Roche when the company was looking for something with CNS activity.

LH: Had methaminodiazepoxide ever been tried in man before?

SK: No, I was one of the first twelve clinical investigators of the drug.

LH: And you were trying it in epileptics?

SK: I was mostly involved with epileptics, trying it in patients who had seizures. The interesting part was that some patients were alcoholics. Actually, a lot of my patients were alcoholics, and I found that during withdrawal from alcohol, patients did very well with Librium; it prevented seizures and DTs. Roche and the University of Texas then sponsored the first symposium on psychoactive drugs, including the anxiolytic Librium, and a drug called Nitoman, which I had rejected, among the four drugs I had studied.

LH: Was that also benzodiazepine?

SK: No, it was a tetrabenazine. I didn't think much of it, but anyway, the twelve of us had a very good symposium. It was published in *Diseases of the Nervous System*.

LH: That meeting was sponsored by Earl Cohen, wasn't it?

SK: He was one of the sponsors.

LH: He's still practicing in Houston.

SK: Is that right? You can give him my regards.

LH: I will.

SK: The meeting was at Galveston. My good friend, Red Tyler, was down there. He had been my Chief during service at Brooke Army Medical Center. He was a great guy, now dead.

LH: So your paper in Galveston was on the use of Librium for alcoholics and in epilepsy?

SK: In epilepsy, not just in alcoholics, but in anyone with seizures. I think eight were epileptics and several were alcoholics. That's where I got into alcohol withdrawal, and using Metrazol activation. In epileptics who had been on Dilantin and other anticonvulsants, I did a base EEG, then Metrazol activation to see what their seizure threshold was, before I would gradually taper them off Dilantin and start increasing the dose of Librium. Then, I would do an EEG, followed by Metrazol activation. I found that in most cases the threshold increased, so that patients were doing better with Librium than they had with their previous anticonvulsant medication. And also, their seizures were decreasing, especially in those involved with alcohol. So we thought we had a good anticonvulsant, as well as an anxiolytic in Librium. We had a patient in status epilepticus, and I found that an intravenous dose or two of Librium would stop the seizures. This was before Valium, which is now the drug of choice for status epilepticus.

LH: But, didn't we use intravenous sodium pentothal for status at the time?

SK: Yes, but it didn't really do a lot, and Dilantin intravenously wasn't nearly as good as Librium. Then, Valium was even better and is now the drug of choice. As Librium was the first of the benzodiazepines, a new class of psychoactive drugs, there was a lot of interest in this symposium. It was picked up as an interesting and provocative new idea in psychopharmacology, and in 1960 I was called up to Central Office in Washington to present my findings to the Research Service. Ivan Bennett had just left; he had been Chief of Research in Psychiatry at Central Office and left to become the clinical research director at Lilly. After my presentation, I was offered his job. I took it, reluctantly, because I'd been in Florida ten years.

LH: So you had to leave Coral Gables?

SK: Yes and I came in time for the blizzard and the Kennedy inauguration. My then wife, Polly, was a hostess for the inaugural committee, and I had to chauffeur her around in all those snow drifts. We had about three feet of snow, and Washington doesn't do well in snow. I think we were the last car on the road, escorting governors to the hotels where they were supposed to stay.

LH: Polly was from Iowa and you went to college in Cleveland, so you knew something about snow.

SK: A little bit, and I had a small Thunderbird, which did very well in snow. Anyway, I became involved in the big research that the VA sponsored, the pioneering cooperative study, which NIMH and many other organizations subsequently followed, carrying out multi-site studies with the new drugs as they came along. I had never been in any of their studies at Coral Gables where I was involved in my own work with the EEG mostly. I'd done a study in 1953 on the EEG in multiple sclerosis and a number of other studies, which I had presented at Harvard, MIT, and other places. But I'd never done a study with the VA collaborative group.

When I came to Central Office, it occurred to me this would be a great opportunity to study alcohol withdrawal, which I had pioneered with Librium. I thought, let's see if Librium will stand up to the older treatment methods. So we studied four drugs, including Librium, in 537 cases at 23 VA Hospitals. Patients on Librium had two percent of seizures and DTs, compared with over ten percent in each of the other groups. Librium has now become the drug of choice in the treatment of alcohol withdrawal. Two psychiatrists at the University of Missouri wrote a very nice paper on the use of benzodiazepines in alcohol withdrawal. They sent questionnaires to 101 hospitals inquiring about the drugs used for alcohol withdrawal, and eighty-two percent were using one of two benzodiazepines, Librium or Valium. When questioned why they had switched from older drugs to the benzodiazepines, thirty-six said, due to my paper. So I feel I did contribute something to American medicine which has lasted, and I am eternally grateful for at least bringing one standard medication to the scene.

LH: Well, Librium detox is still the favorite method for a lot of people.

SK: I think Librium is still used more often than Valium, which I would say is second best. Back in 1967 I was offered the job of clinical research director at a pharmaceutical company. When I told my Chief Medical Director I might be leaving, he said, "You can't do that, Sam; what can we do to keep you here?"

LH: Was this Bill Middleton?

SK: No, this was Hal Engle. So, I told him, "Look, Hal, I've studied alcoholism all these years. A third of my patients have been alcoholics, yet the VA and the military keep denying alcoholism is a disease. I think it's about time we faced up to it. I'd be interested in staying if we could have an alcoholism service". We'd never had one in the VA. In fact, there were all kinds of rules against admitting alcoholics in the first place. They had to have cirrhosis of the liver or some severe complication before they could be admitted. So Engle said, "Okay, you are now the Director of the Alcoholics Service of the VA." I got an office and a secretary!

LH: That was a fortunate stroke, because you became the person who made being an alcoholic acceptable. How many psychiatrists would treat alcoholics in those days? None!

SK: That's right. In 1962, I came to your hospital in Palo Alto and set up a conference to bring together fifty scientists from various disciplines to plan a program of research on alcoholism. You were very kind to me and I used your offices and secretary. Making alcohol research respectable finally opened the doors for alcoholic patients who didn't have cirrhosis of the liver, and that in turn, made it a little easier for the VA to accept my idea of having an alcoholism service.

Subsequently, with the Vietnam War, we were getting reports of opium addiction among our troops. I was encouraged to add drug addiction to the alcohol service, and we then had an Alcohol and Drug Dependence Service at the VA, starting about 1970. I was on a task force at the Pentagon, and also one at the White House about what to do with all these drug problems. The Admiral in charge of the Pentagon task force kept denying it was a problem. He said, "There are only 69 cases of heroin addiction world wide among all American troops." I asked, "Bill, how did you arrive at that?" He replied, "Well, let me call the office." So he calls his office at the Pentagon and says, "69 cases, that's all we have." I said, "Would you define those cases?" "Well, those are the only objective cases, the overdose ones. Nothing else is objective." We already had 2,000 cases at the time in the VA system!

LH: How could somebody be so blind?

SK: We had meetings at the Pentagon almost every week, trying to decide what else to do. We had an edict from Nixon, "Cure these patients within one week." I laughed. All the Admirals and Generals in the office at the meeting kept their heads down. No one dared to look up to laugh. I was home free. I could laugh, because I wasn't in the military. However, this reminds me of another problem I had. In 1966, there was an annual meeting of the American Association of Medical Surgeons of the US in Washington and I was asked to Chair a program on Alcoholism. I ventured to offer a theory that military service contributed to alcoholism. The soldier drinks after duty, the loneliness of being away from home and so on. Well, the AP picked that up. I got "holy hell" from the legal department, and also from the Chief Medical Director. "How can you do this in the middle of the Vietnam War? What American mother now wants her son to go into service? This will destroy the war effort." Perhaps it nearly did; we did not win that war.

LH: No.

SK: Anyway, alcohol was my lead into all kinds of things, but it also led me into lots of trouble. On the drug side, the VA had started a study on LAAM, a long acting substitute for methadone, and I took it on. After the VA study, the Special Action Office on Drug Abuse Prevention headed by Jerry Jaffe and I plotted what next to do with the drug problem. I took him and his lieutenant, Jeff Donfelt, to dinner at my country club and we came up with three research projects to address the problem nationwide. One was to find an effective but non-addicting narcotic as an analgesic. Well, the National Academy of Sciences Committee on Drug Dependence had been looking for that drug for fifty years without success. So, we bypassed that. It's still on the books, but that one, luckily, we let go. The second idea was to find a long acting substitute for methadone, and that was the LAAM project, which I pursued for twenty years. The head of the neuropharmacology section at FDA didn't like addicts. He wouldn't review LAAM. So, I would sit down with him every year and the White House also encouraged him to review LAAM. But he wouldn't budge. Finally, the FDA started a new program on orphan drugs and their first project was LAAM. At the same time, NIDA had started a new program on new drug development. They also picked LAAM. So finally the FDA and NIDA converged behind LAAM and I was brought on as a consultant; they called me the 'Grandfather of LAAM'!

LH: Well, it took long enough to reach maturity. It was almost twenty years from first studies to its final approval, two or three years ago, wasn't it?

SK: It was from 1972 to 1993, twenty-one years. Luckily, the FDA panel had some good people on it, including Bill Martin. Anyway, they finally approved it. One of the questions about LAAM was its long lasting effect. So, in 1981, Don Jasinski, who headed up the Addiction Research Center for NIDA, sent me on a fourteen clinic visit. These were still using LAAM after many years. And I found that no one had died from LAAM; no serious complications or adverse events. The patients liked it; the staff liked it. I brought that report back to Don Jasinski, and still, the FDA wouldn't look at it. Naltrexone had appeared on the scene introduced by Endo, (later part of Du Pont), but it was really in the public domain, it had been around a long time.

LH: Who was the chemist that developed both nalorphine and naltrexone?

SK: Bloomberg.

LH: Harold Bloomberg. I've been trying to think of his name.

SK: My memory isn't great, but, occasionally, a name comes back.

LH: You've got a few years on me, but I'm getting old, too. I've always thought that he didn't get as much recognition as he should have, because they were very important drugs. And about naltrexone, we still don't know the whole story.

SK: That's right. The Academy took it on, reluctantly, as a small multi-site project. You were the Chairman of the committee to evaluate narcotic antagonists. The National Academy of Sciences had never done this before. This was the first time they had taken on a study; usually, they just review other peoples' studies. You were the Chairman of the committee, and I was the Director of the Staff. We recruited five clinics but found retention of patients very difficult, because this is a drug without any positive reinforcement. The patients found no pleasure from it.

LH: Say your excuses and leave, but you can't do that with methadone.

SK: Right. Anyway, the retention rate was not great, but we had no serious problems with the drug. We had a craving scale and it did show that craving lessened while patients were on naltrexone. Also, it reduced appetite. Some drug companies got interested in possibly using it as an appetite suppressant, but I don't think that went anywhere. It's a nasty drug to take, very bitter.

LH: Have you tried it?

SK: Sure.

LH: I wrote a paper some years ago about "Adverse Effects of Naltrexone" and before that Lew Judd had published one. But, you know, if you block the endorphin systems life isn't the same.

SK: I asked that question of Hans Kosterlitz. I said, "What happens to the endorphins when we use naltrexone?" He said, "Endorphins, they're so ephemeral, they last only for a few seconds. Naltrexone is a long acting drug. It isn't going to do much one way or the other." He didn't think it would do anything.

LH: We tried to measure dynorphin using Albert Goldstein's lab, but the data was so fragmentary, we couldn't make sense out of it. Nonetheless, you succeeded.

SK: We did get the project finished, and now people who are highly motivated, can kick their opiate habit with naltrexone; people like doctors, lawyers and executives.

LH: If you've got a lot on the table to lose, you're going to take it.

SK: That's right. Naltrexone is also being tried on alcoholics with some success.

LH: That one puzzles me.

SK: Me too.

LH: You remember Virginia Davis at the VA in Houston?

SK: Yes, I remember her talking about tetrahydropapaverine.

LH: She thought that alcohol dependence was opiate dependence in disguise, but nobody else really believed that, and Seevers took off on her in the worst sort of way. But I don't know how to explain why naltrexone works.

SK: That's one of the evolving mysteries of psychopharmacology; in some peoples' hands, it works. Be that as it may, I still am hopeful that narcotic antagonists will have a place in our armamentarium.

LH: Which way do you think we should go about cocaine dependence? Should we go for the substitutive route like methadone or the antagonistic route like naltrexone?

SK: I would go for the antagonistic route. I think it's preferable, theoretically. Whether it will work is another question. You know, methadone and LAAM do work; naltrexone is an iffy thing still.

LH: Theoretically, it should be perfect.

SK: Yes.

LH: It's perfect but you can't give it away.

SK: Right. Now, there's a question about where do I think we're going in psychopharmacology. You did a good paper on that. I recall at an ACNP meeting, you gave a paper on "The Future of Psychopharmacology."

LH: I did?

SK: It's published somewhere. If you look in your files, you may find it. It was a good paper, I enjoyed it. I would say, judging from my own limited experience with the benzodiazepines, that they are going to play an expanded role in seizure control, either alone or aligned with other anticonvulsants. This is one area I'm almost sure there will be a very good addition to our therapeutic armamentarium.

LH: Why do you think that Roche never picked that up though?

SK: I was at a meeting in San Francisco early on, at the time when Valium was first used for status epilepticus; when I saw, in the insert from Roche, no mention was made of this, I rashly said I was very upset Roche hadn't included status epilepticus as an indication.

LH: Well they can't do that unless they've produced data to the FDA.

SK: Yes. Roche apparently didn't want to open the whole subject up because to prove that Valium is good for that indication, they would have had to do more studies. They felt that physicians have great leeway in using drugs that are proven.

LH: Off-label use.

SK: Yes and they didn't want to go through all the problems that I had with LAAM.

LH: You're not going to sell a hell of a lot of drugs to treat status epilepticus.

SK: That's right. There wasn't a great sales pitch. I don't know if they include it now, I haven't seen a PDR lately. But it is a great drug for status, and I'm sure it saves many lives; and Librium, which I did even before Valium, could be used the same way. So, that's about what I see in the future.

LH: I'm still trying to follow why you think benzodiazepines still have a future, because a lot of people are ready to write them off.

SK: I think that would be very wrong. When I first presented papers at meetings about Librium's use in alcohol, I had eminent alcohol specialists, so called, who shouted me down, "You're going to get these people hooked on benzodiazepines, on Librium or whatever will follow. These are addicting drugs." A drug used for ten days for alcohol withdrawal is not going to lead to addiction, and as far as I know, there is no case reported. It's like someone getting morphine after surgery for two or three days, for post operative pain. He is not going to get hooked on morphine. If a doctor, incautiously, uses it for several weeks, sure. But I don't know of cases after two or three days of legitimate analgesic use.

LH: Medical use of these drugs is very rarely followed by abuse. The Committee on Problems of Drug Dependence is one that I probably feel best about my participation in, and that Committee had begun to question whether the search for the non-addicting analgesic was worthwhile. How many people get addicted to the addicting analgesic, in medical use? None!

SK: You are right.

LH: And, God knows how many potentially good drugs we kept from going on the market by being concerned about addiction.

SK: I spoke to Nathan Eddy about the quest for a non-addicting perfect narcotic. Even he had started to question this whole thing. I remember I was at one of the early meetings of a committee at the Academy that consisted of about a dozen people. We sat around a conference table and Vince Dole was sitting outside waiting to present his first talk about methadone. We had him come in. He spoke to us and we all thought it was a good talk and he had a very good idea. Addiction at the time was treated as a criminal offense, not as a medical problem. And here, we had the first medical treatment for addicts. Henry Giordano was a liaison member of our committee, from the Bureau of Narcotics and Dangerous Drugs. Giordano asked Dole to leave the room and he said, "I'm going to call the police and have that man arrested. He's breaking the law," which he really was, because until that time, doctors were not allowed to prescribe addictive drugs to non-addicts. I was in practice and that's one of the things I knew about. And we had to talk him out of it. We said, "Look, Henry, this guy has a treatment, finally, for the problem. The jails have not cured them. Let's give him a chance." And we finally talked him out of arresting poor Vince Dole and his wife, Marie Nyswander. That's a marvelous thing they did, with methadone.

LH: Oh, yes.

SK: Mary Lasker invited me and Dole to her apartment, to make plans for the future of the drug problem. She was very supportive and Vince and I went over all the possibilities, as I had done with Jerry Jaffe. I'm afraid we didn't come up with any new solutions though. It's a tough problem and it's at a plateau. We have about half a million heroin addicts in the country. We'd probably have more than that in the way of cocaine addicts and multiply that figure if marijuana is included. So, it's still a big problem; new psychotherapeutic agents probably will help us solve some of the problem. What they will be, I don't know.

LH: Well, now that you have brought it up, what do you think of the current efforts to solve the drug problems? We've been on a war against drugs for over twenty years. It doesn't look like we've won very many battles.

SK: It's very disappointing. The anti-addiction program hasn't worked. Jail hasn't worked. The presidential programs have been of limited value. The drug therapies have had some effect, except we reach only twenty percent of addicts at any one time with a drug program like methadone. So we are not winning this battle. It isn't getting much worse. It's on a plateau. I got into it in 1970, twenty-seven years ago. I would say we are about where we were then, in the size of the addict population.

LH: We are with heroin and possibly with marijuana, but I think cocaine has increased quite a bit.

SK: That's correct. Cocaine is now the drug of choice.

LH: Another local specter is ice; methamphetamine is back again.

SK: The ecstasy drugs, is a dangerous area. And prescription drugs are also being abused. So we're in a very precarious situation where we don't have any definitive answers. We're groping but it's a long time to grope. When I was at the Burghölzli, Maier presented a couple who were addicted; this was a wealthy couple who spent all their money on drugs, sold their house in order to get drugs and the wife had even sold her clothes. She came to our meeting in a fur coat and that's all she was wearing. That was my first introduction to addiction. I was very impressed by this as a problem and felt we needed to do something about it.

LH: Didn't you mention that part of your training was at the Institute of Living later on.

SK: I didn't train there, no. I just took that woman patient there. I didn't train there.

LH: For a long many years, that was the place to go if you were famous or a very rich alcoholic, before the Betty Ford Clinic took over the business.

SK: And Burghölzli used to get their share of kings and merchant princes. I had many famous patients while I was there.

LH: I think your campaign, first of all, to make the VA recognize the alcohol problem, and secondly, to make it legitimate as an illness to be treated was a major step forward. You eventually brought the treatment of alcoholism back into the domain of psychiatry, where before it was sort of an orphan, with either general practitioners or internists taking care of the consequences. When you had cirrhosis of the liver you went to the internist, but nobody was much interested in trying to prevent that.

SK: I did have one-recognition for my role in alcoholism. The NIAAA had its twenty-fifth anniversary meeting last year; they picked sixteen seminal studies in alcoholism, and one of them was the one I did on alcohol withdrawal. So I felt I had achieved something in that field. I got one commendation from NIDA for my role with LAAM. It was an interesting commendation, recognizing my historical knowledge of LAAM and my help in furthering its approval. I feel I have accomplished a little bit of something and I am gratified with what I've done.

LH: That's what you need when you get to be our age, some sort of accomplishment before we turn in our chips.

SK: I was thinking this video may prove of some help to my son, Eddy, who is working in the pharmaceutical field; I will let him see the video and he can write my obit from it.

LH: I remember Nathan Eddy used to be notorious for drowsing off during lectures, and yet he could pop up with the most salient question afterwards.

SK: Sounds like you.

LH: I could never pop up with a question. I said to him, "Nathan, rumor has it that you aren't really sleeping, that you're just intently listening." And, he said, "Don't you believe it."

SK: You also knew when a question arose, and the answer!

LH: Perhaps.

SK: I enjoyed my contacts and friendship with you, Klett, Walter Ling, Jim Musser, and so many others in the VA.

LH: That's one of the other satisfying parts to one's career, the people you meet, the friends you make and the really bright people you run into. I can't think of any other career more satisfying. Would you change it?

SK: No. I met Bleuler, Adolf Meyer, Kosterlitz, Goldstein, Jonathan Cole, all the greats in the field. Bleuler was especially a marvelous man.

LH: Well, I've always thought we've been extraordinarily fortunate in medicine and in science, in general, to be doing work we enjoy. I always say, rather than being a member of the "Thank God, It's Friday" club, it's better to be a member of the "My God, It's Friday" club. A week goes by so fast and

you haven't got as much done as you hoped; it's nice to be in that position. Thank you for sharing your thoughts with us. It's awfully good to see
you.

SK: Thanks for having me and I wish you well. You're still in use!

LH: Off the record, how old are you now?

SK: Eighty-five.

LH: My goodness!

A. ARTHUR SUGERMAN

Interviewed by Thomas A. Ban
San Juan, Puerto Rico, December 9, 2002

Tb: This is an interview with Dr. A. Arthur Sugerman* for the historical series on neuropsychopharmacology for the Archives of the American College of Neuropsychopharmacology. I am Thomas Ban. We are at the annual meeting of the college in San Juan, Puerto Rico. It is December 9, 2002. Let's just start from the beginning. Where and when were you born? Tell us something about your education and just go on chronologically.

AS: As someone once said, I was born at a very early age. I was born way back in 1929 in Dublin, Ireland, and grew up as the oldest of four children. I was back there recently on a couple of occasions. The place has certainly changed. I started at a Jewish National School in Dublin, the first such school that opened there. Church and state were not as clearly separated in Ireland as they are here today. There were Protestant schools, Catholic schools, and the one Jewish school. All were supported by the government, provided they taught the Irish language. Schools that did so were given grants toward the school. I did quite well and went on a scholarship at a Methodist high school for four years, from 1942 to 1946. There again, I did very well, especially in mathematics. I again won a scholarship to Trinity College in mathematics. At that point, I had already decided to study medicine. I'm not quite sure why. I could have gone in for engineering, but medicine looked like a better career. I could have been a mathematician, a professor, I suppose. But, anyhow, in Dublin, as in many other British colleges, you take your university and medical degree at the same time. So I got my BA with honors in 1950 and my medical degree in 1952.

TB: What did you do after that?

AS: I did an internship, and since Ireland at that time produced more doctors, priests, nuns, nurses, and dentists than it needed for home consumption, I went to England. I did another internship in London and I was senior house physician at the Brook General Hospital in London. At that time I was looking forward to doing internal medicine. It was 1953 when I arrived in London; the Queen had just been crowned. The decorations were still up. They had what they called the Festival of London. The city was very bright and gay, but the food was terrible, still rationed six years after the war. I looked around, and found during my work in internal medicine, that about half the patients I saw had psychiatric problems. So I thought that might be the thing to do. I was offered a psychiatric residency in the

---

* A. Arthur Sugerman was born in Dublin, Ireland in 1929. Sugerman died in 2007.

Midlands at Darby for six months full-time and then went to Sheffield where Professor Martin Roth had just started his chairmanship. At the same time Professor Erwin Stengel was nearby in Sheffield, and I went to him for lectures. It was a small group. There were four or five of us in this particular program, one in each of the hospitals in the Sheffield region.

TB: So you did part of your training with Martin Roth?

AS: Yes. He was somewhat nervous taking over from Professor Alexander Kennedy, who was a very outgoing guy while Martin was not. As you remember, he was rather reserved, quiet, not demonstrative, while Kennedy was the sort who would hypnotize the whole class to show how it was done. But Martin did quite well; he impressed the faculty of the Royal Victoria Infirmary at Newcastle, not by being a psychiatrist, but with his knowledge of neurology. He was called in to consult on cases; Martin had trained in neurology at National Hospital, Queen's Square in London. Supposedly, he was able to diagnose a brain tumor others had missed in a psychiatric patient and that made his reputation. There were some very good people, e.g., Henry Miller, a neurologist, and John Walton, who later became Sir John Walton, and president of the BMA.

TB: Am I correct that we are in the mid 1950s?

AS: That was from 1955 to 1958. A few years later Martin Roth had a textbook with Eliot Slater and Mayer-Gross.

TB: It was probably just about the time you arrived that Mayer-Gross moved from Newcastle to Birmingham.

AS: I think he was still in Scotland. It was an interesting and exciting time. We had six months of full-time study; the rest we spent in the hospitals.

TB: Was there any research going on?

AS: No. There was not much research going on at that time. I really started with my research later. But I did get a pretty good training in psychiatry with some psychology and statistics. Eventually, at the end of that training. I took a Diploma in Psychological Medicine at the Royal College in London.

TB: What did you do after that?

AS: I finished training and was looking around for what to do. Had I stayed in England, which it really was not the time to do, I would have had to put in time in Her Majesty's armed forces, which I was not too keen on doing. So, I accepted an offer from a member of a team of New Jersey medical directors who were touring England and visited our hospitals. They came to see how the open door system worked after hearing how wards were unlocked in England; all their wards in the States, of course, were locked. Apparently at that time patients were used to taking orders from someone higher in rank; the British knew their place in the social system.

So, if a doctor or a nurse told them to stay on the ward, even if the door was open, they obeyed the hierarchy, the pecking order. In America, if you opened the door and told them to stay in the ward, patients would head down the road as soon as your back was turned. In America, everybody is equal, and people don't take orders from anybody.

So, I headed for the US and found myself in a large psychiatric hospital in Trenton, NJ where people were real friendly. I met some nice people, including my wife. I was there for a year, but then I accepted an offer of a research fellowship in Brooklyn. The medical director at Trenton was very unhappy and wrote a letter of non-recommendation saying I was not dynamic, meaning I didn't subscribe to psychoanalytic principles and the job should be given to an American, not a foreigner. In spite of that, the people who interviewed me, including Dave Engelhardt, were very nice and accepted me and three others for psychiatric research training. That was from 1959 to 1961. So for a year I was in Brooklyn commuting weekends to Trenton to see my wife. We married in 1960, lived in Trenton and commuted in opposite directions because I was doing the fellowship in Brooklyn and she was going for her masters in education in Philadelphia. As I said, I did a research fellowship with Dave Engelhardt. I was interested in Kretschmer's idea, and was testing the process-reactive distinction. I finished my fellowship in 1961; my thesis was on prognostic practices in schizophrenia, a developmental approach.

TB: Didn't you use perceptual tests?

AS: Yes, we did, and besides that, we looked at the whole process-reactive distinction in schizophrenia, and the premorbid history. Phillips was the man who developed a scale for distinguishing "process" from "reactive" schizophrenia using three criteria. Of course, all that is obsolete now since DSM came out. What we were calling process schizophrenia is schizophrenia, and what we were calling reactive schizophrenia is diagnosed as an acute psychotic reaction.

TB: So this work was done in the early 1960s?

AS: This was in 1961 to 1962 and we published several papers on the findings. We were able to show in figure drawings that process schizophrenics had the poorest self concept.

TB: Published when?

AS: In 1964.

TB: What did you do after that?

AS: I looked around for a job, preferably a research job, and there were none to be found. One other factor, of course, was that in New Jersey at that time you couldn't get a license without being a citizen. I couldn't get a license until 1963, so I had to find a job where I could work without a license and preferably do research. After several months of looking I found that not too far away was the New Jersey Bureau of Research Neuropsychiatric Institute where Joe Tobin was director of research. Remember Joe Tobin? He was one of the founders of the ACNP. So I visited and met not only Joe Tobin, but Carl Pfeiffer and Leo Goldstein, who was working in quantitative EEG. So I accepted the job and took over a unit of chronic schizophrenics. I also took over the drug studies that Joe Tobin had initiated and an ECDEU grant which had just begun. And that's how I fell into drug research and met up with several members of the ACNP.

TB: By taking over the grant you became a member of the first ECDEU group?

AS: Yes. I started there in 1961 and the ECDEU grant came immediately after.

TB: Could you tell us something about the research you did and papers published in those years?

AS: The first few papers had to do with the quantitative EEG research I was doing with Goldstein and Murphree in psychotic patients. LSD was popular at that time and they were using it as a treatment for alcoholics.

TB: Did you do any work with Carl Pfeiffer?

AS: Yes, indeed. He was a very interesting man; he was also one of the founders of ACNP, in that first photograph with all the founders, at the original dinner. He is very recognizable with his close-cropped white hair. He had come to New Jersey from Illinois where he had been professor of pharmacology and chairman of the department. I believe he brought Leo Goldstein with him from Illinois. Henry Murphree may have gone down to Emory from Illinois before he came to New Jersey. I know that Murphree graduated from Emory. Anyhow, he had a major heart attack before he came, and was looking for something quieter than university work.

TB: Was Pfeiffer involved in research with trace elements in those years?

AS: That came later. What they were really working on was the brain wave work, and he wanted to look into brain wave variations produced by different drugs. They were giving various drugs to normal subjects and looking at brain waves. But my involvement with them was with schizophrenic patients. Murphree went on to become a member of the faculty of the medical school that is now the Robert Wood Johnson Medical School. When it started it was Rutgers Medical School and he became chairman of psychiatry. Murphee was also a very interesting man since he'd had training in pharmacology but didn't have training in psychiatry until he went to Rutgers, where he moved quickly up to become chairman of the department. He is now retired. And, of course, Leo Goldstein was a lovely man. He had come from France and had great ideas about what to do. He was always better at getting the EEG results he wanted than I was. I used a similar apparatus and a sound proof room to duplicate his work, but I never really succeeded. His results were eventually replicated at several labs in Europe and eventually in the United States. Unfortunately, the method was too simple and you just couldn't get a federal grant. Max Fink got the federal grants. I visited Max and was very impressed with what I saw. He had a lot of support from the state of Missouri as well as from the federal government.

TB: You were in charge of chronic schizophrenics. How many patients did you have?

AS: Well, we generally had about forty. So, we were doing mainly small studies. You know, 6, 8, 10, 12 patients.

TB: Did you always use clinical and electrophysiological measures?

AS: Yes, at the beginning. Later on we used primarily the BPRS and the NOSIE. We were one of the first to use the NOSIE.

TB: Didn't you study some of Paul Janssen's drugs?

AS: Yes. I worked with haloperidol and later with floropipamide. He called it pipamperone.

TB: It was the one he thought has a kind of atypical neuroleptic effect.

AS: True, it did have some atypical effects, but then I thought molindone did also. You know molindone made the patients happier. It didn't cause weight gain or lactation. But that has been largely ignored, unfortunately, and people haven't paid much attention to it. There were many other antipsychotics at that time; it was about the end of the phenothiazine era and the beginning of the butyrophenone era. I also did the first study in this country with pimozide, and with half a dozen thioxanthenes, most of which have not been released for clinical use.

TB: Did you work with thiothixene?

AS: Yes, but that was a Pfizer compound.

TB: Could you talk about your ECDEU grant? You were involved with ECDEU from early on. Can you recall who the other EDCEU investigators were?

AS: That was a very exciting time. Interesting people were involved, and we all got together, as you recall, for very pleasant meetings, generally at some other investigator's base, so we had an opportunity to see where others were working. There was a heavy concentration of people from New York, Nate Kline and George Simpson from Rockland, Hy Denber from Manhattan State, Sid Merlis from Central Islip, Arnie Friedhoff from NYU. Don Gallant was there from New Orleans.

TB: And Mel Bishop.

AS: Bishop, yes. Al Kurland was there from Maryland. He was also one of the early ECDEU investigators.

TB: Max Fink?

AS: Yes, Max Fink.

TB: Dave Engelhardt?

AS: Yes, Dave Engelhart from Brooklyn, and, of course, yourself and Heinz Lehmann from Canada.

TB: Pierre Deniker?

AS: Yes, Pierre Deniker. We had meetings in a variety of places; first it was only the investigators. Then the drug companies found out about it, and sent representatives; it became hard to have meetings of the investigators without the drug companies. In the beginning we had a chance to present our results to each other first. That was a very interesting time when you saw how other people dealt with the drugs you had been testing. We found, for instance, that experience is very important in using rating scales; people who had seen a wide range of pathology rated differently from people who had only seen a narrow range. We showed that psychiatrists and psychologists rated the same way. I remember going to Palo Alto for an ECDEU meeting as well as a meeting in New Orleans. Don Gallant took us for dinner at Antoine's. Oh, we forgot Burt Schiele.

TB: Burt Schiele played an important role in the beginning.

AS: Doug Goldman was also there, involved with the VA.

TB: For how long did you have the ECDEU grant?

AS: I had my ECDEU grant from 1961 to 1972 and after 1972 I think all the ECDEU grants faded away. They were not renewed after that. I was able to do some studies outside of my unit in the state hospital and other facilities. I did a study with haloperidol in geriatric patients at a state supported hospice in New Jersey. I remember studying benzodiazepines on an "addictions unit." There was a study with prazepam and placebo in the treatment of convalescing narcotic addicts in 1971. So, all that stopped in 1972.

TB: What did you do after your ECDEU grants expired?

AS: By that time, the state of New Jersey, like other states, had lost interest in supporting drug research. It happened in the other states too. And when the grant expired, there wasn't much future in doing clinical studies. What happened was that Pete Penick who participated in a VA-NIMH study of lithium at the Carrier Clinic decided he wanted to do a residency in psychiatry. So he asked me to take over that study from him and I went to work part time at the Carrier Clinic. Then Dr. Carrier asked me to join the clinical staff of the Clinic. And after that I spent 20 years at the Carrier Clinic, which included seven years as director of research and four years as medical director. I started in the outpatient department and after awhile I became director of education.

TB: So you started at the Carrier Clinic in the early 1970s?

AS: This was from 1972 until 1990. I started there with the lithium study. We put more manic patients into the study than any of the other participating centers, and some of those patients have stayed with me, so I've been seeing them every three months or six months for thirty years. We also occasionally did drug studies, for instance, one with synthetic TRH in the treatment of depression. I never had the sort of results with TRH that Prange had. He had very good results, and he still thinks it works, but it didn't work for me. I sent him all the data on the study at his request. There wasn't anything there. I have been involved in other types of research including non-psychiatric drug research. I spent 20 years consulting for Squibb on phase I studies. So, what else can I tell you?

TB: What did you do after you retired from the Carrier Clinic?

AS: I've been teaching all along at the Robert Wood Johnson Medical School, first as associate professor, then in 1978 as a clinical professor. From 1990 to 1993 I went full-time with the medical school as director of the addiction services. Then I retired and since then have been part-time in private practice, still doing some teaching of medical students.

TB: Are you still active in research?

AS: I'm still involved in drug studies, but this is just a very small part of my activities. Things have changed so much now. Max Fink wrote about it at length in your CINP series. I don't get much satisfaction from looking at a fragment of a study. In the old days we wrote our own protocols, picked our own measures, saw all the patients and wrote up the results. All of that is gone, we can't cry over spilt milk. There is not much we can do about it, so I don't get involved.

TB: When did you become a member of the ACNP?

AS: I must have become a member about 1964 and became a fellow in 1967.

TB: So, it was about 38 years ago. Have you served on any of the committees?

AS: No, I never volunteered for anything. Actually, George Simpson asked me to be on the ethics committee, and I did that, but I really didn't volunteer for anything.

TB: What do you think was your most important contribution to the field?

AS: It is difficult to point to one particular thing. Apart from drug studies, I was very involved in the brain wave studies with Leo Goldstein and was very impressed with his showing that schizophrenics have low variability in their brain waves. That seems to be pretty clear, although it hasn't really been followed up.

TB: Are you considering that one of your important contributions?

AS: I think that was important. I was very pleased with the various drug studies I did but they are all obsolete now, and there have been a lot of other things that came along since. We did a nice four-year follow-up study with alcoholics when I was at Carrier. That was the biggest study I did there. What we showed was that the treatment didn't work; no matter whether patients were treated there for a week, two weeks or four weeks, the results were the same. One-third of the patients got better, one-third stayed the same, one-third got worse. So I think that was important, but for various reasons it wasn't followed up. What has happened since is that because of insurance pressures, nobody is in the hospital for four weeks for alcoholism.

TB: As director of education you trained probably a number of people. Is there anyone you would like to mention from those you trained or worked with during the years. You have already mentioned a few.

AS: We talked about Carl Pfeiffer, Leo Goldstein and Henry Murphree, and I think I also mentioned Pete Penick. He died young, unfortunately. He was a very athletic man, kept very trim, but after a tennis game he collapsed with a heart attack; that was a great loss.

TB: Is there anything else we should cover? That we left out? What was your last publication? You seem to be still active in your practice, right?

AS: Yes.

TB: Well, let me ask you one final question. Is there anything you would like to see happen in the field?

AS: That's a great question. In the field of psychiatry?

TB: Psychopharmacology.

AS: Coming to this meeting over so many years, you can't but be impressed by the amount of fragmentation that is going on. In the early days of ECDEU one could understand what all the different people were talking about. Now we have wonderful presentations with the latest cutting edge advances in imaging and genetics, and one wonders how much is accessible to people in unrelated fields. I mean, there may be 20 or 30 different fields in basic science being discussed but very little overlap between them. In the old days, we sought out what was going on in related fields and could understand them. The knowledge has expanded so much that most of the work that goes on is beyond the comprehension of most of the people not directly involved with it. So, unfortunately, we're getting a Tower of Babel where people don't understand each other's language.

TB: So you think that communication should be improved across the different areas in the field?

AS: Yes, but I don't know how; you're asking me what can be done, but I really can't think how because it is so inevitable we become more and more fragmented.

TB: This is a reasonable note on which to end this interview. Thank you.

AS: Thank you.

IRWIN FEINBERG

Interviewed by Leo E. Hollister
Kamuela, Hawaii, December 12, 1997

LH: Today is Friday, December 12, 1997, and we're in Kamuela, Hawaii, for the thirty-sixth annual meeting of the American College of Neuropsychopharmacology. As part of our historical series on people who've been in the field of psychopharmacology a long time, we're going to interview, today, one of the long time sleep researchers, Irwin Feinberg.* Welcome, Irwin.

IF: Thank you Leo, it's a great pleasure to be interviewed by you because I've admired your work for so many years.

LH: Oh, my!

IF: And appreciated your friendship and support over the years. It's a great pleasure.

LH: Hearing that from somebody who knows something about a field I have very little experience with, I like that. Tell me when you started in this field?

IF: I started off in sleep research accidentally. I was at the National Institute of Mental Health working in Seymour Kety's laboratory.

LH: When was this?

IF: I went to the NIMH in 1957, my draft number come up and I had the option of going into the Commissioned Corps of the Public Health Service at the NIMH. So I went to work in Ed Evarts' Section of Neurophysiology in Seymour Kety's Laboratory of Clinical Science. Ed Evarts became one of my closest friends and had the largest influence on my scientific development. Ed was a psychiatrist who thought he would learn some neurophysiology because it would be useful for research. By the time I got there he had made many basic advances in neurophysiology. Although I had been hired to help him with his psychiatric work, Ed said "I'm not interested in psychiatry anymore. I'm going to be a neurophysiologist full time, so find something to make your time useful and worthwhile."

LH: Prior to that, you had completed medical school?

IF: Yes, I completed medical school at NYU in 1955. I interned at Boston City Hospital and did my first year of residency at what was then Boston Psychopathic Hospital, later to become the Massachusetts Mental Health Center. Harry Solomon was the director of Boston Psychopathic Hospital when I was there. I think he retired at the end of my first year or shortly thereafter. Anyway, I had only one year of residency training in Boston, because I had to join the PHS.

---

* Irwin Feinberg was born in Brooklyn, New York in 1928.

LH: You received your MD from what school?

IF: New York University Medical School.

LH: And you went into psychiatry right after internship?

IF: I did my first year of residency at Boston Psychopathic Hospital and from there I went into the NIMH with Ed Evarts and Seymour Kety. Both of them had great influence on me scientifically, especially Ed Evarts. I had tremendous admiration for him as well as for Seymour Kety and Louis Sokoloff.

LH: Evarts did a lot of work on the motor system, didn't he?

IF: Yes, he ended up focusing on the motor system. But he also did pioneering work on sleep. He did some of the best early work on differences in neuronal activity in different parts of the brain in REM, NREM and waking, measuring activity in the same neurons in all three states. Part of that work involved pioneering microelectrode techniques for single unit recordings in cats. Later, Ed moved to monkeys when he started to do research on the motor system. There I was, kicking around in Ed Evarts' lab. I was interested in hallucinations, an interest I still have, and was studying them in schizophrenics at St. Elizabeths Hospital when Bill Dement came through the NIH and gave a talk on REM sleep. Having by this time some knowledge of the history of thinking about hallucinations, it occurred to me that I could use REM sleep to investigate Aristotle's hypothesis that hallucinations come about from a disturbance of the mechanism that normally produces hallucinations during sleep, i.e. dreaming.

LH: Hallucinations as a kind of REM sleep awake.

IF: Right. So, I embarked on what I thought would be, at most, a six month study to compare REM sleep in hallucinating and non-hallucinating schizophrenic patients. The reason I had only six months to collect the data was that I was scheduled to spend a year with Piaget in Geneva. I was able to collect the data in collaboration with Fred Snyder and Richard Koresko and then I spent my year in Geneva. When I returned, I found that analyzing sleep EEG records was not as simple or straightforward as the literature led one to expect. So the study I thought would only be a six-month digression took two years before it was finished. It turned out there was no important difference in REM sleep between hallucinating and non-hallucinating schizophrenics. However, there was a substantial difference in the amount of Stage 4 sleep or deep sleep between schizophrenics and normal controls. Fifty percent of the schizophrenic group had no scoreable Stage 4. The other fifty percent had perfectly normal Stage 4 sleep.Therefore, as a group, the schizophrenics averaged half the stage 4 levels found in age-matched controls. What this means is still a very interesting research problem, especially so because the stage 4 abnormality remains the most consistent brain abnormality demonstrated in schizophrenia, even though it is present in only half of the patients. This stage 4 result has since been replicated several times.

LH: Is there any clinical difference between the two groups?

IF: A good question that I can't answer. By the time the data were analyzed and I recognized this finding I no longer had access to the patients. They had gone their various ways. But medication was not a factor. These were essentially un-medicated schizophrenics and that was an unusual aspect of the original study one cannot duplicate.

LH: Not today.

IF: Not at this time. So I had put several years of effort into sleep research. After much effort I now had a negative result with respect to REM sleep in schizophrenia. By this time I was hooked on sleep because I was convinced it must do something important for the brain. Because we often dream about what happened to us during the day I reasoned that REM sleep might be related to memory processing. To study that question, I selected a group of elderly patients with dementia of varying severity and etiologies. I compared their sleep to that of a group of elderly, age-matched normal subjects. In both groups, there was a correlation between the amount of REM sleep per night and independent measures of cognitive function. A positive finding at last! However, this study, in which I used elderly normal controls, led me to assemble data on sleep and aging. I had elderly normal subjects as controls for the demented patients and I had data on normal young adults who were controls for the young schizophrenics. To use these normal data to construct age curves for EEG sleep measures over a broad range I recorded sleep in a small group of children. In graphing these data, I discovered what had already been mentioned in the literature, although less well documented. There are many changes in sleep EEG with aging.

The finding that intrigued me most was that there is a huge amount of deep, stage 4, sleep in children that decreases very steeply across adolescence. Stage 4 then continues to decline, at a very much slower rate, to a plateau in late middle age. I'm now going to skip ahead a decade to the interpretation of the biological significance of the huge decline in deep sleep across adolescence This interpretation turned out to have some influence on psychiatric research. It became evident to me that the change in sleep across adolescence was one component of a major brain reorganization taking place. During adolescence there is a great loss of brain plasticity. This is shown, for example, by diminished ability to recover from brain lesions, particularly notable in lesions that cause aphasia. There is also a substantial decline in cerebral metabolic rate.

In adolescence there are rapid advances in cognitive function that traditionally had been assumed were entirely due to education. But I thought that these biological changes in the brain might contribute as well. I summarized this evidence in 1982–83 and proposed that the brain changes across adolescence might all be explained by a genetically programmed elimination of synapses; a few years before, in 1979, Peter Huttenlocher had demonstrated a reduction in synaptic density in human frontal cortex over adolescence.

LH: That would be a second pruning.

IF: Indeed, that would be at least the second, and one coming quite late, at an age when brain development, except for myelination, was thought to be complete. In this paper, I also proposed that a defect in this late pruning process might cause some kind of mental illness, notably, schizophrenia, which often has its onset at the end of adolescence. This hypothesis was the first modern neurodevelopmental model of schizophrenia and I was led to it by my attempt to understand the enormous change in deep sleep EEG across adolescence. This change remains one of the most fascinating unsolved problems in human developmental neurobiology. One can also state the issue more generally; sleep is very tightly linked to age over the human life span. Inherent in that tight link must be clues to both the function of sleep and the nature of brain aging. So that was one direction my research wandered into.

LH: This was all done in Evarts' laboratory?

IF: No. I have been excessively peripatetic, perhaps, the most peripatetic of sleep researchers. After seven years at the NIH, I went to Downstate Medical Center and worked in Brooklyn for five years, near where I grew up. I then left to go to San Francisco as Chief of Psychiatry at the VA Hospital and Professor in the Department of Psychiatry at UCSF. So this last set of studies I described was done in San Francisco. You mentioned at the beginning that I have been somewhat contrarian in the sleep field. That is absolutely correct. I've taken my own direction in several respects. One example, in which my deviant thinking influenced the field, was my emphasis on the importance of deep or Stage 3 and 4 sleep. This was when sleep research was all agog about REM which had been recently discovered. Although non-REM sleep occupies 75% of total sleep, as compared to 25% for REM sleep, REM was considered biologically more important. This position was maintained even though the priority activity of the brain, in falling asleep, is deep sleep. Most of the night's deep sleep occurs in the first couple of hours after falling asleep. In contrast, the highest proportion of REM is at the end of the sleep period. Among other arguments, I pointed out that if REM sleep were the most important component of sleep, it would come first, because in nature the organism doesn't know how long it will be possible to remain safely asleep.

LH: Yes, but I think the reason that REM caught on, especially at that particular time, was, of course, that Freud made such a big deal about dreams that we could now find out when people were dreaming. Don't you think that was it?

IF: That was a very major influence. Yet another aspect is the physiology of REM which is so dramatic. In REM the organism is asleep but neuronal activity in several parts of the brain, such as the visual cortex and lateral geniculate, is explosively active. The same is true for various brain stem structures that mediate arousal. So not only was REM related to dreaming, almost exclusively it was thought at the time, but there was also a striking paradox; intense neuronal activity, including in the motor system, in a sleeping subject. In the 1960s, Jouvet called REM "paradoxical" sleep, a term that is still used, though mainly in animal research. Again, the paradox is intense activity in many brain structures when the organism is asleep and behaviorally quiescent. Prior to the discovery of REM it was thought the brain simply shuts down during sleep.

LH: At the same time the body was paralyzed.

IF: Right. The body needs to be paralyzed during REM. If it were not paralyzed the intense neuronal firing in the motor cortex would cause movements that produce waking. These dramatic features, along with its relatively recent discovery and apparent relation to dreaming – now known to be much weaker than originally thought – caused the rapidly developing field of modern sleep research to focus on REM and neglect non-REM sleep.

However, there were several considerations that led me, in 1974, to propose that if there is a component of sleep that is homeostatic for the brain, it's much more likely to be slow wave sleep or deep sleep than REM sleep. The most important of these considerations is that slow wave sleep, rather than REM sleep, is correlated with how long you've been awake. If you take a nap early in the morning, you have essentially no deep slow wave sleep, but if you take naps later and later in the day, you have more and more slow wave sleep. If you are deprived of sleep, the amount of slow wave sleep increases still further. This was primarily the work of Wilse Webb and Ralph Berger, who demonstrated the relationship of slow wave sleep to prior waking duration.

In contrast, REM is not related to how long you've been awake. The amount of REM increases the longer you've been asleep. And, if you extend sleep beyond habitual levels in college students as we did by keeping them in bed for 12 hours, they double their normal amount of

REM sleep. But this doubling has no effect on the amount of REM they have on the following night, or on its timing. In striking contrast, the amount of slow wave sleep that occurs in a late nap gets subtracted from slow wave sleep on the following night. These and other considerations led me, in 1974, to propose the homeostatic model of Δ sleep. An essentially identical model was published eight years later, without attribution, by Alexander Borbely in Zurich. Borbely added a circadian factor that controls sleep timing and he also quantified the model, which got it more attention. These two proposals regarding Δ as the homeostatic component of sleep remain the operating models for basic sleep research and theory. Another area in which I was a contrarian was on the issue of REM latency and depression. I was contrarian in two respects; with regard to diagnostic significance and biological meaning. First, I pointed out very early on that short REM latency was not specific to depression but also occurred in schizophrenia.

LH: Narcolepsy.

IF: Right, it occurs in narcolepsy and in many conditions of abnormal or disturbed sleep. To this day I am puzzled by the fact that expensive research projects are being supported under the assumption that early REM onset is a specific marker of depression. My other contrarian position with respect to REM latency is one the field now pretty well accepts. It concerns the biological, as opposed to pathophysiological, significance of REM latency. After all, what is measured in REM latency is the amount of non-REM sleep that occurs prior to the first REM period. If REM latency is abnormally short, does that signify an abnormality of NREM or REM sleep? The assumption had been made, in the context of an overemphasis on REM, that a short REM latency must indicate increased REM "pressure."

LH: It could be the other way around?

IF: Exactly! In fact, we now have very nice experimental evidence that it is the other way around in normal subjects. That evidence, which I alluded to earlier, is that if subjects take a late nap, the slow wave sleep in the nap is subtracted from the slow wave sleep that night. Where does the subtraction take place? It takes place in the first non-REM period by shortening REM latency.

LH: By virtue of the fact that you have less non-REM preceding it.

IF: Precisely! Moreover, you can show this relationship is nicely quantitative.

LH: That's a very important observation.

IF: I agree. Nevertheless, it is still usually ignored by the sleep researchers who currently investigate clinical populations. However, it has not been ignored by some very good sleep scientists, like Kate Benson at Stanford or Mario Guazzelli in Pisa, Italy. Nevertheless, at present, these points are ignored by the majority of American sleep researchers.

LH: Unfortunately, a body of knowledge gets accepted and becomes dogmatic before anybody really tries to test it out. Of course, one of the mysteries about slow wave sleep is that benzodiazepines, in particular, seem to wipe it out. And, if it has a restorative function, why aren't people who take benzodiazepines impaired? I think you found an answer to that too, didn't you?

IF: Yes. This paradox is extremely important, particularly for clinical psychopharmacology. It is also relevant to some of the recent advances that were discussed this morning at the panel on metabotropic glutamate receptors, and I'll return to this later. As you noted, benzodiazepines and other GABAergic modulators like barbiturates, instead of increasing the amplitude of Δ waves in deep sleep, depress these wave amplitudes and decrease or even eliminate visually scored stage 4. Nevertheless, these drugs indisputably promote sleep. They make normal individuals sleepy and they help insomniacs fall asleep. However, they increase total sleep time only slightly, as measured by the polygraph. They increase subjective total sleep time much more strongly; the patient usually feels he has slept much more soundly and awakens more refreshed. So, it remains a puzzle that garden-variety insomniacs, for whom most sleeping pills are prescribed, don't have much of a reduction in total awake time from before treatment when studied in the laboratory. These people report "I still feel I was awake all night long. I remember everything I thought about during the night."

One aspect of sleep is that there is much more mental activity going on during sleep than is remembered. This is because memory systems normally shut down during sleep. That's why we don't tend to remember much of the dreaming that we have during the night; memory consolidation does not take place unless one wakens shortly after the dream.

In 1982, I proposed that inconsistency of subjective complaints of insomniacs with the EEG evidence they get almost a normal amount of sleep could be explained by a failure of insomniacs' memory systems to shut down normally during sleep. Insomniacs therefore remember much of the mental activity that goes on during sleep that normally is not remembered or consolidated. They interpret this as having been awake and this memory is correlated with the subjective experience of un-refreshing sleep. However, the failure of memory systems to shut down is not discernable in the polygraph, which makes it a poor tool to study insomnia. With this background, one can understand why benzodiazepines and other GABAergic brain inhibitors improve subjective sleep of insomniacs. These drugs depress arousal and cause a relative amnesia. They suppress the ability to remember by reducing brain arousal level by increasing cortical inhibition. This improves subjective sleep in insomniacs.

LH: How consistent are the amnestic effects of those benzodiazepines?

IF: Extremely consistent, and one can show this effect by using benzodiazepines to suppress memory in animal learning studies as well. So what had been considered a side effect of benzodiazepines, namely their amnestic effect, appears to produce their therapeutic effect on the sleep of insomniacs.

LH: When you get back to the apparent loss of slow wave sleep you proposed awhile back that you don't lose it; it just shows itself in a different fashion.

IF: Yes, I did show that there's no net reduction in the number of Δ waves. If you measure Δ waves after administration of benzodiazepines with computer analysis, as we showed in a *Science* paper in the late seventies, you may find no scoreable Stage 4. The stage 4 classification requires that Δ waves of criterion amplitude be concentrated in short epochs of sleep.

LH: It's an artificial categorization.

IF: Totally artificial. And if one measures each Δ wave by computer after administration of GABAergic hypnotics, one finds that the number of Δ waves is not reduced. They are simply more spread out so they don't meet the stage 4 criterion.

LH: They don't cluster up so they don't look like Stage 3 or 4.

IF: Right. However, there is a net reduction of Δ wave amplitude due to the fact that these drugs suppress brain metabolism. As you know, if you give a large enough dose, you can induce coma with a profound reduction of brain metabolism and EEG amplitude. With larger and larger doses, the EEG gets almost flat. I'm glad you brought up the question of these effects of hypnotics because this brings us to the most recent work that I've been doing, which has been with glutamate antagonists and sleep. If you think about it, all of our GABAergic hypnotics work by increasing neuronal inhibition. What about the alternative way?

LH: Of decreasing excitation?

IF: Yes, logically at least, decreasing neural excitation should have some of the same pharmacological effects as increasing neural inhibition. One of the first public discussions I've heard of this approach was at this morning's panel on metabotropic glutamate receptors. Our own lab has been doing experiments in this area for six years. It would be laborious to go into the details. In brief, antagonizing glutamate, excitatory neurotransmission has produced huge increases in deep sleep that last for a relatively short periods of time, for three to eight hours. Afterward, the EEG returns to normal. This is not the case with GABAergic hypnotics. The EEG remains abnormal for days to weeks after these drugs. Even a single nighttime dose leaves the sleep EEG abnormal for a couple of days. We believe that reducing brain excitation with glutamate inhibitors is a promising area that may have clinical potential.

LH: Glutamate inhibitors as hypnotics.

IF: Right. As I just mentioned, this possibility was discussed this morning by an investigator from Eli Lilly at the panel on metabotropic glutamate receptors. So this is a very timely issue. That's pretty much the way my career has gone. A lot of it was accidental. For example, I maintained my early interest in hallucinations and schizophrenia, and it was because I retained that interest I put together the pruning hypothesis of schizophrenia in the early eighties. It was because of my work with Ed Evarts that I formulated a model in which auditory hallucinations are caused by a defect of corollary discharge control mechanisms in the motor systems of thought. Briefly, we know that the commands of motor systems are monitored as they're emitted by the brain and this monitoring informs sensory systems and allows feedback to occur even before the action takes place, before the muscles have responded. This is called feed-forward or internal feedback or corollary discharge. Hughlings Jackson emphasized that thinking is simply the most complex of our motor acts. If so, it might maintain the feed forward or corollary discharge mechanisms present at simpler motor levels. These mechanisms might inform the brain that we have initiated a thought. We have always assumed that we know our thoughts are our own because we "will" them. In fact, most of our thoughts are not voluntarily "willed" by us. Our thoughts, usually, just pop into in our minds. Some of those spontaneous thoughts can be quite bizarre but we still recognize that we have produced them. It may be this internal thought-monitoring mechanism that is impaired in schizophrenia. The schizophrenic, after all, has thoughts, voices, or neural activity which he does not recognize are produced by his own brain.

LH: Leading to a totally bizarre experience of reality?

IF: Yes, when the schizophrenic doesn't recognize that these are his thoughts he interprets them as coming from the environment, which may not be unreasonable given the way his brain is functioning. So, schizophrenics interpret voices or thoughts as coming from the TV or from radios implanted in their head. It seems to me that this must indicate impairment in the brain's self-monitoring mechanisms, in the corollary discharge mechanisms that I hypothesize exist in the control systems of thought.

Evolution is conservative. We might therefore expect that efficient control mechanisms known to be present in simpler circuits will be retained as more complex circuits evolve. These ideas were stimulated by the work of Evarts on motor control systems. In any event, I believe that the question of how we know our thoughts to be our own is at least philosophically interesting. I am also convinced that it bears on psychopathology.

LH: How long has it been since the Kales and Rechtschaffen classification of stages of sleep was proposed? That was in 1962 or some distant date, wasn't it?

IF: It was. Your memory is very good. It was 1962.

LH: Is that still operating?

IF: It is still used exclusively by people who don't do computer analysis. But I think there is very little excuse not to do computer analysis which is now quite inexpensive.

LH: That's why I raised the question. Is it time to rethink that classification?

IF: Yes. Visual stage scoring is a grossly inadequate arbitrary classification. I don't blame Rechtschaffen or Kales for this. What they were doing was trying to standardize widely varying visual scoring procedures that different investigators were using.

LH: So all would speak the same language, at least.

IF: Exactly, and that was a very valuable contribution at the time. But today its arbitrary and unsatisfactory nature is grossly obvious. As we discussed, for an epoch to be scored visually as stage 4 it must be made up of 50% of Δ waves with amplitudes of fifty or seventy-five microvolts peak to peak. If the 50% criterion for stage 4 is reached, the entire epoch is classified as stage 4, whether it consists of 100% or 50% of these Δ waves. Much information is being lost. Even more information can be lost when studying age effects with visual scoring. In a child, Δ waves might average 500 microvolts in amplitude, rather than 50 or 75 microvolts. But a stage epoch made up of 50% 500 microvolt Δ waves gets the same visual score as one with 50% of 75 microvolt waves. Visual scoring simply does not recognize that huge biological difference. Another problem with such scoring is poor reliability No matter how hard one tries to train individuals to perform reliable visual scoring, reliability remains limited. Even my very best visual scorer could not reproduce the same scores on the same epochs when I gave her blinded records that she had scored six months earlier. These limitations of visual scoring led me and others to embark on direct computer measurement in the 1970s and this has been an extremely productive approach that has now been adopted by many investigators. The computer is of course almost perfectly reliable.

LH: So, inter-rater reliability with visual stage scoring is very limited.

IF: Yes, and because it was unsatisfactory in the very best of hands, I pursued the development of computer analysis. We now use a fine program written by J.D. March of Δ Software. He's selling it commercially. It is the only program that simultaneously performs both period-amplitude (time domain) analyses and power spectral (frequency domain) analyses. It also manages efficiently the huge volumes of data generated when one analyzes, for example, 1,500 epochs per night with each epoch getting over 100 measurements. Nevertheless, in spite of the strengths of computer analysis, there remains a need for some visual processing of the EEG because computer pattern recognition is still not satisfactory. We still need visual inspection to classify an epoch as REM, non-REM or waking and to exclude artifact. Once the classification has been made, one can perform computer analysis to quantify the EEG in each stage.

LH: That's drastically different.

IF: Yes, but necessary. With this approach, one can determine exactly how many Δ waves are present including their amplitudes and periods. One can do this for all the other waves in the EEG spectrum, and of course, do this separately for REM and non-REM sleep.

LH: Why don't you propose to the Sleep Disorders Association that they reconsider the computer scoring of sleep epochs in view of the technological developments that occurred in the last thirty something years?

IF: That's a very reasonable question. I have proposed this but so far made little headway. There are several reasons. One is that many clinicians have invested in commercial computer systems that do not do wave measurement but try instead to reproduce visual sleep stage scoring. This is what many clinical sleep labs want because it saves money. But commercial sleep scoring systems have never been adequately validated even with respect to stage scoring. Moreover, the best they can do is to produce visual stage scores that lose the information I just described to you. I think the situation will change soon because small ambulatory recorders that do both stage scoring and EEG wave measurement are being developed. But right now the clinical labs are sticking to stage scores.

LH: They don't want to spoil the business, huh? Whatever happened to Aserinsky? I can't think of any situation in science where somebody has been part of a dramatic discovery and walked away from it so quickly.

IF: Well, I don't know the whole story. After Aserinsky discovered REM sleep as a grad student for Kleitman in 1953, he took a job in a physiology department in one of the medical schools in Philadelphia. I don't remember which one, maybe Temple. I would rather not comment on that development because I think Aserinsky may have been treated unfairly. I don't think he walked away from his discovery willingly. But he certainly did make the seminal observation and it was his alone.

LH: Kleitman was the father of the sleep studies and, as I understand it, Bill Dement might have come there at the time they discovered this and he took it up and ran with it and did a tremendous job.

IF: My understanding is that Bill Dement was Aserinsky's research assistant while a medical student and that is how Bill got into sleep research. He made a number of important contributions, including the best first early description of EEG cycles across the night with Kleitman. Bill was also the first to demonstrate REM sleep in the cat.

LH: And, the PGO spikes.

IF: He described the PGO spikes though I think it may have been Jouvet who first discovered them. But Bill used them in several studies and emphasized their importance. A tremendous part of Bill's contribution was as a popularizer, a person who emphasized the importance of sleep to medicine and to basic physiology. However, I believe he went a little bit overboard in the establishment and promotion of sleep disorder clinics.

LH: Overused.

IF: Overused, particularly at a time where costs of medical care are sky-high. And the use of the sleep laboratory is not helpful for many conditions but is always very expensive. Sleep apnea is the most important condition that has been discovered by clinical sleep investigation. The care of patients with sleep apnea is not something that psychiatrists or psychologists are qualified to do. It requires pulmonologists. The field has been too slow in sifting out of what is valuable from what is not valuable in sleep disorders. For example, many sleep disorders clinics would refer patients with a simple complaint of insomnia for sleep laboratory examinations. As I mentioned earlier, most patients with insomnia have fundamentally normal polysomnograms, typically with only a slight increase in the sleep latency. So, these are very expensive tests with limited value for diagnosis or therapy of most sleep disorders. I hope there will be an evolution to a more focused and limited use of sleep laboratory examinations.

LH: I wish you would publish something called, "What I Have Learned in Thirty-Five Years of Sleep Research," because you've had more original ideas than anybody I ever talked to in the field. And yet, your ideas don't get publicized as much as they should.

IF: Thank you Leo. I must confess that has been frustrating to me. It is an example of the need to market research findings. There's a regrettable aspect of modern science; if you have an interesting finding or idea, you are not likely to get recognition if you only publish it once.

LH: Repeat it.

IF: Unfortunately it appears one has to keep publishing it over and over in different forms to maintain priority and get recognition. And I have always found it boring to write a second paper with the same finding. I'm more interested in writing new papers on new things, and that has in the reality of this world cost me a lot.

LH: I expect it has. But I think you're right. I remember, many years ago, I asked a well known scientist "Harry, why do you publish the same damn stuff? Why do you keep repeating it?" He said, "That's the only way to get your ideas across"

IF: That's unfortunately true. Another way one can do it is with a book where you summarize a point of view and an approach. I hope to do a book on sleep and one on schizophrenia, but I keep putting them off.

LH: Well, I have been just a little bit discouraged about the way programs of this ACNP organization are being driven toward neuroscience exclusively. I was going to propose to the Program Committee that they send around an announcement to all the members and say, "Look, if you want to be on the program, send a one page summary of what you want to talk about, either work you have in progress or work you've done for review by the whole field," Something like a summary of what we've just talked about. I think it would be a very eye opening experience for a lot of people.

IF: I would certainly love to do that but I don't think it will happen.

LH: Well, I would change from a top down to a bottom up model.

IF: If you can, I will be happy to be part of it.

LH: I hope you will be. It's been very nice talking to you, Irwin. I knew this was going to be stimulating and it certainly has been.

IF: Thanks a lot, Leo. I appreciate it.

LH: You might call it an eye opener.

J. CHRISTIAN GILLIN
Interviewed by William E Bunney, Jr.
San Juan, Puerto Rico, December 10, 1996

WB: I am Dr. William Edward Bunney, Jr., currently Professor and Director of Research at the University of California, Irvine. I'm interviewing Professor J. Christian Gillin,* who is a professor at the University of California at San Diego. Chris is, in my view, clearly the outstanding sleep researcher in the world. He has that international reputation. He is known for the quality, for the carefulness with which he conducts research. Chris has been a pioneer in the field of sleep research and its relationship to neuropsycho-pharmacology. So, I'd like to start the interview by asking Chris about his training.

CG: Thank you Biff. I was an undergraduate at Harvard College and did my medical school training at Western Reserve in Cleveland. After my internship in Cleveland, I went to Stanford University, where I was a resident for two years in psychiatry, and then in 1969 I went to the National Institute of Mental Health, where I was what we called a "clinical associate" and I initially worked in the laboratory of Dr. Frederick Snyder. But then I had an opportunity to collaborate with you. That went on for some twelve or thirteen years while we were both at the NIMH. Later on, I worked in the laboratory of Dr. Richard Wyatt. These were the two main places that I got my research training: in your laboratory with Dr. Snyder and in Dick Wyatt's lab in the NIMH Intramural Program.

WB: Were there new psychopharmacological agents and drugs of interest to you at that time?

CG: Maybe I should go back to when I was at Stanford, and was developing my interest in sleep research. I had an opportunity to work for about three months in the laboratory of Dr. William Dement. At that time, there was great enthusiasm about the possible role of serotonin in schizophrenia. We had an idea that some of the manifestations of schizophrenia, such as hallucinations, might be related to a dysregulation of REM sleep, that hallucinations might be dreams that somehow escaped the confines of REM sleep. I did a little work with serotonin in Dement's laboratory and some animal studies. Then when I went to the NIMH and was working with Dick Wyatt, we were particularly interested in the role of serotonin and its relationship to schizophrenia. We conducted a number of studies, giving 5-HTP or tryptophan in large doses to schizophrenic patients to see if it had any antipsychotic effect. It didn't really do too much. So that was a line of research that didn't go much further at the time.

---

* J. Christian Gillin was born in Columbus, Ohio in 1938. Gillin died in 2003.

There was an incident when I was a resident that had a major influence on my interest in neuropsychopharmacology. Once when I was on call, I got a call from the emergency room saying that there were four young people who had come in with an anticholinergic delirium. They were crawling the walls and were totally delirious, and I was trying to think what could I do for these kids. Remembering my pharmacology lectures from medical school, I thought if we could give them physostigmine that might reverse the anticholinergic effect of the scopolamine they had taken. It wasn't a drug that was available at that time. But shortly thereafter, by pure chance, I met an army colonel who was on sabbatical at Stanford, and his job in the army was to do research on chemical biological warfare. He had conducted studies in army volunteers given scopolamine-like drugs and had shown that physostigmine was effective in treating them. So I had occasions later on in the emergency room to use physostigmine in some patients and it worked quite well. At about the same time, physostigmine was approved for treatment by the FDA. The cholinergic system has been one of the areas of my research all along.

WB: Why don't you tell us a little bit more about the cholinergic hypothesis of REM sleep?

CG: One of the interests I had when I started research in sleep was to understand what neurotransmitters were involved in the regulation of REM sleep. For a long time, we really didn't have a clue. But as I read the animal literature, it seemed that more and more data supported the idea that cholinergic mechanisms might initiate REM sleep. So we were trying to figure ways to test this, and after some false starts, we found the right dose and right way of administering physostigmine. When we gave it intravenously to normal volunteers during the first non-REM period of sleep we learned that we could turn on REM sleep, and also that these REM periods seemed to be totally normal, i.e., did not differ from naturally occurring REM sleep.

WB: Wasn't this the first demonstration of that?

CG: In humans, yes.

WB: Right.

CG: A lot of this work was done by one of our former students, Dr. Sitaram. At the same time we were doing our first studies on sleep and depression, and one of the key findings we had observed, as Dave Kupfer and others had previously, was that depressed patients had short REM latency. These findings indicated that cholinergic mechanisms were involved. So we tried to figure out some ways to approach that and ended up developing a test we called the Cholinergic REM Induction Test; we gave a cholinergic agonist like arecoline intravenously to either normal volunteers or patients with depression while they were asleep, and would measure how long it took to induce REM sleep. We found that depressed patients entered REM sleep more quickly after receiving this challenge than did normal controls. So that was a line of research, and a number of groups around the world have replicated our findings; Berger's group in Germany has done so on several occasions.

But certainly that's not the whole answer to understanding the basic mechanisms of sleep disturbance in depression, so we've returned to my earlier interest in serotonin, and right now we're trying a variety of techniques to understand how to study the role of serotonin in sleep in normal subjects and in patients with depression. One of the things we are interested in is the tryptophan depletion technique pioneered by the group at Yale, headed by Pedro L. Delgado. We have some very interesting findings, which I think tie serotonin deficiency to sleep disturbance and maybe to the pathophysiology of depression.

WB: Were there other drugs that you were interested in working with?

CG: The two main substances in terms of basic pharmacology have been ace-tylcholine and serotonin, but in the course of our research we've studied many different drugs, including those that affected the dopamine system. We've looked at a whole series of antidepressant medications and had the very interesting finding that MAO inhibitors completely suppress REM sleep in depressed patients. When maintained on high doses, we found they could go for more than a year or so without any REM sleep. We've looked at a whole series of antidepressants in recent years. For example, with John Rush, we found one of the newer antidepressants, nefazo-done, increased REM sleep in depressed patients, contrary to nearly all of the other antidepressants. So it raises an interesting question about whether increasing REM sleep might be good or bad for people. It might be harmful for some, and it may be good for people with, say, abnormal nightmares, such as in PTSD. We are going to look at some of these patients in the near future.

WB: Your lab pioneered looking at the effects of psychotropic drugs, particu-larly the antidepressants, on sleep parameters and, specifically, on REM sleep. Is that correct?

CG: That's true because it was very appealing that we had this electrophysi-ological measure that was basically non-intrusive; we would put peo-ple in the lab, give them medications to see how it affected their mood or their psychiatric condition, and at the same time get some notion of what it was doing in the brain by using sleep parameters as an outcome measure.

WB: You casually talk about doing these sleep studies. My experience working with you in the laboratory is that this is a heroic effort. Why don't you comment on that?

CG: It certainly gives you an appreciation of need for sleep. I know you stayed some long nights in one of the studies we did together, giving L-DOPA infusions to patients with depression and normal controls. It is a very tough life. But as you grow older, you hopefully recruit energetic, enthusiastic young people who don't mind it as much as I do now.

WB: Maybe it's worth going over some of the hypotheses you were involved in creating and designing studies to test them.

CG: What we were doing in part was to move away from a mono-neurotransmitter hypothesis of psychiatric disorders or for the regulation of sleep. It's obviously an interaction of many different neurotransmitters, and we didn't really believe that acetylcholine was the primary mover in depression, even though that had been proposed in the past. What was much more appealing to us was the idea that there was a balance between cholinergic and aminergic mechanisms and that we would never really understand how the brain works or how any of these disorders are manifested if we didn't begin to look at it in a multivariant rather than a univariant way. Using these probes was one approach to overcoming that narrow univariant conceptual outlook. So, we're still trying to develop techniques where we could give both probes to an individual and test the hypothesis of a balance between neurotransmitters. We're doing some studies now in which we are probing people with both cholinergic and serotonergic drugs, and our hypothesis is that there is some kind of correlation between the two; in a given individual you're tipping the balance in the case of depression. It's a bit like the notion of Parkinson's disease representing a balance between cholinergic and dopaminergic mechanisms. The major abnormality is probably on the dopaminergic side, but the cholinergic side is obviously involved.

WB: In addition to clinical research, you've been involved in basic animal research also. Do you want to comment on that?

CG: After we got interested in the cholinergic system, we realized that very little was known about the neuro-anatomical pathways or specific receptor systems that mediate cholinergic effects within the brain. I was fortunate to have a post-doctoral student, Peter Serramonte, who performed one of the first studies demonstrating pathways from the brain stem to the forebrain which mediate cholinergic mechanisms. We did other studies which pinpointed the effects of cholinergic mechanisms in inducing

REM sleep, primarily mediated by muscarinic-M_2 receptors. We've also done studies on the muscarinic-M_1 receptors, both pharmacologically, and more recently, using in situ hybridization techniques to identify the specific RNA message that is expressed in demonstrating which specific muscarinic receptors are involved. I think it's the marriage between basic and clinical studies that is the most attractive way to advance the field.

WB: Are there new technologies that you had to develop, either in your clinical or basic research, which allowed you to move the field ahead?

CG: One of the things that maybe our group played a major role in, was to develop methods for studying cholinergic mechanisms with physostigmine or arecoline, in which we had to give injections intravenously to humans, because the half life of these drugs was so short. We found one of the key variables was at what time during the sleep cycle we had to administer it. It was quite revealing how you would get much faster induction of REM if you gave the physostigmine half way through a non-REM period than at the beginning. Again, this finding hinted at a change in the dynamics of the nervous system.

One other area that also fascinated me over the last ten or twelve years, which involved some of the collaborations with you, is brain imaging. That started when I was at the NIMH and we collaborated with Lou Sokoloff, Charles Kennedy and that group, and did the first credible study using the deoxyglucose technique on non-REM sleep in monkeys. We were able to measure on a quantitative basis in a very rigorous fashion what the rates of absolute glucose metabolisms were during non-REM sleep compared to the waking monkey. We found quite a dramatic drop in overall metabolic rate of glucose throughout the entire period of non-REM sleep. Later on, when your group and Monte Buchsbaum's moved to Irvine and I moved to San Diego, we were able to do a series of studies on humans in PET scanning with fluorodeoxyglucose. We were the first group having a very carefully controlled study with fluorodeoxyglucose of brain metabolism, both during REM, non-REM sleep and wakefulness.

WB: I think there was similar study done before that on one patient in Cologne, Germany.

CG: That's right. Even our study was done in a very small group of subjects. But we had at least ten subjects in each of those three cells, so we were able to use statistical analyses. We also did a study of the effect of sleep deprivation on glucose metabolism in normal subjects. Again, I believe it was the first such study ever done. Another important issue I think has been neglected is the basic mechanisms of sleepiness and what the effect of sleep deprivation is on the brain in performance and so forth.

Human brain imaging will contribute a lot in the future to help understand those mechanisms.

Another interesting part of this story is the "antidepressant" effect of sleep deprivation in depressed patients. You certainly pushed it for a long, long time. I think you are one of the first investigators to really see the potential importance of sleep deprivation used as treatment for depression. We did the first study with fluorodeoxyglucose before and after sleep deprivation in patients with depression. In about a third to a half of patients, sleep deprivation had a significant antidepressant effect. What we found in this particular study was that the patients who responded to sleep deprivation had an elevated glucose metabolic rate in the limbic system, particularly the anterior cingulated gyrus that normalized with improvement. That first study was published by Joe Wu about four or five years ago, and now we've got a larger group and the basic findings, with some modification, hold up quite nicely. It's an extremely strong experimental paradigm. If we could understand how sleep deprivation has an "antidepressant" effect, it would be a very important breakthrough. One could make a lot of generalizations from it for other aspects of the treatment of depression.

WB: I couldn't agree with you more. When did you publish your first paper and what was it on?

CG: The first paper I published was on the use of physostigmine in anticholinergic delirium. Jack Heiser and I published that in the *American Journal of Psychiatry* in 1969 or 1970, as I remember.

WB: How many papers did you publish in the last two years?

CG: Maybe twenty or twenty-five.

WB: I'm trying to make a point that you've had a long career and that you are still active and going full steam.

CG: I still enjoy it.

WB: That's an incredible credit to you.

CG: I hope I'll be able to do research ten years from now.

WB: You're a vigorous role model for people.

CG: Thank you.

WB: Are there other findings we haven't covered?

CG: We covered the major areas. One of the things I've taken a lot of pleasure in, over the years, is working with young people who want to do research. We've had some success in people who've gone through the lab. One of the things we started when I went to the University of California in San Diego was a Fellowship Program for training young psychiatrists to do biologically oriented research, particularly neuropsychopharmacology. We've been able to get funding through NIMH for that. It's been turned over to Michael Irwin recently, who is one of my colleagues, but I am still very much involved with that program. I usually have about five or six people in the lab, who are there as either post-doctoral or pre-doctoral students.

WB: Who are the people who had a major influence on you or you collaborated with during your career?

CG: One person was Bill Dement, who is a tremendously charismatic person, totally committed to sleep research. His enthusiasm always inspired me.

WB: And he made the first discovery with Kleitman about REM.

CG: He was certainly one of the very first people there.

WB: Wasn't he the first?

CG: Aserinsky and Kleitman are given the credit for the discovery of REM sleep, but Dement came in very shortly after that and I think probably was the one who started the field more than anyone else. And Dave Kupfer has certainly been a very important person. He and I have been good friends over the years.

WB: So you've been active from almost the beginning of the explosion of interest in REM sleep.

CG: REM sleep was discovered quite a few years before I even went to high school, but I think I certainly got in as second generation. REM sleep was discovered about 1952 or 1953, something like that.

WB: So, you got in about fifteen years later. But that puts it in a historical perspective. For two thousand years mankind was not aware of REM sleep and then Kleitman came along. If REM sleep hadn't been discovered, it would have been a different world for you, wouldn't it?

CG: My mother certainly didn't raise me to be a sleep researcher and I never heard of the field until I was in medical school. It's certainly been fortunate. The timing was good and I was able to get in a field that was still relatively young, there were lots of exciting questions to be answered.

WB: When you got into it, there were not a lot of people involved.

CG: No, there weren't. The Sleep Research Society had maybe a hundred or two hundred people, something like that, and now there are about thirty five hundred people who belong to the two major sleep societies in this country alone.

WB: It's an order of magnitude larger now.

CG: It has grown enormously, and the whole field of sleep disorders medicine has emerged. There have been tremendous advances in understanding the basic mechanisms of sleep, even in the past decade, in terms of the relationship to circadian rhythms, the basic mechanisms that underlie the circadian clock, the mechanisms that regulate the circadian rhythm of REM and non-REM sleep, and the mechanisms underlying the EEG. These are all major things.

WB: There are really two parallel bodies of scientific inquiry, those about sleep and those about psychopharmacology. You were one of the individuals who put those together and almost from the beginning merged the two disciplines.

CG: It's always been my hope that we could apply our understanding about sleep mechanisms to the understanding of psychiatric disorders, because sleep disturbances are such an intrinsic, prominent aspect of depression, mania, schizophrenia and many other disorders.

WB: And you've employed a new technology, PET scanning, in sleep research. So three fields have been combined in your research.

CG: Absolutely. But I still consider myself primarily a psychiatrist. My goals are really to do something about psychiatric disorders and to understand them better. And I use sleep, as the window into the brain. I am also very interested in understanding sleep as a phenomenon.

WB: Before we finish, who were the major giants in the field of sleep research, regardless whether you did or did not collaborate with them?

CG: David Kupfer is someone who played a major role in drawing attention to the relationship between depression and sleep disturbances. He was the first person to describe short REM latency in depression. Bill Dement, I've mentioned already for his influence on the overall field. There have also been some basic scientists. I would say one of the most important people in my judgment was Allen Hobson, who was a psychiatrist at Harvard. He was interested in the fundamental mechanisms of sleep. He was on the Scientific Board of the Intramural Program at the NIMH and I used to talk with him a great deal. Bob McCarley was in that group and I think he's played a very important role in the development of my thinking.

There are several neuroscientists around the world like Barbara Jones, Mircea Steriade, Michel Jouvet, Dennis McGinty, Jerry Siegel, and Michael Chase, just to mention a few, who have been very important in the development of my thinking. Alexander Borbely from Zurich, Switzerland has been a close friend and a collaborator in a number of projects; he has a very broad view of sleep, neuropharmacology and its relationship to psychiatric disorders. R.H. Van den Hoofdakker from Holland was one of the first in the mid-1970s to study the effect of sleep deprivation in depressed patients. He has played a major role in the development of my thinking; he has also been a good friend throughout the years. I probably don't remember everyone I should give credit to. But there have been a lot of people who've helped along the way. One of my collaborators was

Wally Mendelson. He's now a member of the ACNP and professor of psychiatry at the University of Chicago.

WB: What you are telling us illustrates that like any field of science, there is a network of scientists working in the same area of research. You've been totally plugged into that network for many years and that has helped in developing your ideas.

CG: Yes, and certainly it was a very exciting time when we were at the Intramural Program of NIMH. One of my role models is Jules Axelrod. I was not fortunate enough to have the opportunity to work with him, but I was always very intrigued by the way he thought about problems and how he was always turning out ideas. We were able to utilize some of those ideas in our own research. Irv Kopin was a critical thinker; and Dick Wyatt a very imaginative person. We collaborated with Tom Weir and Norm Rosenthal on several projects. And Tom, Norm, and Anna Wirz-Justice taught me a lot about chronobiology that was important for my work. Since I've been at San Diego, Lew Judd has been a great leader and supporter of our research. I also have had the opportunity to work with a lot of interesting and bright people there.

WB: What would you select as your single most important contribution?

CG: I see my contributions more in linear progression. I have been interested from the beginning in the relationship between sleep and psychiatric disorders and the effect of pharmacological substances on both. It's not one of our studies but the cumulative effect that contributed to the development of the field. I'm very pleased I had an opportunity to work with functional brain imaging and to use that for studying sleep. We were among the first to study sleep deprivation with brain imaging and that area of research was also very exciting.

More recently I've had the chance with Mark Shuckit at USD to do some research on alcoholism and sleep. This was an area that hadn't been studied for twenty years or so. Mark is one of the foremost clinical authorities in alcoholism and he set up a beautiful system that allowed us to track people longitudinally. It's a carefully designed study that was done in carefully diagnosed patients. We were able to show for the first time that the sleep measures in the very early phase of the treatment, like the first week of hospitalization, are good prognostic indicators. We could predict in non-depressed alcoholics with about eighty percent accuracy those who would relapse and who would stay sober three months after discharge.

WB: Are you happy with the way things are going?

CG: In general, yes. My career has been very satisfying. I've enjoyed the people I worked with. I still get excited by new ideas. On the negative side, we all face the uncertainties about whether there will be enough money or public support for research in the future or whether we're going to be able to attract the bright young people into the field that we need. But I hope I'll be able to keep working for a good many more years.

WB: What's going to happen in the future? Where is the field going? Will the field of sleep research connect with psychopharmacology and brain imaging? Tell us realistically and also your fantasy.

CG: I can see progress in several important areas. I hope we'll have a much better understanding of the neurophysiologcal basis of sleep and the neuropharmacology of sleep to use sleep as a sort of window for understanding psychiatric disorders. I think this research could be married with functional brain imaging, so that we would get more precise localization of which neurotransmitter systems and what physiological areas might be involved in the regulation of sleep in health and in disease.

From a public health point of view, I think understanding sleepiness in the context of circadian rhythm disturbances is a very challenging area. We are living in a twenty-four hour a day society now, where a very large proportion of the population is chronically sleep deprived partly because of work schedules and pressures, jet lag, work shifts, and I think it should be possible to play a role in helping people adjust to their schedules. Melatonin, for example, might be used to shift the clock in a desirable way, and there might be other ways that could be exploited. I would also be very interested in understanding the effect of sleep deprivation on cognitive processes, on our thinking and feelings. Another exciting area is the use of sleep as an outcome measure for neuropharmacologic probes. We can measure the effect of drugs on the brain in depressed patients and we might be able to use sleep as a way to tell whether a drug has an effect on the serotonergic system. We studied recently in a group of dysthymic patients maintained on SSRIs, the effect of tryptophan depletion and found that the REM-suppressing effect of SSRIs was removed without any effect on mood, i.e., without an exacerbation of depression.

WB: By the year 2005 we're going to have the human gene sequenced. Is that going to have an impact on understanding sleep mechanisms in normal subjects and psychiatric patients?

CG: The genetic approaches have not been applied successfully as yet in sleep research. But hopefully they will help us in two different diseases. One of these is narcolepsy. We know that narcolepsy is partially a genetically determined disorder in humans and in dogs, and there is some preliminary evidence that there are genetic markers, related to the HLA markers in the DR2 region, that may be related to narcolepsy. The other is a disease called fatal familial insomnia, probably one of the prion diseases, in which molecular genetic approaches will help.

WB: There can be psychotic symptoms in familial insomnia.

CG: There can be psychotic symptoms when it becomes a generalized disorder involving degeneration of the thalamus, primarily. Donna Giles' group is now doing a longitudinal study with some very promising preliminary data suggesting that can be used as a genetic marker of depression. They found short REM latency in non-affected family members of patients with bipolar and unipolar depressive disorders. There is currently a series looking at c-fos activation as soon as animals enter into REM sleep or into non-REM sleep. I think we are going to see more and more studies of this kind.

WB: Chris, what have I left out? Are there any issues around your career, your experiences, your view of the general field that you want to comment on?

CG: I think we are living in an exciting time. I'm happy that in all the different research areas in our field we are working together. I hope that it'll continue. Our greatest challenge is whether we can continue to attract bright young people into our field and whether we can get the necessary public support to make progress. I think the opportunities are there; there are much more opportunities than ever before. If we look back on the field of psychiatry it has become much more sophisticated since the time we entered the field. And we have much more to offer to patients. We have scientific tools that weren't there before.

WB: I've been interviewing a pioneer in the field of sleep research, Dr. J. Christian Gillin. From this interview, one can get a feel for the breadth and intensity of his knowledge and understanding of our field and especially of the interactions of sleep research and neuropsychopharmacology. It's been an honor to interview him. Thank you.

ERNEST HARTMANN

Interviewed by Thomas A. Ban

San Juan, Puerto Rico, December 9, 2002

TB: This will be an interview with Dr. Ernest Hartmann* for the Archives of the American College of Neuropsychopharmacology. We are at the Annual Meeting of the College in San Juan, Puerto Rico. It is December 9, 2002. I am Thomas Ban. Let's start from the beginning. When and where were you born?

EH: I was born in Vienna, Austria in 1934. My family is Austrian and Swiss. My father was a psychoanalyst, a student of Freud. As a matter of fact, I met Sigmund Freud when I was two years old. He was eighty and I was two.

TB: How old were you when you came to the United States?

EH: I was seven.

TB: Could you tell us something about your education?

EH: I lived in New York and went to school in Chicago. On the one hand, I wanted to be a theoretical physicist. But, on the other hand, I was also a poet. Medicine was a compromise. I found psychiatry or neurology the most interesting but since my father was a well-known psychoanalyst I felt that would be too much following in his footsteps. I was at Yale Med School and I got involved in cancer research for my dissertation. After med school I spent a year at the Institut Gustave Roussy, in Paris, doing some early research with immunoelectrophoresis in cancer.

TB: When was that?

EH: From 1958 to 1959. After my return to the US I did a residency in psychiatry at Harvard at the Massachusetts Mental Health Center. I had three very important mentors there: Elvin Semrad, a psychoanalyst, Milton Greenblatt, an early psychopharmacologist, and Jack Ewalt, who held things together as an administrator.

TB: So, one of your mentors was Milton Greenblatt?

EH: Yes.

TB: What did you do after your residency?

EH: I spent two years in the Intramural Program of NIMH, where I worked with Lyman Wynne, and Fred Snyder, an early sleep researcher. I'd always been interested in dreams, including my own. I completed a project on dreams with Justin Weiss, a well-known psychologist, while I was still in my residency. We studied whether a dream induced by hypnosis, was similar or different from a night dream. Of course the EEG's are quite different.

TB: Did you publish your findings?

---

* Ernest Hartmann was born in Vienna, Austria in 1934.

EH: We published only an abstract.

TB: When did you get interested in sleep research?

EH: I got interested while still in my residency, when Chuck Fisher, a psychiatrist and psychoanalyst, reported that some patients who developed schizophrenia had over four hours of REM sleep per night. His findings seemed to fit with theories about the relationship between dreaming and schizophrenia. Although it turned out that Fisher's data were completely wrong, they got me interested in REM sleep. I followed up his findings at the NIMH. In a long-term, controlled sleep study with dream collection we found that the amount of REM sleep is changed in mental patients.

TB: When was this research done?

EH: In 1963 and 1964.

TB: Were you involved in psychoanalysis in those years?

EH: Well, I became involved with psychoanalysis after I went back to Boston in 1964. I had a career investigator development award from NIMH that helped to support my research, and also paid for psychoanalysis.

TB: Could you tell us more about your research at the NIMH?

EH: I was involved in many studies. In one of these investigations, for example, we studied the changes in the sleep pattern of patients with manic depressive illness. I published a long paper with Biff Bunney on a manic-depressive woman who had forty-eight hour cycles, shifting from mania to depression or depression to mania every 24 hours. The switch from depression to mania always occurred in sleep. She generally woke up manic every other day. A few times she woke up from a nap manic in the daytime. On one occasion, I was able to demonstrate that the switch to mania clearly occurred after a long REM sleep period.

TB: You did this research with Biff Bunney?

EH: I worked with Lyman Wynne and Fred Snyder, and also Biff Bunney. Biff took overall care of our patients. He was in a sense my Chief Resident. He ran the ward, but he was also starting his depression research.

TB: Any other research you did at NIMH?

EH: I also did some studies at NIMH on how the mind is organized during REM sleep, by giving people psychological tests just after awakening from REM and NREM sleep. These studies were recently redone by Bob Stickgold at Harvard who found the same thing, with much better equipment. The finding was that the brain is organized differently during REM sleep; connections are being made more broadly, more loosely, than in NREM sleep.

TB: You told us that you had a career investigator development award after you left NIMH. Could you tell us about the research you did after you returned to Boston?

EH: I was hooked on sleep research and I was undergoing psychoanalysis. I was interested in connecting basic biological research with psychoanalysis, and psychiatry in general. I actually wrote a paper in 1970 entitled, "The Biology of the Mind." I was interested in what might underlie primary process thinking, defense mechanisms and so on. I followed it up with a number of research papers, but I'm not sure how much impact it had.

TB: Did you go back to work at the Massachusetts Mental Health Center?

EH: I went to work with Milton Greenblatt at the Boston State Hospital. He was wonderful. I met with him every week or two and we found connections between my interests and his, and he always asked wonderfully perceptive questions. And, then, Jon Cole took over from Milton Greenblatt at Boston State. He was an excellent director too.

TB: Did they have a sleep laboratory at the hospital?

EH: No, there was no sleep laboratory there when I came. I set up the sleep laboratory at Boston State. I did human studies, and studies on rats as well. But now that you've refreshed my memory I remember that I did test some specific neurochemical hypotheses about changes in norepinephrine and serotonin after REM deprivation in rats. These convinced Danny Freedman at Yale to work with me on the project. I used to go down to New Haven with a research assistant, and we deprived rats of REM sleep. We found interesting changes in serotonin and norepinephrine levels but not exactly the changes we expected.

TB: Would it be correct to say that you used REM sleep as a means to test relationships between psychoanalytic concepts and neurochemical changes?

EH: Yes, you could say that, though it's a big leap. I am not a neurochemist, but I worked with people who measured biochemical changes. I did long term sleep studies in schizophrenics, and I did long term sleep studies with psychotropic drugs. I did a study that involved twelve hundred nights of recorded sleep, in which we studied the effect of five prototype psychotropic drugs and placebo.

TB: Could you name us the drugs?

EH: Chlorpromazine, reserpine, amitriptyline, chlordiazepoxide, chloral hydrate, and placebo. Each subject received each drug for a month and each month of drug administration was followed by a one-month drug free period. Thus twelve months for each subject. Long study!

TB: When was this study done?

EH In 1968, 1969 and 1970. By then I was a member of the ACNP.

TB: When did you become a member?

EH: After Milton Greenblatt left and Jon Cole became the superintendent of Boston State. He was very interested in pushing research, and he was also very enthusiastic about the ACNP.

TB: You did some of the classical studies in sleep.

EH: I did studies that I don't think are specifically psychopharmacological, but which are considered to be classical studies in sleep. I studied the effects of sleep deprivation on REM; then I compared REM sleep in short, ordinary, and in long-sleepers.

TB: What did you find?

EH: I found huge differences in REM sleep but not in Stage 4 sleep, between the long, short and average sleepers. Then we studied the relationship between sleep and psychological functions. We found that short sleepers were smooth, efficient, well organized people and if they had any psychopathology, it was hypomania. Long sleepers were the opposite; they were worriers and took life very seriously. They worried about everything. We hypothesized that people who worry a lot need more REM sleep than people whose life is smooth. We tried to put it in computer terms, that short sleepers seem to be pre-programmed: their lives are organized, and run efficiently, whereas long-sleepers are weakly programmed and need to re-organize their lives every day. Thomas Edison was a well-known short sleeper; he was very well organized. He prided himself not just having ideas, but also of being able to put them into practice immediately. Albert Einstein, much of his life, was a long sleeper. He was a deep thinker, and he worried a great deal, about humanity, war, etc.

TB: When was REM sleep first described?

EH: In 1953 Aserinsky and Kleitman in Chicago conducted the first REM studies. I was at the University of Chicago at the time but did not know much about their work. However, a good friend of mine was one of their first subjects.

TB: So research in REM sleep started in the fifties.

EH: It was started in the mid-fifties and really became known in the late fifties. When Dement and Fisher published papers on the effects of dream deprivation in the early 1960s, that was when it really took off. I was one of the first people involved. There's some dispute about who gets credit for what. But certainly, it was Dement, Jouvet and I, who came up with the idea that the dreaming state, the D-state (now called REM-state), is not just a different kind of sleep, but it's a third state of existence. Waking, non-REM sleep and REM sleep are totally different states in many ways. I was very involved in pushing the idea that each state was different. I published a summary of the differences in 1962–63. In waking we have overall high activation and good feedback and in the REM state we have high activation with very poor feedback.

We have very good studies by Rechtschaffen as to why animals die of REM deprivation – rats die after extended REM deprivation – but the best he could come up with was that temperature regulation goes off. I believe thermoregulation is just one of the homeostatic systems that are restored during REM sleep.

TB: Could you elaborate on norepinephrine and sleep, both in animals and humans?

EH: I came up with the summary idea that medications which increase norepinephrine levels in the brain decrease REM sleep, and conversely those that decrease NE act to increase REM. It's very hard to increase REM sleep, but I found it persuasive that decreasing norepinephrine would increase REM sleep. This, with other research, led to a whole theory of the functions of REM sleep.

I also did studies with tryptophan that seemed to be very important at that time, and did turn out to be important, clinically more than theoretically. I just walked in to a session here at this ACNP meeting today and someone said to me, "Oh, are you the Dr. H. who did all the tryptophan studies?" Some people know me just from those studies. For years in the 1970s and 1980s, I worked with tryptophan. It turned out that tryptophan was a good sleeping pill and, of course, it was a "natural" sleeping pill. This was in the late 1970s and early 1980s. In some countries, tryptophan is on the market and used as a sleeping aid. I think it is on the market in Canada, but I'm not quite sure.

TB: In Canada it was also used as a mood stabilizer.

EH: Right. I showed that it reduced sleep latency. I had patients who did very well on tryptophan. Then tryptophan ran into problems in the United States; some patients developed eosinophilic myalgia and the FDA thought it might be due to tryptophan. Much more likely it was due to a contaminant, but as you know, tryptophan was removed from the market. It's still almost impossible to get in the United States. I had some patients who would go to Canada regularly to get their tryptophan.

TB: When did you get back to your research in dreaming?

EH: In the 1980s, I again became interested in dreaming, partly because my clinical patients with schizophrenia often had a period with intense nightmares before they became psychotic. I also had some patients and some friends who told me they had nightmares every few days for years. So I did a study in which I interviewed many people who had life-long nightmares.

TB: What did you find?

EH: These people had "thin boundaries" in terms of thinking and feeling, and in numerous other senses. Some people never let their feelings get in the way of their thoughts. But these people had the opposite. They asked me how one could possibly imagine a thought without feeling. So I developed my concepts about "thin and thick boundaries." I wrote a book about *Boundaries in the Mind* and many papers.

TB: What is the title of your book?

EH: It's called *Boundaries in the Mind*.

TB: When was it published?

EH: The book came out in 1991. And that was very exciting. There have now been over two hundred papers published on boundaries, and we have a 138-item Boundary Questionnaire about different kinds of boundaries. We have done a lot of work with that.

In the last years, I've been doing not so much laboratory sleep research, but research on dreaming. I've done work on dreams after trauma and dreams in stressful situations.

TB: Stresses of everyday life?

EH: No. Stresses of people whose house burned down or people who were raped, attacked, robbed or who lost someone close to them. There are emotional concerns clearly involved in dreams, but most dreams are so complicated. I can't blame some people for thinking that dreams are just junk thrown together. But I never believed that dreams were just random.

The easiest place to look at that question would be in those people who have just experienced a trauma. The feelings in those people's minds is: I am scared; I'm terrified; I'm overwhelmed. So, what do they dream about? Sometimes the dreams are about the actual event; but the most common finding is that they don't dream about the event, or dream about the event only once or twice. Then they have a dream something like; "I was on a beach and was swept away by a tidal wave, or a whirlwind". It's amazing how common those kinds of dreams are. I've heard that many times. I have statistics showing that those dreams are more frequent following the trauma. See, most dreams you don't remember. So much stuff is being thrown away or thrown together in dreams. But here, you have someone who has just escaped from a burning building in western Massachusetts, who hasn't been anywhere near the ocean in many years, and whose dream is; "I was on the beach and a huge tidal wave swept me away." For me, that is very important, and I have been studying that. Such a dream is a paradigm: obviously the man is not dreaming about the events themselves that occurred. He's picturing his emotion; "I am terrified; I am overwhelmed".

It's not easy to study dreams; you have to work with what people tell you. But I have found people who write down all their dreams, like me, and who are willing to share them. I've done several interesting studies on dreams including one that's about to be published on dreams before and after 9/11, 2001. All of us were traumatized, or at least stressed on that day. There are studies showing that some symptoms of trauma occurred more often if you lived in New York City than if you lived in California. We found 44 people who had been recording all their dreams every morning, for years. Each sent me twenty dreams; the last ten dreams in their records before and the first ten dreams after 9/11 and we did a series of dream analyses.

TB: What did you measure?

EH: We selected the Central Image, the tidal wave for example, and measured its intensity in these dreams with our rating scale. There were slight, but not highly significant differences in content before vs. after 9/11. The highly significant difference was in the intensity of the Central Image. What we found was that after 9/11, people had more intense Central Images in their dreams. And, insofar as we can generalize, we all had more powerful dreams after 9/11. When we are emotionally aroused, we dream more intensely. But we do not dream specifically of the events: there was not a single dream of planes hitting towers, or anything close to that! So, that's what I have done recently.

TB: Are you still fully active?

EH: Yes, I'm active; I'm practicing part-time and I'm doing dream research part-time. I don't have a sleep research laboratory and I don't have a big grant.

TB: So, you don't have grants any longer?

EH: But this kind of dream research, you can do with students and people interested in dreams.

TB: What kind of practice do you have?

EH In the past it has been long-term psychoanalytic therapy, but in recent years it is mostly sleep disorders medicine. I see some psychiatric patients, but I have to admit the ones I'm most interested in are patients with nightmares or psychiatric patients with sleep problems. What I see most commonly at the sleep center is people with sleep apnea and sleep problems.

TB: So you see patients mainly with sleep problems.

EH: Well, as I said, in the last years it's been more sleep disorders. For a time, I saw some long-term patients in therapy and I did some psychopharmacology. It was never a major interest of mine.

TB: Still, you have contributed to the field. Could you tell us more about your research in psychopharmacology?

EH: Let me think. Well, the tryptophan research involved many different studies. It led to studies of other amino acids, especially the ones that compete with tryptophan. We did several in normal subjects, and have shown that tryptophan produces a daytime tendency to sleepiness, whereas phenylalanine produces the opposite effect. I did one psychopharmacological study on nightmares in the 1970s. It was a fairly small and not very impressive study; but it is the only placebo controlled psychopharmacological study of dreaming.

TB: Could you tell us more about that study?

EH: My hypothesis was that dopamine had something to do with nightmares. It was done in a group of normal subjects. Each person went through two nights in which they were given L-DOPA and two nights in which they were given placebo.

TB: What was the dose of L-DOPA that was given?

EH: It was five hundred milligrams of L-DOPA, given twice during the night, timed so that it would have its effect at the next expected REM period. We found that dreams after L-DOPA were more vivid, detailed and exciting. We also found more nightmares after L-DOPA compared to placebo.

TB: Any other studies in psychopharmacology you would like to talk about?

EH: I studied over-the-counter sleeping medications, antihistamines, as well as analgesics.

TB: You have published many papers in the past decades.

EH: I've written and published about 310 papers.

TB: And several books.

EH: Nine books. I like writing books. The first book was *The Biology of Dreaming.* One early book was on adolescents in a mental hospital. That had nothing to do with my sleep research. In my book on *The Biology of Dreaming* I summarized my early phylogenetic studies: I did sleep studies on the elephant, on rats and on humans. Others had studied cats and mice. I wanted to study elephants, which are obviously at the opposite extreme from the mouse in terms of size, metabolic rate, etc. These studies were cited a great deal. I demonstated that the dream-sleep cycle (REM non-REM cycle) is a basic cycle of the mammalian body. I did some studies, published a paper and a book, in which I showed a clear correspondence across species. We find the same shaped curve – covering data from the mouse to the elephant – in the pulse cycle, respiratory cycle, gestation period, and in the REM/non-REM cycle. The longest cycle is always seen in the elephant and the cycle length is inversely related to the resting metabolic rate of the species. That was published in several papers and in *The Biology of Dreaming* (1967). Then, *The Functions of Sleep* (1973) was an important book of mine summarizing many studies leading to a theory of the functions of sleep.

TB: What do you think the function of sleep is?

EH: Overall, we don't fully know. But I put forth a number of hypotheses, which are still being debated. I believe that sleep, especially REM sleep, is involved in the restoration of norepinephrine-dependent systems, which are necessary for feedback regulation in the central nervous system and in the entire body (homeostatic systems).

TB: What about functions of dreaming?

EH: There is no consensus on the functions of dreaming. I believe that dreams are hyperconnective, making connections that are guided by the dreamer's emotion. I believe that dreams weave in new material, integrating it with existing memory systems. Among other things, this weaving-in of traumatic material for instance makes a subsequent event less traumatic.

TB: How about your work on "boundaries"?

EH: My group has done a great many studies on *Boundaries in the Mind* and we developed the Boundary Questionnaire taken by over 10,000 people. Many psychologists are using my concepts about "boundaries" and I would like to get some brain imaging people to study the difference in people with "thin" and "thick" boundaries, to see what the differences are. I would expect major differences, but I haven't done the experiments.

TB: Is there anything else you would like to talk about?

EH: I have a feeling I've talked too much. You got me reviewing my work and I have a feeling I've tired you out.

TB: We covered many areas in your research from psychoanalysis to psychopharmacology. Let me ask you: Did you use the sleep EEG in screening for psychotropic drugs?

EH: No, I didn't use sleep EEG for that purpose. Fink did a lot of that kind of work. I pride myself that I have almost never done any research for a pharmaceutical company.

TB: Never?

EH: Almost never. Once, I got some money for doing research with tryptophan.

TB: What's your opinion of ACNP?

EH: I think ACNP is a wonderful society. The meetings are exciting. I always learn something new. However, I think there is too much influence by the pharmaceutical companies, especially in recent years.

TB: Were all your research projects supported by NIH or NIMH?

EH: Almost all.

TB: Didn't you do research in narcoleptic patients?

EH: Yes, a bit. Narcolepsy in most cases begins at the age of sixteen, seventeen or eighteen, but is not diagnosed until age twenty-five or later. I suggested that the onset of nightmares in adolescence can be an early sign of narcolepsy.

TB: Didn't you do research also with cocaine?

EH: I don't think so. However, I did several studies on amphetamine addiction. We studied norepinephrine, dopamine and serotonin and their metabolites in people addicted to amphetamines, and we did sleep recordings while people were on amphetamines and after they got off.

TB: Let me shift and ask you about your membership and activities in societies.

EH: I have been very active in the Sleep Research Society. I have sometimes presented papers at meetings of the American Psychiatric Association and several psychoanalytic associations. Since 1985, I've also been very active in a new society, called the Association for the Study of Dreams, that's a pure Dream Society. I'm trying to push that society to become more research oriented.

TB: Have you been active in the ACNP?

EH: Yes, somewhat. I was on several committees, including the Credentials Committee.

TB: Is there anything you would like to see to happen in the future in your area of research?

EH: That's a very good question. Here's one area; As mentioned, I've done a great deal of work on "Boundaries." We've gone all the way from psychological boundaries in individuals to how nations get along with each other. People who have "thick" psychological boundaries tend to think in terms of "thick" boundary peace; whereas, people who are a little more loose and flexible can think of "thin" boundary peace. I would love to have people with equipment to do brain imaging collaborate with me in this research on psychological boundaries. I am certain we would find clear differences in the spread of activation in the brain, especially in the cortex.

TB: So, I think on this note we should conclude this interview with Dr. Ernest Hartmann. Thank you very much for sharing with us this information.

EH: Thank you very much. You really got me talking!

PHILIP S. HOLZMAN

Interviewed by Thomas A. Ban
San Juan, Puerto Rico, December 9, 2002

TB: This will be an interview with Dr. Philip Holzman* for the Archives of the American College of Neuropsychopharmacology. We are at the annual meeting of the college in San Juan, Puerto Rico. It is December 9, 2002. I am Thomas Ban. Let's start from the very beginning; when and where were you born? Tell us something about your childhood, education and move on in chronology.

PH: I was born in New York City on May 2, 1922. My father was an accountant, and my mother was a painter who loved Millet and would spend time in the Metropolitan Museum of Art copying his art. She loved the peasant scenes he drew so beautifully and poignantly. My mother died when I was 22 months old. I was reared by my mother's parents, in New York City. My father remarried about two years after my mother's death and chose to have me stay with my grandparents. So essentially I was reared by older parents and have never ceased to have a fondness for older people. I went to public schools in New York. My high school was Townsend Harris High School at 23rd Street and Lexington Avenue, to which I had to travel on what they then called the Inter-borough Rapid Transit, the IRT. It was about a 25-minute ride that gave me time to do the homework I had not completed the night before or to read either the *Herald-Tribune* or the *New York Times*, which one could buy on the news stand for 3 cents.

After graduation from high school, I went to the College of the City of New York and didn't have the foggiest idea what I wanted to do. One summer evening in 1939, it must have been about a month before Sigmund Freud died, I heard a heated discussion between two people in their early 20s. It was about Freud and psychoanalysis. I couldn't understand what they were talking about. The arguments that I used to hear in my high school and in the college cafeteria had to do with collective security versus isolationism, with Stalinists versus Trotskyites that left me rather cold. I could not quite get involved in that. But this argument somehow intrigued me because words floated by such as dreams, the unconscious, instincts, sexuality. My goodness, sexuality! You know, for someone who was in the late teens at that time, this was very seductive. After hearing that argument I went to a bookstore and bought a copy of A.A. Brill's translation of several papers of Sigmund Freud. It included the "Three Contributions to the Theory of Sex" and "The Interpretation of Dreams," but when I started to read them I was more bewildered than before. I later

---

* Philip S. Holzman was born in New York City, New York in 1922. Holzman died in 2004.

understood that A.A. Brill, while a passionate acolyte of Sigmund Freud, did not know either German or English well. His language was Yiddish. So he used an amalgam of languages.

Psychoanalysis didn't capture my interest until my second year in college when I took my first course in psychology. My instructor was a man named J.E. Barmack, who had us read a number of wonderful works, such as Kleinberg's *Race Differences*, and the *Introductory Lectures to Psychoanalysis* by Sigmund Freud, translated by Joan Riviere, who certainly knew English. And this was quite revealing. I found that Freud was a master expositor, and was totally taken in by his arguments in this interesting psychological discourse of what the inner life is presumably all about. So I resolved to study psychology, and I majored in it. Before that I didn't know what I wanted to major in. At the time I wanted to be a journalist but I quickly changed course. And the odd thing is that what captured me was experimental psychology. I took two courses in experimental psychology, one in physiological psychology. I was captivated by the idea that by experiments you could tease apart one variable from another in mental life. This was a revelation to me because Freud was an expositor; he laid out "This is the way it is," while in experimental work we ask, "Is this the way it is?" I thought, "That's the way I would like to go." Then I was inducted into the army. It was World War II.

TB: So we are in the early 1940s?

PH: This was 1943. The United States had been in the war since the end of 1941, December 7th, and that was the end of my education up to that point.

TB: So you studied psychology and physiological psychology?

PH: Yes.

TB: Did you graduate by then?

PH: I had a bachelor's degree, but no more. I was in the army for a bit over three years and discharged in late August of 1946. I was in the Pacific and ready to invade Japan if it had come to that.

Since I didn't know what I was going to do after my discharge I wrote to a professor, Gardner Murphy, who had been the chairman of the department of psychology in college. He was an erudite man who could give lectures and, if you were to transcribe them, you wouldn't have to change a word or a comma. And yet we knew that he didn't write them out, because he would walk to the lecture hall with an envelope in his hand and a pencil and he would be jotting down some words as he walked and those were his notes. But the lectures came off mellifluously, as Hamlet said, "Trippingly off the tongue." I wrote to him, and I said, "I've been gone for over three years, and I don't know what's happening in academia and in psychology. What do you recommend?" I didn't hear from him. But I did get a letter from the Menninger Clinic, from Margaret Brenman, who said that Professor Murphy had recommended that they get in touch with me, that I might want to be part of their training program.

I had read everything I could get my hands on in psychology while in the army, including several influential works. One was *Diagnostic Psychologic Testing*, by David Rapaport, who had come to the United States as a Hungarian refugee during the Hitler era, and who was, I think, a genius. At that time Gardner Murphy had sponsored him, and he got a job at the Ossowatomie State Hospital in Kansas. While there, he would attend case conferences at the Menninger Clinic and became known to Karl Menninger. Menninger was another person whose works I had read. I read *The Human Mind* and *Man Against Himself* while in the army. And the two, *Diagnostic Psychological Testing* and Karl Menninger's works, were as different as day and night. One was a popularizer, and the other one would brook no nonsense from anybody. I decided these were the two people I would like to learn from. So I applied to the Menninger Clinic, and after being tested by Rapaport himself with the Rorschach test, an intelligence test and a word association test – I guess to see if my head was screwed on OK – they accepted me.

In the meantime I was very much in love with the young woman I had been dating before I went into the army, and we decided to get married before going to Topeka. As a New Yorker, the furthest west I had been was New Jersey, until I was in the army. So, Topeka was a revelation to both of us, to my wife Ann and me. To understand what follows I need to tell you that after the war ended in Europe, General Omar Bradley was put in charge of the Veterans Administration. He was a five-star general, and he had his medical deputy go around the United States and find the best places to start hospitals, particularly psychiatric hospitals. The deputy was a man named Arthur Marshall. He was a full colonel in the European theater, but he was now back in the United States. He stopped in Topeka to visit a cousin who was a resident at the Menninger Clinic, and the cousin, whose name was Maimon Levitt – we used to call him Mike – arranged an interview for him with Karl Menninger. Both of these people, Arthur Marshall and Karl Menninger, were enthusiasts. And the two of them began to spin a fantasy of how it would be to have a residency training program for psychiatrists in the middle of the country, in Topeka, perhaps even in a wheat field. And when Karl Menninger said, "Well, we could take 10 residents," Marshall said, "Well, how about 20." The bidding continued until it was 100. And the first residency class consisted of 100 residents, MDs either fresh out of the army or fresh out of medical school, and 18 psychologists fresh out of their baccalaureate degrees, including me. And there we were, influenced by these two giants, David Rapaport and Karl Menninger.

They couldn't have been more different if one were to compare the deserts of Arabia with the tropical forests of Africa. One was a Midwestern Presbyterian who breathed good works, hope and optimism. One of his statements was, "With good psychiatric treatment, you can be 'weller' than well," whatever that means. The other was a Jewish Talmudist who pored over texts trying to discern their meaning, and if you could discern one meaning, there had to be multiple meanings. These two people were my teachers. Now, Rapaport was thoroughly involved in psychoanalysis; that was the Zeitgeist then, the reigning doctrine. There was no other treatment.

TB: Are we talking about the mid-1940s?

PH: This is 1946. Deniker and Delay had not yet appeared on the international scene. We certainly didn't have phenothiazines at that time. We had no treatments for mental illness, except to talk to people. And the folks at Menninger did a good job of that. They spoke to patients. They got ideas about their lives. They even made up wonderful stories about how they became ill in the way they were. You could, retrospectively, construct that story. It was a beautiful thing.

But, I grew a little restive with the idea this is the way it is. The Freudian meta-psychology, which Rapaport was thoroughly involved in, seemed to be too much of a fait accompli, and the more I examined it, the more it occurred to me that this was truly a one-way street. One of my wonderful teachers, George Klein, a psychologist, first used the phrase – you could see from the meta-psychology what was happening to a person, but what was happening could not influence the meta-psychology. It was like the Torah or the Koran. It was not changeable, even though you knew that one day one might come across contradictions. At the same time, I began to see there were such things in the psychoanalytic world as apostasies. I always thought that apostasies were reserved for the religious world so I was uncomfortable. But Karl Menninger was an extraordinary man. He allowed experimentation to occur at the Menninger Clinic. I teamed up with George Klein, an experimental psychologist interested in psychoanalysis at that time although he had his PhD from Columbia University and studied with Salig Hecht, a very distinguished physiological psychologist.

TB: What did you team up to study?

PH: We were interested in studying perception. Not the laws of perception, but the laws of perceivers. The way in which they see the world, in which they organize their world. We produced several experimental demonstrations that there was internal consistency in the way people see things. And we gave these consistencies names that have persisted in the literature; cognitive styles, cognitive controls, perceptual attitudes. We even used the German Anschauung; the way of looking at things and organizing them, the person's point of view. And we took this as far as we could, because we couldn't go further than to demonstrate there were these consistencies within a person. I was disappointed we couldn't take it further but then I didn't realize what we needed was a new brain science. And brain science, at that time, was neurology. Neurology was almost like psychiatry, a despised stepchild of medicine. There were jokes made about neurologists. They would give you perfect diagnoses, which were totally useless.

TB: Are we now in the late 1940s?

PH: Yes.

TB: So, we are just before Moruzzi and Magoun published on the reticular activating system.

PH: Just before Moruzzi and Magoun's discovery of the ascending activating system, before recognizing that there is something in the brain that has to do with attention. Before that, attention was an amorphous concept which Freud called "cathexis." But now Moruzzi and Magoun showed that something was happening in the brain. That was an awakening. And that was one of the things that made me realize one could take psychology just so far, and then one needed something else. But I didn't know what else. After Moruzzi and Magoun entered the scene I thought that one needed beyond psychology, neurophysiology. I also thought it could be chemistry or cell biology, I didn't know. But I knew that those disciplines were beyond me because I was a behavioral scientist at that point. I had published a number of papers on cognitive styles and a number of papers critical of psychoanalysis.

I neglected to say that I had received full psychoanalytic training and became a practicing psychoanalyst, which I enjoyed immensely, while also realizing psychoanalysis wasn't the full story. One could learn from psychoanalysis how to talk to people who were in trouble and about people who got into trouble but I knew from my contacts with people who had serious mental disorders like schizophrenia or major depression that something more was necessary. Talking could help a little bit, but it couldn't do the complete job.

TB: What was your first paper?

PH: My first paper was on cognitive consistencies.

TB: When was it published?

PH: In 1948.

TB: Where was it published?

PH: It was published in the *Journal of Psychology*, and there was another one about the same time that was published in another psychological journal. My first presentation at a national meeting was also in 1948, or it might have been in 1949, at the American Psychological Association meeting.

TB: So your first papers and presentations were in the late 1940s?

PH   Yes. Within those three years, and up to the time that George Klein left Topeka, which was in 1951, I must have published about seven or eight papers. And in those days, one didn't multiply publications. I was one of the extraordinary ones because people tended not to publish. They published when they might have been startled by something a patient said. Or in psychology, they would publish a theoretical paper. But experimental papers were rare, and there were very few experimental journals. There was the *Journal of Psychology*, there was the *Journal of Abnormal and Social Psychology*, which was founded by Morton Prince in 1909, but there were only a very few journals that published experimental literature. The *Journal of Experimental Psychology* was one of them. Today, there's a geometric progression in the number of journals, and you simply can't keep up with the literature. You read the table of contents and maybe a few papers on topics you are interested in.

TB: When did you get your BA, in 1943?

PH: Yes.

TB: And when did you get your PhD?

PH: I got my PhD in 1952 from the University of Kansas. I was in Topeka working full time, seeing patients, doing research, and then at night I was traveling to Lawrence, Kansas, taking courses from wonderful people who were giants in the field at that time; people like Fritz Heider, Martin Scherer, Eric Wright, Herbert Wright and Raymond Wheeler all very well known in Gestalt psychology. So I got my PhD then.

And as I mentioned before, I also began to write critical articles on psychoanalysis. What was my beef with psychoanalysis? It was a love-hate relationship. The beef was that it was a one-way street that you couldn't correct, and if you tried to correct it you were called an apostate. And I thought this is no way for a science to behave. I mean, the science is psychology, the science is behavior, and every science moves by correcting and changing, even the great science of chemistry. My work became known because of the cognitive styles work.

Things began to deteriorate a little bit at the Menninger Clinic, and I began to look around. Offers for jobs had come in almost every year, but

I never paid any attention to them. I would politely decline. But one came through from the University of Chicago, through Daniel X. Freedman. And he called me, and told me that there was a position. Then he corrected himself. He says, "No, I'm going to create a position at the University of Chicago for a professor of psychoanalysis." I thought he was going to ask me for suggesting possible candidates but he said, "Would you be interested in looking at it?" I said, "Well, I think you ought to know that although I am a psychoanalyst, a card-carrying one, I'm rather critical of it, and even if I still think that in the history of ideas it's a very important landmark, and one has to regard Freud as one of the major figures in psychology, I'm interested in schizophrenia now."

I forgot to mention one thing. In 1966, I got a telephone call from Charlie Shagass who was setting up a meeting of the American Psychopathological Association in New York together with Joe Zubin, and they asked me to present a review paper, on perception and psychopathology. Since I had been working in perception since 1948, and certainly knew psychopathology because I was seeing all kinds of patients every day, I accepted the invitation. And when I began to review the literature I was appalled at what I had seen. I was impressed by something George Klein noted in 1949. When we tried to study perception in schizophrenia, we gave it up because of the huge variances we found in patients. We didn't realize that this was a characteristic of schizophrenia. I was reacquainted with this finding in my review of the literature, and also came across several consistent results. One was reaction time. Finger lifting reaction time was always longer in schizophrenia. The second consistent finding was that people, particularly from European countries, Poland, Czechoslovakia and France, had reported diminished vestibular nystagmus in schizophrenia. This was also the only biological finding that Hoskins found in his study at the Worcester State Hospital, diminished vestibular nystagmus. How interesting, I thought, a real biological finding. You can't fake that. The third consistent finding was a raised resting autonomic activation. And another one was the fact that specific responses to autonomic stimuli were diminished. So you had a raised resting level and diminished reactivity in specific responses. The last one was all of these findings, except the diminished vestibular nystagmus, could be mimicked by phencyclidine administration. So I said to Danny, "I'm interested in schizophrenia. I've found some things that are consistent, and I'm going to present it at the APPA." He said, "Let's meet in Washington." I was on an NIMH study section at that time, and he was on another. So we met for dinner, which was hosted by Bert Boothe.

TB: Who was Bert Boothe?

PH: Bert Boothe was a professor of English literature who was hired by Karl Menninger to become the Dean of psychiatry at the Menninger Clinic, because they had 100 residents and 18 psychologists, and needed somebody to organize the program. Bert Boothe also gave courses in English Literature, on Shakespeare and the Elizabethan poets. After awhile he started an NIMH supported career scientist program. I think Danny was on that study section, and Bert was the executive secretary who was in charge of it all. So Bert raised my name in becoming part of that program. Danny and I just hit it off; a kind of chemistry took hold. So I went to Chicago.

TB: Are we now in the mid-1960s?

PH: We are in 1968.

TB: You mentioned the consistent finding of diminished vestibular nystagmus in schizophrenics that had a great impact on your future research. When was the first paper on that published and by whom?

PH: The first paper was published in 1921 by Pekelski and the second one by the Detroit group, Luby, Rosenbaum and others.

TB: Did Luby's publication have an impact on you?

PH: It did have a great impact. When I got to the University of Chicago, I began to establish a way to work on vestibular nystagmus. I went to the department of otolaryngology, found a guy named Fernandez who was an expert in the vestibular system of lower primates, and told him about these studies. By that time, there were about 12 studies showing diminished vestibular nystagmus in schizophrenia. And he said, "You know, it's very interesting, but I'm so busy I can't do this. But there is a man coming from Detroit who might be interested. His name is Leonard Proctor. He's an otolaryngologist, and he's coming as an associate professor." So as soon as Proctor made his appearance, I got an appointment with him. I showed him the articles from Pekelski on vestibular nystagmus, and he was interested. He said, "Well, let's see if it's true." And he showed me how to test vestibular nystagmus by caloric irrigation.

Then I called Roy Grinker who was the chief of psychiatry at the Michael Reese Hospital at the time, and made him interested in this idea. I said, "Here are some clear findings. Let's see if it's true." Roy jumped at it. He said, "I'll send you five schizophrenics," and we examined their vestibular nystagmus response to caloric irrigation. Now, to show you that science proceeds at times by error, because you misunderstand something, here was a monumental error we made. We thought nystagmus consisted of a slow eye movement in one direction and a rapid eye movement back in a sawtooth pattern, so we looked at each of these components separately to see which was impaired. I went to the fishing supply section of Sears

Roebuck, bought some fishing line and a sinker, and knowing the law of the pendulum I measured how long the pendulum should be in order to go back and forth in a cycle of about 2.5 seconds. We had the person follow the swinging sinker suspended from the fishing line. And then we put two dots up on the board, and we would have the person look at the two dots, back and forth, as rapidly as they could. We didn't know that vestibular nystagmus is regulated mostly in the cerebellum and following a pendulum is more of a cortical function. So what we found was that all five of the patients that Roy Grinker had sent to us had perfectly normal vestibular nystagmus, but their smooth pursuit eye movements were abnormal, as judged by the two observers. We recorded these eye movements on a polygraph.

Now, why did we get normal vestibular nystagmus? Because we thought we were controlling all the variables that could affect nystagmus. We knew, or Proctor knew, that attention and staring affect eye movements. Now, every ballet dancer and figure skater knows if you fixate as you twirl around, you diminish nystagmus, and pilots know this as well. So when people test nystagmus, they give them little insignificant attentional tasks, like asking them what did you have for breakfast, or to name all the countries that start with the letter C so they have to think of the answer. Going back to that old literature, most of the patients were catatonic and notorious for staring. Their attention is somewhere else. So if they don't pay attention, and they stare, they diminish nystagmus. What we did was prevent them from staring by having them keep their eyes open and putting on goggles – Frenzel lenses. When we asked them distracting questions normal nystagmus resulted. However, the smooth pursuit eye movements were abnormal. This impressed me. I couldn't understand it.

I went to Danny and said "five out of five is unusual in anything, especially in schizophrenia. I'm not sure I believe it. I think we're lucky. But I need money." So he went to a man named Goldblatt who owned several retail stores in Chicago, who gave me $10,000, with which I bought a polygraph and hired a research assistant. We began to test schizophrenics for smooth pursuit eye movements and for vestibular nystagmus. And we found that smooth pursuit eye movements were disordered, not to the extent that we had first found, but quite a lot of schizophrenic patients showed it. We then used this preliminary data to get an NIMH grant. Previously my application was turned down because they thought that my proposal was crazy and would never work, but now I had more than pilot data, so I got the grant. In our study we found that in recently admitted schizophrenics, what people called acute schizophrenics, the abnormality was present in about 50%, and in the dilapidated schizo-phrenics at the Manteno State Hospital outside of Chicago, over 80%. Can you imagine how lucky we were? We would have pursued the proj-ect even if we had found just a few with abnormal smooth pursuit eye movements.

TB: Were you relying on the hospital diagnosis of schizophrenia?

PH: The hospital diagnosis. If these people were in the hospital so long, the likelihood was that they were schizophrenic. That was before *DSM-III* was introduced.

TB: Are we in the late 1960s?

PH: We are in the late 1960s and 1970.

TB: Ten years before *DSM-III*.

PH: Another thing I got from Topeka and took with me was that when I talked with patients, I also talked with family members who came to visit. And I was impressed that some of these family members were strange indeed. Some of them, although they were not clinically ill, spoke elliptically, but then so did Danny Freedman. But Danny knew what he was doing. And many of them misused words. Some of them were even funny looking, which today we would refer to as having craniofacial dysmorphic fea-tures. So when I got these findings, I thought I must test the relatives for abnormal smooth pursuit eye movements. We found in recently hospital-ized schizophrenics, there were about 52% with abnormal pursuit eye movements, and about 40% of first degree relatives of the patients also had abnormal movements. We couldn't get the relatives of those at the Manteno State Hospital. At this point in our research we started to test the patients for formal thought disorder as conveyed in verbalization, in the way I learned from David Rapaport.

TB: In the processing of ideas?

PH: Yes, we looked past the content to the form of thinking. Now all of us are taught to look past language to the ideas. So we developed a systematic way of scoring formal thought disorder. Now other people have done this too, it was not unique. We don't claim that our test is the best, but ours showed that thought disorder is not a unitary thing, that there are many different kinds, ranging from peculiar use of language and words to neologisms, coining new words, to confabulations and to fusing two ideas with each other. There were 23 formal thought disorders we could identify.

TB: So you developed a method for identifying formal thought disorder and differentiating between different kinds of formal thought disorders?

PH: We developed a scoring system you could use. For example, we could take the transcript of our interview and rate it for formal thought disorder.

We used the Rorschach test; the person was asked to respond to what they saw in ten amorphous forms in a standardized way, but not as a Rorschach test. And it has been quite successful. It allowed us to distinguish schizophrenic from manic thought disorder, and from the kind of thought disorder that one would see after right hemisphere damage.

TB: You supplemented the clinical diagnosis with a formal thought disorder score?

PH: Yes. And at McLean Hospital, there were physicians who would call on my associate, Dr. Deborah Levy, to give this Rorschach to differentiate schizophrenia from bipolar or other disorders.

TB: By using this test you knew the patient had a schizophrenic type of formal thought disorder?

PH: Yes. In the first paper we published in *Science* we suggested that smooth pursuit eye movements are disordered in schizophrenia. The second paper was in Danny's journal, the *Archives of General Psychiatry*. In this paper we showed that the relatives of patients also showed the abnormality. Then we classified patients on the basis of their thought disorder index. And the association between the abnormality and the thought disorder was even stronger than with schizophrenia, although today this would not necessarily be the case. In those days, we didn't have DSM-III. We also did a number of studies trying to disprove that the abnormality of smooth pursuit eye movement was pathognomonic of schizophrenia. We knew that brain stem lesions, hemispheric lesions, Parkinson's disease and multiple sclerosis could also produce this abnormality. But the relatives of someone with Parkinson's or a brain stem lesion do not show the abnormality.

TB: So again, in what percentage of chronic schizophrenics did you find abnormality in smooth pursuit eye movements?

PH: In over 80 percent. There were still a few schizophrenics who showed perfectly normal smooth pursuit eye movements, just like a 15-year old normal kid. We then had to demonstrate that the abnormality is genetically determined, by showing that randomly chosen families didn't show anything. As our dear departed member, Seymour Kety used to say, "Silverware runs in families." So we went to Norway to team up with Einar Kringlen in a study of smooth pursuit eye movements in twins who were discordant for schizophrenia. Now, Kringlen had published in a 1966 monograph that between 25 and 38% of monozygotic twins were concordant for schizophrenia, and about 11% of dizygotic twins were concordant for schizophrenia. These were the lowest concordance rates found at that time with the exception, I think, of Tienari's. Remember, Frans Kallmann found concordance rates in the 80% range. So I felt this was a good opportunity to get the discordant twins. I convinced Kringlen to work with us, and Leonard Proctor, Deborah Levy, and myself tested these twins all over Norway. We found that in spite of the discordance in clinical diagnosis, there was concordance in monozygotic (MZ) twins, as if you had an autosomal dominant trait.

We then wanted to go further. We thought let's test the offspring of the affected and unaffected twins. As you can see we were always trying to disprove something. We found our predictions about how many should have schizophrenia and how many should have abnormal pursuit eye movements came out the way we had predicted.

Let me go back to my early childhood, because I omitted one important fact. My mother's brother was a physician, and his name was Philip, the name that I have. He was a physician who was treating young patients, pediatric patients, at the Willard Parker Hospital in New York City. And, according to family legend, one of his young patients had a convulsion and bit him. The patient had scarlet fever. My uncle contracted scarlet fever and died. This was a cautionary tale in my life: don't become a physician, you can die. And so, I always avoided the path to medicine, even though, as I tell you about my gravitation toward physiology, it seems I should have been a physician. But you can see my interest in the individual person as well as in physiology.

Now, we've kept going further and further in our research. I won't tell you more about the other traits that we looked at. But by this time we have called smooth pursuit eye movement dysfunctions a co-familial trait, because it tends to run in families. We then thought we should use this trait to tell us something about the genetic transmission of schizophrenia. So we teamed up with colleagues, Josef Parnas and Fini Schulsinger in Denmark. Fini is no longer active, so we are now working with Josef only. We identified five large families with schizophrenia, with close to 500 people, and we have tested smooth pursuit eye movement dysfunction in them. And although schizophrenia was relatively rare in these families, about 6%, smooth pursuit eye movement abnormalities are about five times more frequent. So looking for smooth pursuit eye movement abnormalities can increase the power of looking for genetic linkage. We have formulated a model with my colleague Steven Matthysse, who is a mathematician as well as a psychologist. In this model we have a gene that codes for a latent trait – we don't know exactly what – that expresses itself in at least two different ways, i.e., as schizophrenia and as smooth pursuit eye movement dysfunction. These are independent expressions of this latent trait, so they can occur together or separately. Then this latent trait will tell you whether or not there is a genetic component. That is the model we used in looking at the Danish pedigrees.

Independently from us, a man named Volker Arolt in Hamburg, Germany, found linkage between eye tracking dysfunction and a locus on chromosome 6P21-23. We have independently confirmed that. So even though there is a plethora of findings about linkage, this is not just to schizophrenia. This is to eye tracking dysfunctions that occur in a family in which there is schizophrenia. We think that this is a powerful tool for further investigation. So that's the genetics.

The physiology has captured us again. What is there in smooth pursuit eye-movements that is disordered? To make a very long story shorter than it really should be, we think that what is wrong is that the capacity to judge speed, to judge velocity, to judge almost any motion is impaired. We know that vision is modular and in the cortex there are a number of regions that have to do with different aspects of vision: contrast, slant, color, movement. Now, how fast one judges a target to be moving or the direction in which it is moving is important, and it's regulated there before it's all put together as a visual percept. We've got a number of studies I would call psychophysiological, indicating that eye movements are impaired when the person makes errors in judging speed. So we've done psychophysical judgments of how fast something is moving. We've found that the threshold, the Weber fraction, is impaired in schizophrenics and in relatives who are judging the speed of targets. And that is highly correlated with impairment in smooth pursuit eye movements.

TB: What about the effect of drugs on the dysfunction of smooth pursuit eye movements? It is a trait, so drugs shouldn't influence it. Is this correct?

PH: Drugs do not influence smooth pursuit eye movements. They do influence the clinical condition of schizophrenia, they reduce the symptoms, but they do not cure the disease. Now we have another finding, Tom. One of the control conditions we use is to have the person judge the relative brightness of two things. We found there are no differences in the judgment of contrast between normal controls and schizophrenics or their relatives. We got the idea that maybe drugs could affect the contrast discrimination of patients from the findings of a man named Bodis-Wollner at Mount Sinai Hospital in New York, who tested Parkinson's patients and found that contrast detection was impaired. Since contrast discrimination has to do with dopamine, probably retinal dopamine, we thought we should take a look at our patients and divide them up by the kinds of drugs that they take, i.e., typical or atypical antipsychotic drugs. And, lo and behold, we found six patients who for the last two years were on no drugs. They took themselves off all antipsychotic drugs, and were doing relatively well without. What we found with those who were on no drugs was they had the lowest contrast detection thresholds. They were highly sensitive to contrast, much more so, than normal subjects. Those who were on typical antipsychotic drugs, on Thorazine or Haldol were up near the Parkinsonian range. Those who were on atypical drugs were normal. When you average them all, they're all normal. But here drugs make a real difference. And this relates, you remember, Tom, to the old literature which reported high sensitivity of acute schizophrenics or even chronic schizophrenics to the environment. Things bother them. They are readiy distracted. Bleuler attributed this to a poor modulation of attention. And these six patients who were on no antipsychotics at all were highly bothered by everything. I am willing to wager it has to do with dopamine regulation, and doesn't have anything to do with attention.

TB: So you are trying to identify the molecular substrate involved in the dys-function of smooth pursuit eye movements?

PH: Yes.

TB: So you have information on the molecular genetics but are still trying to find out more about its neurochemistry.

PH: Yes.

TB: Let me switch to something entirely different. When and how did you get involved with ACNP?

PH: That was through Danny Freedman. I had been invited to give a talk at an annual meeting, I forget what it was on, and I saw Danny holding court here, and I liked the people. I liked the activity. I liked the knowledge-exchange that was going. It was exciting. I thought, I want to be part of this. Danny said, "Not yet. You're not ready." But then I became ready, and I was so pleased to become a member and then a fellow. It has been of enormous importance to me.

TB: Did you become a member in the early 1970s?

PH: Yes.

TB: We talked about your early papers. What was your most recent publication?

PH: Well, the last one was on contrast detection. We've done some other studies on thought disorder. There is a paper that came out last summer in the *Journal of Abnormal Psychology* that has to do with working mem-ory I had worked with Patricia Goldman-Rakic on her paradigm, applying it to schizophrenic patients. And in this paper we report that both object working memory, i.e., memory for what things are, and spatial working memory, i.e., memory for where things are, are disordered. We used a Bayesian model to help us determine whether they were both impaired to the same extent or one was more impaired than the other. And the answer is, we couldn't tell. So we have to do more studies.

TB: Would you like to mention a couple of people you worked closely with and /or trained?

PH: Well, my close associate at McLean in our lab is Deborah Levy. Martha Shenton, who I think has just become a member at the ACNP, was trained by me. So were Martin Harrow, Dara Manoach, Bob Freedman and Sohee Park.

TB: You trained many people.

PH: If I was asked to write the list there are about 40.

TB: And there are many people working with your model everywhere in the world.

PH: Many people, but surely not all were my students.

TB: What would you like to see happen in the future in your area of research?

PH: Well, of course, schizophrenia is the cancer of mental disease. I would like to see it obliterated. I originally thought it was a simple matter, but now I realize it is not. And I have realized also that you can't do it by trying to obliterate the gene, because our latent trait hypothesis indicates that there are so many components to this disorder which are not the malignant part of it.

TB: Well, we should probably conclude with this. I would like to thank you very much for sharing all this information with us. Thank you very much.

PH: Thank you, Tom.

Laboratory Research

PHILIP B. BRADLEY

Interviewed by Thomas A. Ban

London, England, January 21, 2002

TB: This will be an interview with Professor Philip Bradley,* for the Archives of the American College of Neuropsychopharmacology. We are in London, Egland. It is January 21, 2002. I am Thomas Ban. Let us start from the very beginning. If you could tell us first where and when were you born? Say something about your childhood, early interests and education.

PB: Well, I was born in Bristol in 1919. My parents were quite poor; it was just after the end of the First World War. I had three brothers and two sisters, all of whom were considerably older than me, so I was the baby of the family. I went to a number of schools in Bristol. None of them would be well known, except possibly Cotham Grammar School where I took my matriculation examination before moving to Bristol University to study Zoology and Chemistry. For financial reasons, I could only get a place at university because I was given a grant from the Ministry of Education, which committed me to take a teaching post after graduation for four years. However, the Second World War intervened, and because I failed a chemistry examination, I was obliged to join the army. At the time science students were exempt from military service, but because I had failed this exam, I was no longer exempt.

I spent six years in the army, and at one time I was posted to Brighton Technical College as an army instructor to teach electronics, which was a rather strange thing as I knew very little about it! I thought afterwards it might have been because I had studied Physics for my Higher School Certificate. So I was teaching electronics to army students and had to learn it very quickly. After two years, I went on to various other posts in the army which involved working on radar repairs and maintenance and being in charge of radar and wireless workshops. Eventually I went back to Bristol to complete my degree. Because of this wartime experience in electronics, I then became interested in electrophysiology and my research project in zoology was to record nerve potentials in insects.

TB: So, you continued your studies in zoology after you got out from the army?

PB: Yes, I went back to finish my degree in zoology and chemistry.

TB: What year did you get your degree in zoology?

PB: That was in 1948, and I was then looking for employment. I was offered a post with the Colonial Service to work as an entomologist in East Africa. But before I accepted that offer, I heard about a vacancy at the University

---

* Philip B. Bradley was born in Bristol, England in 1919. Bradley died in 2009.

of Birmingham in the Department of Pharmacology. They were looking for someone with my experience and I had an interview with Joel Elkes and Alistair Frazier, who was then head of the Pharmacology Department. They offered me a post as a Research Fellow that I accepted. I was to work with Joel and study the effects of drugs on the brain, using electrophysiological techniques.

Because of this, I took a course in electroencephalography (EEG) at the Burden Neurological Institute in Bristol with Dr. Grey Walter who, with Lord Adrian, had developed electroencephalography in England. When I arrived in Birmingham, I started work on recording the electrical activity of the brain in animals and studying the effects of drugs on the EEG. At that time, there were not many drugs available with known actions on the central nervous system. So I worked with atropine and physostigmine, which were used clinically at the time. The only treatment then for schizophrenia seemed to be sedatives and surprisingly, amphetamine, which had a dramatic effect on catatonic stupor.

Shortly afterwards new drugs appeared. The first was, I think, LSD-25, and then we heard about chlorpromazine being used in Paris. This was a very exciting time, because we received samples of chlorpromazine and Joel Elkes and his wife Charmian did the first clinical trial of chlorpromazine in the UK on schizophrenic patients and I was a member of the team, doing the EEGs. My own work was primarily on animals. The idea was to develop techniques for recording the EEG in conscious, unrestrained animals, which at that time I do not think had been done. It was Joel's idea for me to do the EEG course at the Burden, so that I would have some expertise in human EEG and I used that subsequently.

After taking part in the clinical trial of chlorpromazine in schizophrenic patients, I worked in collaboration with another psychiatrist in Birmingham, Peter Jeavons. We studied the sedation threshold in schizophrenic patients, using the EEG. I was also invited to work with the neurosurgeons in Birmingham, who realized that recording the electrical activity directly from the cerebral cortex would be helpful in delineating tumors and epileptic foci on the exposed cerebral cortex. They did not have suitable equipment of their own, and I used to trundle my equipment across to the hospital where we sterilized the electrodes and other bits of equipment that came into contact with the patients. Occasionally, I accompanied Eric Turner, the neurosurgeon I was working with, to London to watch neurosurgical operations performed at the Maudsley Hospital. I also worked in collaboration with the Professor of Neurosurgery, Professor Brodie Hughes, recording the activity of single cells in the caudate nucleus, using stereotactic techniques. Brodie

Hughes was interested in Parkinson's disease, and at the time, the condition was relieved by lesions of the caudate nucleus. It may sound illogical, but that's what we were doing. So I did have some experience using the electrophysiological techniques I had learned at Burden, and I think that was quite valuable.

TB: Did you by that time develop your technique for recording electrical activity of the brain in unrestrained conscious animals?

PB: Yes, I had to develop the technology for animals as up to then recordings had been made in anesthetized animals, and apart from the effects of the anesthetic obscuring changes in the EEG, we also wanted to see the effects of the drugs on behavior. Therefore, I developed techniques for implanting electrodes in animals, in order to record the activity of the brain at the same time as observing the behavior. This was the work I did for my PhD.

TB: So your PhD was in neuropharmacology.

PB: No, it was in pharmacology, neuropharmacology as a subject did not exist then.

TB: Then, you got your DSc, your Doctor of Science?

PB: That was later, and that was in Neuropharmacology. I got my PhD in 1952, at the time when Joel Elkes went off to spend a year to Washington. When he came back, he established a new department called Experimental Psychiatry, in which he took responsibility for the clinical work of the department and I was in charge of the basic research, which also included neurochemistry.

TB: When did you do the research with barbiturates and amphetamines?

PB: That was in my PhD work.

TB: So, it was done between 1948 and 1952?

PB: That sounds about right. I worked initially with the drugs that were available at the time, i.e., atropine and physostigmine, to modify cholinergic function in the brain, and amphetamine and barbiturates to modify levels of consciousness. Later, when chlorpromazine and LSD became available, I studied those as well. In 1949, after Moruzzi and Magoun published their seminal paper on the reticular formation of the brain, I devised a series of acute experiments using lesions at different levels in the brain.

TB: Before telling us about your findings with lesions could you elaborate on Moruzzi and Magoun's influential paper?

PB: They showed that stimulating the reticular formation, a diffuse structure in the tegmental region of the brain stem – comprising mainly short axon neurones and distinct from the main afferent pathways and the cranial nerve nuclei – with a relatively high frequency electrical stimulus (300 c/s,) produced an arousal response as observed by changes in the electrical activity of the cerebral cortex.

TB: What did you find with lesions?

PB: We were able to show that a lesion which transected the midbrain cutting off the ascending influence of the reticular formation blocked the stimulant effects of amphetamine; whilst, on the other hand, the effects of drugs with actions related to cholinergic mechanisms in the brain were unaffected by this lesion. So, we made some rather naïve predictions about the possible site of action of these drugs.

TB: At what levels did you have the lesions?

PB: I adopted the techniques of the Belgian physiologist, Bremer. One of the lesions was at the C-1 level in the spinal cord, which produced what he called the encéphale isolé, an isolated brain but with an intact blood supply. This preparation showed periods of wakefulness and sleep, as judged by the activity of the cerebral cortex and responses to sensory stimuli. Another lesion was at the midbrain level which resulted in the cerveau isolé, or isolated cerebrum and this preparation showed permanent sleep activity, presumably as the result of the removal of the ascending influence of the reticular formation. Our studies in these acute animal preparations showed that both transsections of the spinal cord and of the midbrain did not modify the effect of cholinergic drugs, physostigmine producing an alert pattern of activity in the EEG and atropine, sleep-like activity, i.e., the reverse. However, transsection at the spinal cord level appeared to block the alerting effect of LSD, and lesions of the midbrain blocked the alerting effect of amphetamine.

TB: What about chlorpromazine?

PB: Chlorpromazine seemed to have very little effect in these experiments and we were unable at the time to localize its effects to the brain stem.

TB: Didn't you find that chlorpromazine interfered with the response to afferent stimulation?

PB: Yes. With my colleague Brian Key who was a PhD student at the time, we devised an experiment in which we measured the threshold for arousal to electrical stimulation of the reticular formation and the threshold for arousal produced by afferent, auditory stimulation. This work was done with acute encéphale isolé preparations and was supported financially by the US Air Force. We found that sedative drugs, such as the barbiturates, blocked the effect of the stimulation in the brain stem very quickly, whereas amphetamine had the opposite effect: it reduced the threshold although this was very difficult to measure.

We also tested the arousal response to afferent stimulation and found that chlorpromazine had little effect on the threshold for arousal produced by brain stem stimulation, but depressed afferent-induced arousal. LSD on the other hand had the opposite effect, facilitating the afferent-induced arousal. So we put forward the hypothesis that drugs which affect levels of consciousness probably act directly on the reticular formation either by stimulating or depressing it, whereas others, such as chlorpromazine and LSD seemed to have less direct effect on the reticular formation but influenced the effects of afferent stimulation either by depression, as chlorpramazine, or stimulation, as LSD.

TB: Was anyone else at the time involved in similar research?

PB: Well, I think that some of the experiments that the Killams were doing in Los Angeles at the time might have been similar.

TB: How did the scientific community respond to your findings?

PB: Not very well, I must say. My recollection of presenting papers to the Physiological Society in London was that they were met with quiet acceptance, without much discussion. What we were doing was probably not considered proper physiology. On the other hand, because of my training in electroencephalography I was a member of the EEG Society and I gave papers at their meetings. These were received quite well by the audience, which consisted largely of psychiatrists and neurologists, and even some physiologists.

TB: You mentioned before that while doing your research for your PhD you worked with drugs like atropine and physostigmine. Did you do the research with anticholinergics that showed dissociation between the changes in the EEG and behavior, before or after Wikler published his findings?

PB: I would say that it was about the same time, because I met Wikler and we discussed his work on dogs where he showed the dissociation of the EEG from behavior, and we were able to demonstrate a similar phenomenon in other species, cats and later on rhesus monkeys.

TB: So you showed that some drugs would produce dissociation between behavior and EEG in the cat?

PB: That's right. The most striking dissociation was with atropine, but large doses of the drug were needed. It wasn't what you would regard as a normal dose of atropine in either animals or man for that matter but we noticed no untoward effects.

TB: Do you remember the research you did immediately after you got your PhD?

PB: I did some work on the effects of DFP, diisopropylflurophosphate, an irreversible cholinesterase inhibitor. I had a student working with me then and we became interested in a technique developed by Feldberg for injecting drugs into the ventricles of the brain. These experiments produced some interesting results but their interpretation was difficult especially as it became apparent that the CSF-brain barrier was as potent as the blood-brain barrier.

TB: Could we review again briefly your findings on the effects of drugs? Barbiturates and amphetamines have . . .

PB: A direct action on the reticular formation on the brain stem, barbiturates depressing and amphetamine stimulating.

TB: LSD and chlorpromazine?

PB: Well, it seemed from our experiments with the measuring of thresholds for arousal to afferent auditory stimulation, compared to thresholds for arousal to direct electical stimulation of the reticular formation, that the effects of LSD and chlorpromazine were more likely to be related to the afferent inputs, i.e., afferent collaterals, into the brain stem, this being the mechanism by which afferent stimuli produce arousal. At a meeting in Geneva in 1964 I proposed the hypothesis that chlorpromazine had an action in the brain stem similar to that of de-afferentation, and this could explain its clinical actions but it did not arouse much interest.

TB: This was the first hypothesis about the mode of action of chlorpromazine?

PB: I think it might have been, but I'm not sure.

TB: It was an important discovery because it showed that the mode of action of chlorpromazine is different from the old sedatives. It also showed that the mode of action of LSD is different from the mode of action of anticholinergics.

PB: Yes, the hypothesis was that the anticholinergics and cholinergic agonists act more diffusely. Their actions are not restricted to a particular area as you would expect from the distribution of cholinergic receptors in the brain, based on studies of the distribution of the enzymes choline acetylase and acetylcholinesterase, which showed a fairly even distribution throughout the brain.

TB: You were also one of the first to show dissociation between behavior and electrical activity in the brain after the administration of anticholinergics.

PB: We observed the phenomenon in the cat and also in primates, rhesus monkeys, whereas Wikler's observations, which I think were concurrent with ours, were in dogs. So it seems the dissociation is not species-specific. I have to say that my friend Vincenzo Longo, working in Rome, never agreed that the dissociation existed, and I think he tried to disprove it at the CINP Meeting in Tarragona in 1968, but I couldn't be bothered to get into a dispute as I had then moved on to other things. I thought it was the sort of thing anybody could reproduce if they wished to.

TB: The finding about the dissociation has kept lingering on for a long time.

PB: I suppose so, because nobody has ever really examined the phenomenon in detail, and we still do not know what it means. It seems strange that an organism can show sleep-like activity in the EEG while it is fully alert. You could say it shows the irrelevance of the electrocorticogram to behavior, but I don't think that's the sort of generalization we should make. But it is clear that the electrocorticogram is not always a good indicator of the behavioral state of the animal in terms of wakefulness and sleep. I believe other examples of dissociation have been found more recently.

TB: Let's get back to your activities after you got your PhD. Did you become involved in teaching?

PB: My first involvement in teaching was, strangely enough in neurology. The head of Pharmacology, Alistair Frazer, was of the opinion that only medically qualified staff should teach medical students. Those ideas did not last very long. There were some aspects of neurology I did not know very well, and again I had to learn quickly. However, I was able to give lectures on the reticular formation and on the EEG where I also gave demonstrations, using student volunteers.

TB: Any other important events in those years?

PB: There was the Neurochemistry Conference in Oxford in 1954, which Joel Elkes organized and I assisted with the administration. That was my first involvement in organizing meetings and the experience proved useful in later years, particularly with the early CINP meetings. It was an enjoyable experience and I met some interesting people.

TB: Can you tell us something about the Oxford meeting?

PB: It was a very mixed group, mainly biochemists, some physiologists and anatomists. I can't tell you much about the scientific aspects of the meeting as I was working behind the scenes and looking after people's problems. One of the problems I had was that the organizers had invited a number of speakers from the Soviet Union but had received no response. Then, half way through the meeting, this group of Russians arrived and I had to receive them, as everyone else was busy. They had an interpreter with them, a lady, but I subsequently found that they could all speak English, so the role of the interpreter was not quite what we thought. Everybody was staying in the colleges, Magdalen College being the main one, but the Russians refused to stay in a college and we had to find them a hotel!

TB: They were probably obliged by their government to stay in hotels.

PB: I think that is true, but it all ended amicably; they were very friendly and participated well in the meeting.

TB: Was that the first International Congress of Neurochemistry?

PB: I think it was. After the meeting it was decided to set up the International Society for Neurochemistry, and later on there was a Journal. Brian Ansell, who subsequently joined me in Birmingham, was one of the founders. He also became Chief Editor.

TB: It was held at the time when emphasis on the transmission of impulses in the brain began to shift from electrical to chemical.

PB: Yes, the person who was most influential was the physiologist Sir John Eccles who had been a strong proponent of electrical synaptic transmission, but in a series of lectures in Oxford described, somewhat dramatically, how he was converted to a belief in chemical transmission, i.e., that the nerve impulse crossed the synaptic junction as a result of the release of a chemical. It was about the time that the physiologists Hodgkin and Huxley were studying transmission in peripheral nerves and the neuromuscular junction. That was a very active period, but those working on peripheral nerve transmission didn't think about the brain. I have a feeling they didn't want to think about the brain because it was an extra complication.

TB: It was in those years that the presence of norepinephrine was detected in the brain.

PB: That was the work of Marthe Vogt and von Euler. Marthe Vogt published an important paper in 1953 on the levels of adrenaline and noradrenaline in the brain, showing that these substances were concentrated in the midbrain and brain stem regions, which fitted in nicely with our theories. But there were other things happening at that time. Joel went off to America in the early 1950s and when he came back he established this Department of Experimental Psychiatry; I was appointed to a Lectureship in Electrophysiology, and joined him.

TB: It was the first Department of Experimental Psychiatry in the world.

PB: Probably so. Some time later, I was offered a Fellowship by the Rockefeller Foundation of New York and told I could choose where to study. The options were the Department of Anatomy at UCLA with Magoun or the Institute of Physiology at the University of Pisa with Moruzzi.

TB: And you chose Pisa.

PB: It was a difficult choice, but in the end I went to Pisa because they had developed a technique for recording the activity of single neurons using microelectrodes. My feeling was that analyzing EEGs was probably not going to get us very far and that further advances were likely to be made by studying the activity of single neurons in the brain and how their activity was affected by drugs.

TB: Before continuing with your experiences in Pisa could you tell us something about the Department of Experimental Psychiatry. Where did the support come from?

PB: There was support from a number of places and there seemed to be a lot of money available. The main source was the Rockefeller Foundation which provided my Fellowship. There was government money from the Ministry of Health and there was a mental health research organization, subsequently taken over by the Medical Research Council. But all these were grants for a limited period. I was not aware of any funding from the pharmaceutical industry at that time.

TB: Was it an independent department?

PB: Yes, it was an independent department of the University.

TB: Who were the people in the department?

PB: Joel's wife, of course, Charmian, and there was a psychiatrist, Felix Letemandia. There was also a psychologist, Tony Harris, and an experimental psychologist, Malcolm Piercey. In addition, there was a biochemist, John Crammer.

TB: How many people were in the department, about half a dozen?

PB: Probably more. In the basic research section there was a biochemist named Archie Todrick, and a pharmacologist, Heinz Ginzel. There were also people on short-term contracts.

TB: Wasn't Mayer-Gross a member of the team?

PB: Mayer-Gross had worked at the Creighton Royal Hospital, in Dumfries, Scotland. He had already retired when Joel consulted him about recruiting a fairly senior person to take charge of the clinical work of the department. I was told that when Joel asked Mayer-Gross whom he would recommend, Mayer-Gross said "What about me"?

TB: Can you tell us something about Mayer-Gross?

PB: He had been Professor of Psychiatry at Heidelberg University in Germany and left in the 1930s for Scotland. He was co-author of a textbook of psychiatry but I didn't see a lot of him in Birmingham.

TB: But you had some interactions with him, didn't you?

PB: Yes. That was when I returned from Italy in September 1957. Joel had already left and things were pretty chaotic as there was no one in charge. Mayer-Gross and I did not see eye-to-eye; he did not approve of what I was doing.

TB: But he was on the team.

PB: Yes, he was one of the team.

TB: There was also Brian Key.

PB: He was one of my PhD students. He did most of the experiments on measuring thresholds and we published that work in the *EEG Journal* and the
British Journal of Pharmacology.

TB: Was he your first PhD student?

PB: No, my first PhD student was a man named Jim Hance. He was a zool-
ogist, as was Key. They were both Birmingham graduates; in fact the
Professor of Zoology, Otto Lowenstein, was very helpful in finding students for me. Hance did the experiments with intraventricular cannulae,
injecting drugs into the cerebral ventricles and observing the effects on
the EEG and behavior. This was work for his PhD. After I came back from
Pisa, I attended a meeting in Brussels. Magoun was there and invited
me to work in his laboratory, but as I'd just had a year off and things in
Birmingham were a little difficult, to say the least, I had to decline. But I
ended by saying there was someone from my laboratory who could be
interested. So Hance went in my place and stayed. He worked with the
KIllams, and moved to Stanford with them and then on to Davis. I visited
him and his wife Ann in Los Angeles, and later on he helped me to find
a house to rent on the Stanford campus. Then they moved to Davis and
I saw him again when I visited the Killams. After that I am afraid we lost
touch.

TB: Actually, Keith Killam died. Eva Killam is still around. I saw her at the last
ACNP meeting.

PB: Oh, dear. I did not know about Keith. I last saw them both at the
Pharmacology Congress in London when we had dinner together.

TB: Where was the Experimental Psychiatry department located?

PB: The department was housed at the University of Birmingham Medical
School. The Medical School and the general hospital, the Queen Elizabeth
Hospital, were on the same site. Most of the clinical work of the department went on at the mental hospital, All Saints, which was some distance
away and that is where I used to do EEG recordings on patients. There
were psychiatrists at the Queen Elizabeth Hospital but I don't think there
was a University Department of Psychiatry.

TB: And the director of the Department of Experimental Psychiatry was
Joel. I read somewhere that at the time there was no other Professor of
Psychiatry in Birmingham.

PB: That's right.There was no Professor of Psychiatry but there was certainly
a Professor of Neurology, Philip Cloake, whom I knew very well. However,
there were two psychiatrists in the hospital who were consultants. I was
with them at a meeting, and after giving my paper, one of them said it
didn't matter how a drug worked as long as it had an effect on the patient.
I think their attitude was one reason for Joel deciding to leave. I don't

know what he would say about this but certainly it wasn't lack of financial support. There were other psychiatrists in Birmingham who were more supportive. There was a day hospital in Moseley, Uffculme Clinic, which was an outpost of All Saints Hospital where the medical superintendent, Dr O'Reilly was very helpful and provided Joel with facilities for clinical trials. I believe the MRC Unit would, at least partially, have been established at Uffculme Clinic.

TB: Do you remember the visit of Ernst Rothlin?

PB: I remember it very well. Rothlin was Professor of Pharmacology at the University of Basel and Director of Research at Sandoz where LSD had been discovered by Albert Hofmann. Rothlin gave a lecture on LSD which I found quite fascinating although not much was known about its pharmacology at the time. Also, Rothlin had brought us a sample of LSD, and perhaps foolishly, we did experiments on a group of about 12 normal volunteers, including ourselves and other members of staff of the Medical School and All Saints Hospital. The experiments were supervised by Joel's wife, Charmian, and I did the EEGs; we recorded everything we could think of, including manual dexterity and reactions to various images. The results weren't very striking, but were, I suppose, pioneering, because it was the first experiment in normal subjects, apart from those of Hoffman and Stoll. There were changes in perception but the EEG changes were relatively slight, in the direction of increased alertness. The drug appeared to exaggerate underlying personality traits in subjects, so people who were slightly obsessive became more so, and subjects who were slightly paranoid showed increased symptoms. Personally, I think it was a mistake to use colleagues and friends as subjects in these experiments. Perhaps medical student volunteers might have been preferable although this could have had its dangers as some years later I was approached by a medical student who said he understood we were studying LSD and he could supply some! I thanked him and said "No" as by then possession of the drug was illegal and I had the only legitimate supply.

TB: Did you encounter depression in any of the subjects?

PB: No, but we did encounter some severe reactions. There was one colleague who did not seem to be responding to a dose of 25 micrograms. Joel came in and Charmian asked if we should give him some more but Joel said "No." So we waited and soon after he got a very strong reaction, which went on for two days. People who were still showing the effects of LSD after the experiment had finished were given a small dose of a sedative, usually chlorpromazine. However, this particular subject's wife was a doctor and she said, "Nobody is going to treat my husband," so she refused the sedative and the effects of LSD persisted for two days. So, these were interesting times.

TB: Could you tell us something about Rothlin?

PB: Ernst Rothlin was a very nice man and I got on well with him. During his visit we discussed the idea of a new international organization devoted to Neuropharmacology and both Joel and I said that we would be enthusiastic supporters. Rothlin said he would discuss the proposal elsewhere and let us know the results.

TB: You were instrumental in opening up the field of Neuropharmacology?

PB: Somebody referred to me once as the "Father of Neuropharmacology" but I do not think that's true and it was probably just a joke.

TB: You pioneered research in neuropharmacology, using microelectrode techniques.

PB: Yes, but I thought of neuropharmacology as a branch of pharmacology.

TB: Still, you were one of those who opened development in neuropsycho-pharmacological research.

PB: That is probably true, and I think I held the first formal appointment as a Neuropharmacologist in 1958; that was the year I was awarded my DSc for studies in the field of Neuropharmacology. I did think it was unnecessary to have both, "psycho" and "neuro" in the name of the new organization, CINP, because what is "psycho" if it isn't also "neuro"? However, some people, such as psychologists, would prefer to have both in the name.

TB: What would you have preferred?

PB: Just Neuropharmacology, but then others would prefer just Psycho-pharmacology, and I am a Founder Member of the British Association for Psychopharmacology. I think the combination Neuropsycho is a bit cumbersome but we all have to compromise.

TB: I think it was during Rothlin's visit to Birmingham that the idea of having an organization in neuropsychopharmacology was first discussed.

PB: It was, and I believe Joel pursued the idea and talked to other people. In fact, Rothlin might have asked him to do so. A lot of people seem to have suggested it was their idea.

TB: Am I correct that the night before you went to Pisa, Joel told you that he might be leaving?

PB: That's true. How do you know this?

TB: I learned it from one of your or his publications.

PB: It wouldn't have been in any of my papers. He'd been back in Birmingham for some years but was still visiting Washington frequently, and it was the night before I was due to leave for Pisa we had dinner at the Cafe Royal in London when he broke the news and said he hoped I might eventually join him. I had been attending a meeting at the Institute of Psychiatry at the Maudsley Hospital and Denis Hill, who was in charge of the EEG Department there, offered me a job. I was in turmoil and didn't know what to do. I thought the department in Birmingham might break up. Anyway, I turned down the job at the Maudsley as I knew it wasn't a very happy place. I knew Sir Aubrey Lewis quite well as I had been advising him on setting up a new laboratory for electrophysiological research. There had been occasions when I was lunching with Aubrey Lewis in the refectory and other people whom I knew would come in but would not join us. It seems petty but I did not think there was a very good atmosphere at the Maudsley Hospital so I turned down the job and went to Pisa, and continued with my research. I subsequently had my opinion of the atmosphere at the Maudsley confirmed by others.

TB: When did you go to Pisa?

PB: It was in 1956. I went by train on a first class sleeper from Paris and it was a pleasant journey. I had taken a supply of drugs and was a bit worried about going through Customs. It was fortunate I did take them as there was nothing at the Institute of Physiology in Pisa. My purpose in going there was to learn to use the technique of the floating microelectrode, with which they were recording the activity of single cells in the brain. I thought it would be very complicated, but it was not. Essentially it consisted of a piece of fine enamelled wire, pushed gently into the brain until the activity of a single neuron was picked up. The other end of the wire was clamped but a loop was formed so that the recording tip was floating and would follow movements of the brain. I learned this technique very quickly and worked with an Italian, Dr A. Mollica, who was Moruzzi's first assistant. We worked hard, including on Saturdays which was the system in Italy, and we obtained some very interesting results which were published in Moruzzi's journal, the *Archives Italiennes de Biologie* (Archives of Italian Biology). I believe it was the first time such experiments had been performed. However, we were injecting the drugs intravenously and since there were changes in blood pressure when the drugs were injected, we could not decide whether the effects observed were due to an action of the drug on the neuron, or some indirect effect via a change in blood pressure. I realized that this technique wasn't going to get us very far and began to think about alternatives. Nevertheless, I persevered for my year in Pisa and enjoyed the Italian sunshine and the culture.

Two events occurred during my stay in Pisa, both of which were important. The first was an invitation to attend and present a paper at a symposium, *The Reticular Formation of the Brain*, at the Henry Ford Hospital in Detroit in March 1957. It was a great experience and my presentation was well received. There were only two other participants from the UK, Geoffrey Harris from London and the neurosurgeon, Sir Geoffrey Jefferson, both of whom I got to know well. It was also an opportunity to visit other centers in the US, including Harold Himwich's at Galesburg, and Magoun's laboratory in Los Angeles. I also visited Washington where I was offered a post in Joel's laboratory at St. Elizabeths Hospital. The second event was an invitation to attend and present a paper at a meeting on Psychotropic Drugs to be held in Milan in May 1957.

TB: Could you tell us something about that meeting?

PB: The meeting was sponsored by the Institute of Pharmacology in Milan, the head of which was Professor Emilio Trabucchi. But Trabucchi was a retiring kind of person and liked to remain in the background so the meeting was organized by Silvio Garattini, whom I already knew, and Vittorio Ghetti.

TB: Later on Silvio published the proceedings of that symposium with Ghetti.

PB: I had my first wife and two children with me in Pisa, and we all went to Milan and stayed in a very nice hotel. There was also a visit to La Scala, where I heard the tenor Guiseppi de Stefano for the first time. Scientifically the meeting was a great success with an opportunity to meet people working the same or related fields. During the meeting I received an invitation from Rothlin to attend an informal meeting to discuss the proposed organization on Neuropharmacology.

TB: How many people participated?

PB: I think about a dozen.

TB: Can you remember who was present?

PB: Rothlin, Radouco-Thomas, de Boor, Denber and others whom I can't remember.

TB: In the records of the CINP history committee, both Corneille Radouco-Thomas and Wolfgang de Boor independently suggested to Trabucchi prior to that meeting the founding of an international society in Neuropsychopharmacology.

PB: I don't think that's true but I am not sure. Trabucchi was a very modest, retiring man. I think he liked to facilitate things and gave his support to the meeting, but I am not sure of who proposed it. Personally, I do not think it is important who had the original idea. We all have ideas from time to time and do not pursue them, and then someone else takes them up. As far as I am concerned, I first heard mention of an organization which eventually became the CINP, in Birmingham in 1954 or 1955 during Rothlin's visit, not in Milan in 1957.

TB: The question is whether it was Trabucchi or Rothlin who inititated that meeting during the Milan symposium and whether it was Trabucchi or Rothlin who chaired it?

PB: As far as I know, it was Rothlin, and it was certainly Rothlin who chaired it.

TB: Do you remember anyone else who participated? I think Hanns Hippius was there.

PB: He might have been there, although he was not a participant in the Symposium. But I know Rothlin chaired the meeting that led to the founding of the CINP.

TB: What about Deniker?

PB: Deniker was there and also Denber and I think Bente. We had quite a long discussion but the decision to found the CINP was deferred in Milan until the Second Congress of Psychiatry in Zurich, which was to take place in September 1957. In my opinion, this was not a good idea because most of the people who would become members of the organization were already in Milan and, apart from psychiatrists, very few were likely to attend the meeting in Zurich. However, Rothlin maintained that as pharmacology would be included in the title, it would be wise to consult the International Union of Pharmacology (IUPHAR) and get their approval; it would be a bad move to go ahead without their agreement and he was probably right. There was also discussion about a journal, which turned out to be *Psychopharmacologia*. Rothlin had been in discussions with a publisher but did not disclose very much information.

TB: Now, the story goes that in Milan there was another important luncheon meeting relevant to the founding of the CINP in which you participated. Do you remember?

PB: I remember the meeting and that we had lunch, I think at Trabucchi's department as I remember talking to him, but precisely what it was about I can't remember. I should think it was probably a preparation for the meeting in Zurich but cannot be sure.

TB: Were you involved in the preparation of the inaugural meeting in Zurich?

PB: No, I had other problems at the time. I had received a message that Joel Elkes had already left Birmingham, so I returned from Pisa a month early, in August, to find out what was happening. Things were pretty chaotic and the finances of the department were in a mess. Then the University appointed me Acting Head of the Department and the Vice-Chancellor, Sir Robert Aitken, said to me, "This is your opportunity." In retrospect, I have sometimes wondered if Mayer-Gross had expected to take over from Joel. I was probably lacking in experience and not very good at handling people.

The main problem was that the three staff members Joel had recently recruited, Letemendia, Harris and Crammer, who were all medically qualified, were on short-term contracts and the money was running out. I was told by the Rockefeller Foundation that they would not be renewing their grant and I knew that the people at the MRC were not very happy as they set up a Research Unit with Joel as director and with some staff, but he abandoned it at very short notice. Not many people knew about this, but I saw it written on headed notepaper about the Unit. Mayer-Gross accused me of getting rid of good people and destroying what Joel had built up, but I had no choice as the finances were in a mess. I probably did not handle Mayer-Gross very well. He was a nice man but very dominating and famous, whereas I was at the beginning of my career. There was one other factor I considered important, and that was, as I did not have a medical qualification, I did not feel I could be responsible for the work of medically-qualified staff. Perhaps Mayer-Gross and I ought to have found a way of working together but it would have been very difficult. It was probably a mistake for him to come to Birmingham after he had retired.

Another important event that year was that I was invited to meet Sir Harold Himsworth, the Secretary of the MRC in London. We had an interesting discussion as a result of which I was asked to present my research findings and future plans to the MRC's Clinical Research Board. I know that discussions went on behind the scenes with the Vice-Chancellor, and the MRC decided to establish a research unit in Birmingham, the Neuropharmacology Research Unit, with myself as Honorary Director. This was my first official appointment as a neuropharmacologist. Eventually, the university appointed a Professor of Psychiatry.

TB: Who did they appoint?

PB: Professor William Trethowan from Australia. It was clear that there could not be two departments of psychiatry and I was quite happy to change the name of mine. I would have preferred Neuropharmacology but the Professor of Pharmacology, Alistair Frazer, would not accept that so as a compromise, we became Experimental Neuropharmacology. I must say that Trethowan and I got on extremely well and he was vey supportive of our research.

TB: But in spite of all the problems you had at home you went to Zurich to attend the inaugural meeting of the CINP.

PB: Yes, I went to Zurich for the 2nd World Congress of Psychiatry. I felt that as I had been involved in neuropharmacology from the beginning, I should be there.

TB: That meeting in Zurich was organized by Rothlin and included invitation to a dinner.

PB: The dinner was in the first class restaurant at the Zurich railway station.

TB: Insofar as we know there were 33 people at that dinner, right?

PB: I think so. From the UK, apart from myself, there was Michael Shepherd, Sir Aubrey Lewis and Derek Richter. Humphrey Osmond was also there.

TB: What about Linford Rees?

PB: I don't think he was there, but I cannot be sure.

TB: Some people say he was, but others say not. It was a very distinguished group.

PB: Probably. A lot of people felt motivated to make speeches. At the end, there was a formal proposal from Rothlin that the CINP should be founded and this was agreed unanimously. Rothlin became its first president and various people were proposed for the committee.

TB: You and Deniker became the first councilors.

PB: Yes. I was proposed by Aubrey Lewis. I think that Rothlin wanted another pharmacologist on the committee, which seemed sensible. But he also wanted a representative from the UK.

TB: Another version is that it was Denber's suggestion that you and Deniker became councilors because of your contributions to the new field.

PB: It is possible that Denber supported my nomination but I know it was Aubrey Lewis who proposed me as he was sitting next to me. Anyway, the CINP was established and I was a member of the Council. Our immediate task was to organize the first meeting in Rome in 1958, which was in 12 months' time. I thought it was crazy, but we did it!

TB: What was your role in organizing that congress?

PB: I was asked to organize one of the symposia. It was the first Symposium, "Methods and Analysis of Drug-induced Behavior in Animals". As I was also the first speaker, it was chaired by Rothlin and Jules Masserman.

TB: Could you tell us who were involved in organizing the congress?

PB: Both Rothlin and Trabucchi were involved. I think Trabucchi made most of the local arrangements as Chairman of the Local Organizing Committee, whereas the program was the responsibility of the Executive Committee, chaired by Rothlin.

TB: In addition to Rothlin and Deniker could you tell us who the others were on CINP's first executive? There were two secretaries. . . .

PB: Yes, Radouco-Thomas and Denber.

TB: And the treasurer was Stoll.

PB: That's right. It was dominated by Europeans.

TB: Could you tell us something about the Rome congress?

PB: It was a very successful meeting. We tried to put together a program which covered all the different scientific disciplines contributing to neuropsychopharmacology and I think we succeeded. Certainly a number of people who attended told me later how successful it was. There was an excellent social program as well, although I was obliged to miss the audience with the Pope as I needed to prepare my talk. Apart from the opening symposium in which I participated, I persuaded my colleague, Brian Ansell, who had just joined me in Birmingham as Lecturer in Neurochemistry to give a lecture on "The Present State of Neurochemistry."

TB: Didn't you edit the proceedings?

PB: The Executive Committee met on the last day of the meeting and decided that the proceedings should be published. Myself, Deniker and Radouco-Thomas were appointed as editors. We had a difficult task as many people were already leaving and had not been asked to prepare a manuscript, and there was no publisher. However, we succeeded, and the Elsevier Publishing Company proved to be very co-operative. I think Radouco-Thomas had already been in touch with them. Inevitably some contributions were missing as we could not delay publication for too long. I think that the book was well received. This was my first venture into publishing and it prepared me for the future.

TB: How many people attended the congress?

PB: There were over five hundred. Some people came because this was something new. There weren't many from the UK at the inaugural meeting in Zurich and my impression was that the bulk of the psychiatric population in the UK wasn't terribly interested. However, when they heard about the success of the Congress in Rome, many more became interested and eventually joined the CINP.

TB: Could you tell us something about your research after you returned from Pisa?

PB: It was some time before I could get back into experimental work. As I was in charge of a department that had been abandoned by its previous head, I had a great deal of administration to contend with and was lacking in experience. There was also a good deal of planning to do. Fortunately, research funds had not dried up completely, in spite of the Rockefeller Foundation not renewing its grant. I think that was a personal grant to Joel anyway. I still had my funding from the US Air Force which was generous, and the University provided a number of new appointments, including a Lectureship to which Brian Ansell was appointed. Eventually, the MRC established its Neuropharmacology Research Unit under my direction, occupying accommodation provided by the University.

During my absence in Italy the electrophysiological research had been kept going by two postgraduate students who were in touch with me by mail. Now I had a new student working with me making micro-electrode recordings of single neurons in the brain. I had heard about iontophoresis being used by some people at University College London and I visited them. A similar technique was being used at John Eccles' laboratory in Canberra. Then, at a meeting of the Physiological Society, I met John Wolstencroft who was working in Leeds. He was planning a visit to Moruzzi's laboratory in Pisa and wanted my advice. Our discussions led to the discovery of many mutual scientific interests and we both concluded that the use of microiontophoresis to apply active substances on single neurons in the brain, whilst recording their activity, was the way forward for both of us. I was able to persuade the MRC to create a senior appointment for John in the unit and he moved to Birmingham. This was the beginning of a very exciting time for both of us.

The equipment we were using at the time was very primitive and the experiments very time-consuming. Because of electrical interference in the Medical School during the day, although we were using a Faraday Cage, we had to work at night when the lifts could be switched off. Also the only way we could record the action potentials was by photographing onto 35 mm film. Then, after the film was developed, one of us would take it home and count the activity usually over a 10 second period. Eventually, we designed electronic equipment for recording and counting the neuronal activity that provided a printed output. The people working with iontophoresis in London and Canberra were studying neurons in the spinal cord, and as far as we knew, no one had used the technique in the brain. We obtained some exciting results. Using putative transmitters, such as acetylcholine, noradrenline and serotonin, we were able to classify the brain stem neurons into different types according to their responses. Thus, when acetylcholine was applied, some neurons showed a pattern of excitation whilst others were inhibited, and a third group was unaffected. A similar pattern of activity was shown by the other two substances, noradrenaline and serotonin. Furthermore, some neurons responded to just one substance, some to two and, rarely, some to all three and the pattern of responses could be a mixture of excitation and inhibition. From this complex pattern of responses, we attempted to classify neurons in the brain stem, and although this classification was somewhat crude, it was a beginning.

We then started looking at interactions with centrally acting drugs, for example chlorpromazine, LSD and amphetamine. One interesting finding was that LSD antagonized the actions of serotonin (5-HT) which supported the hypothesis put forward by Gaddum in 1956, based on studies on peripheral nerves. At the time some workers in the Physiology Department in Birmingham had isolated a substance with oxytocic properties, which was released from the cerebral cortex in response to stimulation of peripheral nerves. John Wolstencroft was very excited about this and wanted us to test it in our experiments. I was not keen as we knew nothing about the chemistry of the substance, only that it was oxytocic. Nevertheless, we did some experiments and found the substance had some activity on brain stem neurons but the results were difficult to interpret. Later on the substance we were using was shown to be a prostaglandin, which has an important role in platelet aggregation. We also did some experiments with a "sleep-inducing" substance discovered by Monnier working at the University of Basel in Switzerland. He sent us samples and we collected them at the airport and rushed them to the lab. Again very little activity was found and I was not pleased when I discovered that Monnier was sending us placebos as well without telling us which was the active sample and which was not.

TB: You said, if I understood it correctly, that you were involved in classifying neurons according to their response to neurotransmtters, and if I remember, you also studied interactions between neurotransmitters and drugs by using iontophoresis. Could you give us an idea what you actually did?

PB: We used multi-barreled microelectrodes which consisted of glass tubing, drawn out to a fine tip. We invented a device in which the glass tubing was held vertically and a weight attached to the bottom end. In the centre was a circular electrical heating element. When the current was switched on, the tubing was heated and the weight pulled out the glass to a very fine diameter. By adjusting the weight and current we were able to achieve the size of tip we needed, usually 5 microns diameter. With this size we were able to isolate single neurons in the brain stem. A number of these tubes would be glued together, usually five but I have heard of people using electrodes with up to eight barrels. The central barrel was filled with saline solution and used for recording the activity of the neuron and the other barrels were filled with aqueous solutions of the substances we wished to test. Clearly only substances that ionized in solution could be used in this way, and we were lucky that most of the substances we were interested in did so. By passing a very small electric current through the relevant barrel, the substance under test was released close to the neuron being recorded. Usually one of the barrels of the electrode was filled with saline to test the effect of the current alone on the activity of the neuron. We assumed that the amount of substance released from the tip of the electrode would be dependent on the strength of current passed.

Some time later one of my colleagues did some tests using radio-labeled compounds to measure the quantity released with different current strengths and confirmed that our assumption was correct. We seemed to be developing a new area of CNS research and I thought it might be interesting to make it known to a wider audience. Since I was a member of the organizing committee for the 3rd CINP Congress to be held in Munich, I proposed that there should be a session on studies on single neurons and this was accepted. John and I put together a program to include those who were working in similar or related fields; these included Salmoiraghi who was working at Joel's new unit in Washington and Krnjevic, who had worked with Eccles and was then in Cambridge. The session was held in a fairly small auditorium which we thought would be adequate, but we were completely wrong as we had people queuing at the door to get in and others listening from the corridor outside. I was pleased with the reception we received.

TB: Weren't there some problems with the CINP in those years?

PB: I am afraid there were. Rothlin was not an impartial chairman. He would lead the discussion and expect other people to agree with him. When a topic came up for discussion, there was no way in which members of the committee could present their own views before a conclusion was reached. I think it was Denber, one of the secretaries, who objected vociferously and I felt obliged to support him although I had some sympathy for Rothlin having visited him at home and at his retreat on the top of the Rigi. I thought he did not know any other way to behave in such circumstances, and I realized that the universities in Switzerland must have been run on very autocratic lines, as were those in the UK at one time.

TB: What was it about Rothlin's actions that created the problem?

PB: Well, it was really about the way decisions were made because Rothlin wanted to have his way in everything and it was impossible to get him to listen to reason.

TB: Was there any real issue?

PB: I don't think so but maybe you should talk to other people who were there. Have you talked to Denber?

TB: He died.

PB: Did he? I'm sorry to hear that.

TB: I talked to him about it some time ago but he didn't say very much.

PB: He would probably sit on the fence for diplomacy's sake.

TB: Am I correct that you supported Denber?

PB: I did, because I felt it was necessary; although I appreciated Rothlin did what he did because it was the only way he knew how and one couldn't change that.

TB: Some people told us that it was about finances.

PB: I don't know if that is true. However, I felt that Denber had a point. Then Seymour Kety told us to pull together, which we did.

TB: I understood from some people that it was a rather difficult situation.

PB: It seemed the CINP might collapse and it was probably saved by the intervention of Seymour Kety.

TB: Some of the founders, Denber and Radouco-Thomas resigned.

PB: Yes, but my memory isn't terribly good, one tries to forget unpleasant things.

TB: The important thing is the CINP survived and by the 3rd congress everything was fine.

PB: Yes it was.

TB: The fourth CINP meeting was in Birmingham. Wasn't it?

PB: Yes, it was the meeting I hosted.

TB: It was a great meeting.

PB: Was it? Good.

TB: Yes; it was the first meeting I attended.

PB: At the end of the week, we went to a performance of Henry V in Stratford and I fell asleep during the battle scene! So it must have been pretty exhausting.

TB: It had an excellent program. It was also interesting in terms of organization. Everyone stayed on campus in the student halls of residence.

PB: Oh yes, but we hadn't much alternative. There wouldn't have been enough hotel accommodation in Birmingham at that time. There probably is now. I thought it was a disaster at the time, because people were in rooms without wash basins. The student accommodation was quite Spartan. It has improved considerably since.

TB: There was one bathroom for about ten rooms.

PB: Not ideal for people used to better things. However, I think the meeting was successful scientifically.

TB: I remember that Max Fink delivered one of the plenary lectures on clinical neurophysiology, on the new science, pharmaco-EEG.

PB: Yes he did and it was well received.

TB: And there was also a lecture by the president . . .

PB: That was the Austrian, Hoff.

TB: Can you tell us something about the budget and finances of the Birmingham meeting?

PB: I believe we covered our costs. I don't think the University was quite as helpful as it should have been although we were provided with the accommodation we needed, including a large lecture theatre for the plenary sessions. We had adequate financial support, some from the United States, and most of the pharmaceutical companies I contacted gave us generous support.

TB: So the meeting didn't cost CINP any money?

PB: Not as far as I am aware. I don't think the CINP had much money at the time. There was a bank account in Basel and the subscriptions were going in but there did not seem to be much money available.

TB: So, there was no money from the CINP.

PB: No. The meetings were supposed to be self-supporting. We were able to cover our expenses and pay the speakers but there were no large grants.

TB: Is there anything else you would like to say in relation to the Birmingham meeting?

PB: During the meeting there was discussion at the Executive Committee as to who the next president might be. I thought it was time we had someone from the UK and suggested Sir John Gaddum who was Professor of Pharmacology at Edinburgh and well known internationally. Unfortunately, when I approached him he was obliged to decline the invitation as he had developed esophageal cancer. It was also in that year I had been nominated for a professorial chair. Prior to that, I had been appointed to a Readership which was the most senior non-professorial appointment in the University and was usually awarded for distinction in one's research field. However, the Vice-Chancellor said to me, "It's time we gave you a Chair." The appointment should have been made in October, but he pushed it forward, so that I had professorial status in time for the meeting.

TB: Before that you were Acting Head?

PB: They made me Acting Head of the Department, but without a Chair. At the time I was the only non-medical head of a department in the Faculty of Medicine but that did not seem to matter and I got on well with my colleagues.

TB: It was after the Birmingham meeting that you became treasurer of CINP.

PB: It must have been then. I had served for six years as Councilor and thought it was time for new faces on the Committee but they invited me to become treasurer and I accepted.

TB: And you continued to be treasurer for six years.

PB: Was it as long as that?

TB: I think it was.

PB: I can remember at the Washington meeting having to go to the bank to draw out a large sum of money in order to pay the speakers' expenses. Why we had to do it in that way I don't know and I was concerned at having to travel across Washington in a taxi with such a large amount of cash. Perhaps I should have had an escort! I made the payments from my room in the hotel. I think it was the Sheraton, wasn't it?

TB: Yes, it was at the Sheraton.

PB: Max Fink and I were invited by the Program Committee to organize a Symposium at the Washington meeting.

TB: What was the symposium on?

PB: The topic was "Anticholinergic Drugs".

TB: Yes.

PB: I still had an interest in that area at the time.

TB: Would you like to say something about your symposium?

PB: I think it was successful. It was certainly well attended; we invited a number of distinguished speakers, including Wikler, Votava, Herz, Longo, Domino and Jacobsen.

TB: In those years there was still interest in publishing the proceedings of meetings.

PB: I had been involved in editing the proceedings of a number of CINP meetings. I had formed a good relationship with the Elsevier Publishing Company who had a series of books, called *Progress in Brain Research*, which later became a journal. They proposed to Fink and I that our proceeding should be one of these volumes.

TB: I think you were involved in editing the proceedings of the 1st, 3rd, 4th and 5th congresses.

PB: Yes, but with different collaborators each time. I should have stopped but I enjoyed doing it.

TB: You co-edited the Washington proceedings with Brill, Cole, Deniker and Hippius.

PB: That's right and that was quite a big volume, wasn't it?

TB: Yes.

PB: They were getting too big, I think.

TB: Yes.

PB: Well, I have enjoyed all the CINP meetings I have attended.

TB: By the time of the Washington congress in 1966 you were also involved with Mimmo Costa editing a journal in the field.

PB: In the early 1960s, at a meeting in Milan on "Adrenergic Mechanisms" held at the Mario Negri Institute, Costa asked me if I would be interested in co-editing a journal with him. Before that, Elsevier, who had published all the CINP Proceedings up to then, told me that they would be willing to publish a CINP Journal, taking all responsibility, including financial. This would have meant publishing the proceedings of meetings in the journal rather than as books which were getting rather large. However, when I put the proposal to the CINP Executive Committee, it was rejected. This made me more sympathetic to Costa's approach. It is interesting that the CINP did later start a journal and I think it has proved successful.

TB: What was the name of Costa's journal?

PB: It was the *International Journal of Neuropharmacology*, which had been founded a few years earlier by Radouco-Thomas and Brodie. I knew about it as Radouco-Thomas had discussed the proposal to found a journal with me. I was already a member of the Editorial Board. Later on Costa and I thought it would be better to simplify the title so we changed it to *Neuropharmacology* which it still is.

TB: And you have been editor of that journal until . . . ?

PB: Only until 1993.

TB: About 10 years ago.

PB: Yes, I retired from my university post in 1986 and I thought editing was something I could do in retirement. Also, Costa wanted to give up at that time, so for a while I was sole editor. Costa and I had hoped to appoint our successors as editors but that was not to be. The journal was published by Pergamon Press which was owned and run by Robert Maxwell with whom I always got on well. He stated he would never sell Pergamon Press as it was one of his earliest ventures. However, when he ran into financial difficulties shortly before his death, he did sell and the new publisher wanted to appoint his own choice of editors. So I resigned. I think it was time, although I enjoyed doing it.

TB: So you kept the journal but gave up your CINP activities by the 1970s.

PB: That is correct. I was attending too many meetings and that is why I dropped out of the CINP. I used to enjoy the meetings, but I had to think about where to present my work, particularly as I was working on single cells. I was also getting involved with the British Association for Psychopharmacology and the International Union of Pharmacology.

TB: When was the British Association for Psychopharmacology founded?

PB: In the early 1970s.

TB: Aren't you one of the founders?

PB: Yes I was, but it was a difficult birth.

TB: Why?

PB: Some of us in the UK had been discussing the possibility of establishing a British psychopharmacology group along the lines of the ACNP. People such as Roger Brimblecombe, Hannah Steinberg and others were encouraging me but I had too many commitments elsewhere. Then a letter appeared in the *Lancet* which proposed much the same thing except that it would include only people who were doing clinical work. I had no choice but to get involved. There was a meeting at the Royal College of Medicine in London where there was a somewhat heated discussion. Eventually it was accepted there were people in biochemistry, psychology and pharmacology who were making a significant contribution to psychopharmacology. Our opponents seemed to think that psychopharmacology should be purely clinical. The most difficult person was Max Hamilton, Professor of Psychiatry at Leeds. He and I had a big bust-up during the

CINP meeting in Paris in 1974. But eventually we won the day and the BAP was founded along the lines of the CINP with an equal balance between clinical and non-clinical members and alternating chairmanships.

TB: So the difficulties were resolved and the Association was founded.

PB: Yes.

TB: And some years later, you became President.

PB: Hamilton, of course, became the first President. That was inevitable. Then he was followed by Coppen, although it should have been a scientist, and I became President in 1978.

TB: Could we shift back to your research after the 1950s?

PB: As I have already indicated, I was becoming less interested in behavior and more interested in what was happening at the single cell level in the brain. I felt that I could leave behavioral studies to other people. So, I recruited a psychologist, Ian Stolerman to my department and he did psychopharmacological experiments with animals.

TB: When did you do your work on opioid receptors? Wasn't it in the late1970s?

PB: No, it was earlier than that. I had another sabbatical when I was offered a one-year Fellowship at the Center for Advanced Studies in the Behavioral Sciences which was located on the campus of Stanford Universty in California.

TB: When was that?

PB: It was in1967. It may seem strange, since at that time I was relinquishing some of my interests in behavioral studies. Still, it seemed to be an opportunity not to be missed.

TB: And what did you do in Stanford?

PB: It was a "Think Tank," where people went mainly to think and write. There were no laboratory facilities, but I could probably have arranged to work in the Department of Pharmacology at Stanford Medical Centre as I knew a number of people there, including the Killams. I decided to spend my time writing, which was what most Fellows at the Centre were doing. And, of course I received many invitations to visit other laboratories and give talks. I had been asked to write a chapter on the phenothiazines for a book which I think was the *Annual Review of Pharmacology*. I spent some time on that as I decided to make it as comprehensive as possible; I covered the history, chemistry, pharmacology and clinical uses. I was told later that my chapter has been useful for teaching! I also wrote another chapter for a book whilst I was at Stanford, and I started planning a book of my own.

TB: After your return to Birmingham from Stanford I suppose you were mainly involved with research.

PB: I had hoped to be, but again it was a difficult time. Having left my department in the hands of my colleague Brian Ansell for a year, with the MRC Unit being looked after by John Wolstencroft, there were many administrative matters to deal with. There was also the journal which a friend and colleague, Ted Marley at the Maudsley Hospital in London, took charge of during my absence. I was lucky to have such reliable people stand in for me, but it took time to pick up the threads. In addition, I had heard whilst I was still at Stanford that the teaching of pharmacology to medical students in Birmingham had virtually collapsed and the students were complaining. I won't go into the reasons for this but after consulting my colleagues I went to see the Dean of the Medical School and offered to put on a course in pharmacology for the preclinical medical students. My proposals were accepted and we became involved in establishing the course, bringing in people from other departments where necessary, including clinicians. I had done a limited amount of teaching from the time I received my PhD, but I had felt for some time that we should be doing more. There were also political and financial considerations. I found myself on many committees, both university and NHS, some of which had no relevance to my own subject, but as a senior academic it was considered a duty.

At the time, I was the only non-medical head of a department in the Faculty of Medicine which meant I was frequently asked to serve on NHS consultant appointment committees. They were obliged to have a university representative and I was told they preferred to have someone non-medical who would "have no axe to grind!"

TB: How much interaction did you have with the drug industry?

PB: I did some consulting but not very much. I did not find it very interesting although I made some good friends in industry.

TB: Was there any particular drug that you had been involved in consultation?

PB: No, the work was more general. I would be asked to look at particular types of research and advise whether it should continue or stop. I was attending a meeting in Basel on one occasion and received a call from Hugo Bein who was head of research at Ciba-Geigy, and also a friend. Over lunch he invited me to be a consultant at the firm and after discussing my role, I accepted. Unfortunately, before my first visit, Bein had left and new people had taken over with completely different ideas so I did not continue for very long. I also consulted from time to time with UK firms such as ICI, Wellcome and Glaxo, and supervised research workers in industry who were allowed to work for a higher degree. That was quite rewarding.

I've always had good relations with the pharmaceutical industry and was happy to advise them from time to time on appointments.

TB: You trained many people. Would you like to mention the names of a few?

PB: Well, I have already mentioned Brian Key and Jim Hance, who eventually went to California. Brian remained in Birmingham and was a Senior Lecturer when I retired. There was Tony Nicholson, who was medically qualified and finished his PhD whilst working at the Institute of Aviation Medicine at Farnborough. During my stay in Stanford he visited me, accompanied by a senior RAF psychiatrist. I acted as their guide and accompanied them on a visit to NASA where I was allowed to try landing a 747 on the simulator! Then there was Malcolm Roberts, who went to Edinburgh to work with John Smythies and then moved to the Physiology Department in Cardiff. There was also Gill Samuels, who did research on prostaglandins for her PhD. She went into industry, ending up at Pfizer, where she became a vice-president for research and involved in the development of Viagra. Ian Phillips went to Ohio University where I visited him; he is now head of a department at the University of Orlando, Florida. Another was Andy Dray who worked on opioid receptors. Peter Keane was offered a Royal Society Fellowship to work in Lyon and stayed in France with Synthélabo. There were a number of others who went mainly into the pharmaceutical industry as academic jobs were getting hard to find.

TB: Could you tell us about your work with opioid receptors?

PB: It came about from a conversation with Hans Kosterlitz from Aberdeen. He admired our work but asked why we had not investigated morphine. I said that we thought morphine was not suitable for iontophoresis, but I was wrong and when we tried it morphine produced striking effects which we were able to antagonize with naloxone applied iontophoretically. Then came the discovery of enkephalins from the Aberdeen group which aroused world-wide interest and we received one of the first samples to test.

TB: So, the research was focused on classifying opioid receptors.

PB: Yes.

TB: Didn't you also do some research with serotonin receptors?

PB: We worked quite a lot on serotonin receptors.

TB: What did you do?

PB: We examined the distribution of neurons that responded to the application of serotonin and its agonists and antagonists.

TB: Weren't you doing also some research with anesthetics?

PB: We were involved in looking at some new anesthetic drugs of the Fentanyl type. They were rather strange drugs and we did not get very far with the investigations which were supported by a grant from a government department. Those drugs are extremely potent and some are now used clinically. One of them was interesting because it blocked respiration without affecting consciousness, yet respiration started again voluntarily.

TB: Any other research you did that you would like to mention?

PB: None that I can recall at the moment.

TB: It seems that by the 1980s you shifted almost completely to receptor research, right?

PB: Yes, and that continued until I retired.

TB: When did you retire?

PB: In 1986.

TB: Didn't you publish a book around that time?

PB: Yes, it was the book I had started planning when I was at Stanford twenty years earlier but when I returned to Birmingham there was little time to finish it until after I retired.

TB: So that was in 1986?

PB: It was published in 1987.

TB: Can you tell us something about the book?

PB: It was called *Introduction to Neuropharmacology*. In my teaching activities, which had developed significantly and included not only medical students, but also dental students, anesthetists working for their primary exams and postgraduate toxicology students, I felt there was need for a basic text. That is what the book was intended to be, an introductory text which could also be read by the intelligent layman. Unfortunately, I was let down by my publishers. The original publishers I approached were well known for publishing medical books and very keen to have my book after consulting their advisors and staff. Sadly, they were taken over by a much larger organization, which although major publishers of science books, were not very interested although they promised to fulfill the contract. I cannot complain about the production and I was pleased with the result, but I do not think the book received adequate publicity. Not many people had seen the book or an advertisement for it. I do not think many copies were sent for review although I received some letters of congratulation including one from a professor of anesthesiology and another from a psychiatrist, both of whom said it would be useful in teaching.

TB: It sold quite well. I read somewhere it sold about 9,000 copies?

PB: I am not sure it was as many as that.

TB: If it was, that was not bad.

PB: I had expected more but it certainly wasn't a bestseller! There was probably too much competition as everybody feels motivated to write a book these days.

TB: It was probably one of the first introductory books on neuropharmacology.

PB: I think it was.

TB: Do you think it could still be used?

PB: I would like to hope so. Some parts, in fact most, are still valid but it would have to be brought up to date and new sections added. I wouldn't want to do that now.

TB: Was it translated into any other languages?

PB: I don't think so. As I said, the new publishers weren't terribly interested. They fulfilled the basic contract and that was it.

TB What did you do after the book?

PB: I was still editing the journal, *Neuropharmacology*, and when Costa resigned I was sole Chief Editor. There was quite a lot to do as I did not have any secretarial help. Previously, I had two secretaries and an editorial assistant plus various other people to help me. Then I was asked to join a newly formed International Committee on the Classification of Drug Receptors, under the auspices of the International Union of Pharmacologists. This came about because in 1984, two years before I retired, we had a meeting of the British Pharmacological Society in Birmingham and the day before the main meeting started, I organized a Symposium on Serotonin Receptors, inviting everyone who had worked on serotonin, including its discoverers, Rapport and Erspamer, neither of whom unfortunately was able to attend. We had an excellent meeting and I arranged for the proceedings to be published as a supplement to *Neuropharmacology*. During the discussions, it was suggested that a small group might meet regularly to discuss receptor subtypes, including not only 5-HT but dopamine and opioid receptors.

Subsequently, at the International Pharmacology Congress in Sydney in 1987, which I was unable to attend as I was in hospital, a proposal was made to set up an international committee on Drug Receptor Classification and I was proposed as one of the UK delegates. The committee was small at first and not very active. The chairman was not keen to continue and eventually Paul Vanhoutte took over. After that the committee expanded rapidly and became much more active, producing a series of reports. I was asked to lead a working party on the classification of opioid receptors. It took a long time and involved many people, and at one time, for health reasons, I was obliged to hand it over to someone else. Eventually, we published a comprehensive report which I think was well received. At one time the Committee was looking for somewhere to publish its reports when I was the BPS representative on the editorial board of *Pharmacological Reviews*. I managed to persuade them to take on the task, so that is where our report on opioid receptors was published.

TB: This was in the early 1990's?

PB: Yes.

TB: Who were the people on the committee? Was Solomon Snyder on it?

PB: No, he wasn't. There was Trendelenburg who worked on adrenaline.

TB: Was Sol Langer on it?

PB: Yes, he was. I used to meet him with his wife. He was moving from South America to Paris to be head of pharmacology at a drug company.

TB: Later on he moved from France to Israel. Anyone else on that Committee you remember?

PB: There was Colin Dollery from London, Eric Barnard from Cambridge who did a lot of work isolating receptors and their constituent proteins, Pat Humphrey from Glaxo, Tom Bonner, Godfraind, Dhawan from Lucknow and Rudolfo Paoletti. These are the people I remember best but there were many others and the membership of the committee changed frequently.

TB: Could you tell us something about your activities on international organizations. We already talked about the CINP. Haven't you been involved with WHO?

PB: It must have been in the early 1960s, that I was invited by the World Health Organisation to join a Working Group on the Major Tranquillisers. When I arrived in Geneva I was met by the Deputy Director of WHO, a Dr Medvedev who took me to his apartment and plied me with vodka, after which he asked me to be the Rapporteur of the meeting. I was reluctant to accept as I had done nothing like it before but could see no way out. In the event all was well and we had a very successful meeting. I received a lot of help from the other members, including John Smythies. The only problem was that I spent every evening after dinner going through the typed transcripts of the previous day's discussions. Lehmann was the Chairman and the only other members I can remember well were Deniker and Freyhan. There was also a man named Lapin, a psychologist from Leningrad, who was very friendly and interested in my work but I never had time to talk to him as I was so busy preparing the report. I don't think Michael Shepherd was there, as I knew him well and would have remembered him. Eventually, our report was published by WHO with the recommendation that the term "Neuroleptic" should be used world-wide and I think it has been. I was on another WHO committee which was concerned with amphetamine derivatives which were being made illegally and were popular with drug users.

TB: Could you name one?

PB: One of them was ecstasy. Do you know it?

TB: Yes.

TB: Was this in the 1950's?

PB: I think it was 1958 but it could have been later.

TB: Who was director of the mental health unit at the time?

PB: I don't know. A Dr Chruschiel, if that is the correct name, was working with us on one of the committees, but I don't remember who the director of the unit was. It seemed that staff at WHO changed frequently, but I remember Nakajima who eventually became the Director. I first knew Nakajima when he was working with Thuillier in the 1950s in Paris. What happened to Thuillier?

TB: He's still alive and writes books.

PB: I think he wrote a book on the history of psychopharmacology but I have not seen it.

TB: I think that at a certain point of time he was involved with the drug industry.

PB: He visited Birmingham on one occasion and gave a talk and showed a film of his circling mice. He had this compound which, if injected into mice, caused continuous circling. I asked him a number of times if he had had it analyzed chemically and if it was optically active but I never knew what happened. It was like Monnier's sleep-substance in that respect. He was a very generous man and looked after me extremely well when I visited Paris to meet Delay. Thuillier was a gourmet and took me to some excellent restaurants in Paris.

TB: He was certainly a very talented person: a writer, a pharmacologist, a psychiatrist.

PB: Yes.

TB: Weren't you also on a WHO committee on psychotomimetics?

PB: I don't remember, but I served on a British Government Committee on hallucinogenic drugs. The Chairman was Bill Paton who was Professor of Pharmacology at Oxford and both Ted Marley and I contributed to the report but what happened to it I never knew. As with so many things connected with government, there was never any feedback.

TB: In the course of your career you have been involved, in addition to research, in all kinds of other activities.

PB: Yes, writing, teaching, editing, administration and even broadcasting, both live television and radio.

TB: You had to take care of people in a rather large department.

PB: It was not that large; but we had many students. Quite a lot of the teaching involved lectures, tutorials and practical classes and there were postgraduate students to supervise.

TB: We already talked about your book that was published after you retired. Was that your last publication?

PB: My last paper was "Classification of Opioid Receptors" which was the report of the working party I had originally led for the IUPHAR Committee on Receptor Nomenclature and Drug Classification. As I was unable to continue due to ill health, the final version was written by M. Hamon who was a good friend. It was published in *Pharmacological Reviews* in 1996. The other thing that happened was that I was awarded the Pythagoras Prize from the University of Cattanzaro in southern Italy, which you have probably never heard of.

TB: I read about that Prize in Mimmo Costa's autobiography.

PB: I am afraid that at first I did not take it very seriously but then I was at a meeting in London and talking to Pepeu from Florence. . . .

TB: Is he a pharmacologist who did a lot of work with cholinergics?

PB: That is right. Anyway, he said I ought to go, as did Costa who had received the prize earlier. It was a long journey but I enjoyed my visit and learned more about Pythagoras who lived in that area of Italy for some years with a group of students. He was, of course, a philosopher as well as a mathematician.

TB: What would you think was your most important contribution to neuropharmacology?

PB: It is difficult to think of any one thing. I like to think that we made a number of contributions, perhaps only minor ones, in many areas.

TB: So you think they are equally important?

PB: I would like to think that the introduction of the microiontophoresis technique for the study of single neurons in the brain is one, and. perhaps our work with opioid receptors and their classification is another.

TB: What about your early contributions about the structures involved in the mode of action of psychotropic drugs?

PB: Yes. I think I made a contribution there, small though it was.

TB: Don't you think that work should have been followed up?

PB: I had hoped it would be. It would have been nice if somebody had done that and I thought one of my students might do so, but people like to do their own thing, and why not?

TB: Has research in neuropsychopharmacology in the past decades moved in the direction you would have liked to see?

PB: I'm not one of those people who like to foresee what is going to happen or has plans for far ahead. I did what I thought was important at the time and what I was interested in. The main thing, I think, is to enjoy what you do.

TB: And you did enjoy it?

PB: Yes, I did. Also, I think I got on well with the people I worked with; but I don't know what they thought! When I retired, a group of my former postgraduate students entertained my wife and myself to dinner at the RAF Club in London and I shall never forget the student who, when I suggested that he should publish his latest research under his name alone, said "No," he wanted my name on his paper in recognition of the help I had given him. I also valued my stay in Pisa, not just for the facilities and the opportunity to learn microelectrode work, but also because of my contact with Moruzzi.

TB: Could you tell us something about Moruzzi?

PB: Moruzzi was a very nice quiet man. He did not shout as so many Italians do when they get excited but was very charming, and was an excellent physiologist. There was an unusual atmosphere in his institute which is difficult to describe. The Italian system involved people moving from one center to another for promotion, Rome being the pinnacle. But I don't think Moruzzi wanted to move from Pisa as it had everything he wanted and he had an international reputation. He sometimes asked me to read his papers before sending them for publication but I found there was nothing I could contribute; his English was better than mine!

TB: Did you maintain contact after you left?

PB: For a while and then, when he was retiring, they organized a symposium for him in Pisa I attended. I met some old friends like Herbert Jasper and Mary Brazier from the early days of EEG.

TB: He was also involved in research on the reticular formation.

PB: Yes.

TB: And in conditioning.

PB: I believe so.

TB: He was working in Montreal. Didn't you also have some contact with Ted Sourkes, the biochemist from Montreal who wrote a book on the *Biochemistry of Mental Disease*?

PB: Yes, I knew Ted Sourkes very well. He spent a year in Birmingham at Joel's invitation. Is he still around?

TB: Oh yes, he is retired, but has remained very active. He is editor of a journal on the history of neuroscience.

PB: That's interesting. Ted used to tell us stories about the institute in Montreal where he worked and about Ewen Cameron.

TB: But, of all the people you were involved with, it was Joel who had the most important impact on your career?

PB: Yes. He gave me my chance; he started me off in what was then a new field, relating behavior with the electrical activity of the brain and he introduced me to a lot of people, especially at the neurochemical symposium in 1954 in Oxford. It meant that my work became known quickly, perhaps too quickly. He made suggestions from time to time but otherwise left me to get on with it. It took me a little while to get used to this way of working and we had our ups and downs. I was inexperienced and I think

I resented it when I heard he was talking about my work to groups I had never heard of. However, he had a way of putting things over much better than I could have done and the support came in as a result. When he left Birmingham for Washington I felt neglected, especially as things were in a bit of a mess, but it did me good in the end and was an excellent, if traumatic, experience. Had he stayed in Birmingham, I would probably have become frustrated and moved somewhere else where the facilities I had in Birmingham would not have been available and I should have had to start again.

TB: Just one last question. Is there anything you would like to see happen in the field?

PB: There has been a trend recently to measure activity at different sites in the brain by means of blood flow. This development is both interesting and important but it would be nice to see the findings correlated with electrical activity. I had always hoped that someone would extend and improve the techniques which we developed, but so far that has not happened.

TB: On this note we conclude this interview with Professor Bradley, one of the pioneers of neuropsychopharmacology. Thank you very much, Philip for your contributions to the field and for sharing this information.

PB: I've enjoyed it. I didn't expect to, but I have.

TB: Thank you.

KEITH F. KILLAM & EVA KING KILLAM
Interviewed by Keith F. Killam & Eva K. Killam
San Juan, Puerto Rico, December 11, 1994

KK: This is Dr. Eva King Killam and I'm Keith.* We're both retired professors of pharmacology at the University of California, Davis. We have worked most of our professional lives together, and we were asked whether we would prefer someone else interview us, but we thought it would be easier if we simply talked about what we have done over the forty-odd years we have been married and working together. Eva, where did you go to undergraduate school?

EK: I went to an undergraduate Arts school, called Sarah Lawrence College, where everybody but me, majored in the Arts, and from there I went to Mount Holyoke for a Master's degree. Then I went to Yale University for a year thinking I would do a PhD in Zoology, but my father had a stroke and I went home to help until the shocking initial problem was over. I looked for a job so I wouldn't be sitting in the house all the time and went to work for a wonderful pharmacologist, who was running the Burroughs-Wellcome Laboratories near my home. He said, "If you're going back to school, you simply can't go back into zoology. You're going to have to be a pharmacologist."

KK: Was that Debier?

EK: Yes, he decided the only thing for me was to be a pharmacologist, and that's what really turned me into one, because a graduate of an Arts college doesn't usually hear about pharmacology as an option. But I was interested in the nervous system; I worked on various drugs, particularly central "muscle relaxants," when I was in graduate school. While trying to find out where muscle relaxants acted I got interested in a scientist named Horace Magoun in California who discovered areas of the brain which, when stimulated, changed reflex activity. I thought if I stimulated those brain areas and put the drug in, I could tell if it was acting on the brain or the spinal cord, depending upon which reflexes were affected. This kind of thinking introduced me to the field, so when I graduated, Dr. Magoun offered me a place as post-doc in his laboratory. He was working on the reticular mechanism for arousal and sleep. In his lab, as a pharmacologist, I worked on barbiturates and anesthetics, depressant compounds, and how they affected the brain stem and arousal mechanisms.

KK: After you worked with Debier, you worked at the Army Chemical Center for Amadeo Marazzi. Tell us about him.

---

* Keith F. Killam was born in Hollywood, Florida in 1927. He died in 1998. Eva King Killam was born in New York, New York in 1920. She died in 2006.

EK: I worked for Marazzi because I was looking for a job near home. Amadeo Marazzi was interested in brain synapses, and especially how neurotransmitters affected them. He was a very bright man. From other members of our college working with him, I learned he had a reputation for being rather difficult, which I never quite understood, because he and I got along very well. He had no patience with small talk or for people saying "I don't know what to do next, tell me what to do." Being young and brash and not knowing very much, I was willing to tell him what we ought to be doing. I was always into some project, so we didn't get into any trouble, and we remained friends all his life. I saw him at meetings and we always remained friends.

KK: Now you are in transition from then until we met. Where did we meet?

EK: In graduate school in pharmacology at the University of Illinois in Chicago. Graduate work was at the medical school, and I went to work with Dr. Klaus Unna, who was a very important member of this society. He was one of my mentors, and he had me doing work on the site of action of muscle relaxants. I was alone in the department, working by myself. It was on the strength of my thesis in that area that Magoun, who had seen my papers at American Physiological, Psychological and Pharmacology Societies, wrote me when I graduated and asked would I visit him and, perhaps, take a job. Things were different in those days. You weren't invited with fanfare and given tours in a new job. You were lucky if you were offered a job and you took it, sight unseen. But, I was a little nervous about that. So, I went to Dr. Snyder, a great neurologist at Northwestern, and said, "I'm thinking of traveling from Chicago to California. What do you think of this man I met at a meeting and who offered me a job"? He looked at me and said, "My dear, he's the only person I know who hasn't got feet of clay." So I took the job and never was sorry, because he started me on my career. He aroused my interest in drugs and how to use neurophysiological methods to localize where and how they had effects on the nervous system. I worked on stimulation, sleep and depression with a brand new compound which was just being introduced, called chlorpromazine. It was there Keith and I crossed paths, because I graduated ahead of him by one or two quarters. I had known him at the University of Illinois but he had left the State. Tell them when you got your degree and what you did.

KK: I began my training during World War II as an ASTP student. If you remember back in the dark days of World War II, these were the groups that were going on to medical school, engineering, etc. As the war progressed, I was rapidly shuttled into the infantry, being big enough to carry a Browning automatic rifle, until I was attached to the Medical Corps, became a medic and ended up running a clinical laboratory. When I came out of the army I finished my degree at Tufts University, and through some familial connections I was offered a job at Smith, Kline & French (SK&F) in Philadelphia.

SK&F, at that time, had synthetic chemistry laboratories on Wharf and 5th Street in Philadelphia, and the pharmacology was done at Temple University in the Department of Pharmacology. There were technical people like myself, who were paid by SK&F and woven into the faculty at Temple. It was during that period that SK&F became a so-called ethical pharmaceutical house; their new building was at Spring Garden Street. During the three years I was with SK&F I was steeped in classical pharmacology. They had a Fellowship within the company to commemorate the former director of research, Carr, and at the end of three years, they appointed me a Carr Fellow at the University of Illinois, where I got my training. During summers I had to go back to SK&F, and it was one of those summers that we worked on a drug called SK-525-A, which potentiated a variety of substances, mostly central nervous system drugs. It was because of that property of SKF-525-A the company was looking at chlorpromazine and eventually became, together with Rhône-Poulenc, a leader in developing CNS drugs.

Following my graduate work, I returned to the company for six months, and during that time Eva and I married and started to think about whether we should live on the east or west coast. As you know, the west coast won out. We began our work at UCLA in Ted Magoun's Brain Research Institute, and had a very productive six or seven years there before we moved to Stanford University where we spent nine years. Finally we moved to Davis, where I was founding Chair of Pharmacology in the School of Medicine, from where we just retired. With respect to the scientific interests we've had, we were very early in the game with chlorpromazine. On one of those days, Eva brought me an abstract from Joel Elkes, Philip Bradley and Jim Hance almost directly in line with what we had been doing. Can you say a few words about that?

EK: We were quite surprised to see the work in Birmingham was close to what we had been developing in our lab. So we wrote to them and they decided to send Jim Hance to visit our laboratory. That began a long and fruitful friendship, both with Jim and also with Phil Bradley and Elkes.

KK: Eva and I have been known for keeping many scientific balls in the air rather than honing into one particular area. In my thesis, I noted that when you deplete the brain of GABA, spontaneous seizures occur. It was actually the first description of that. By coincidence we found that Gene Roberts, who had first described the appearance of GABA in the nervous system, was in Pasadena at the City of Hope, in East Los Angeles. So during the time that we were at UCLA, we did some collaborative work between our laboratories. Most of our research up to that time had been on acute preparations: we induced anesthesia, administered a variety of agents and looked for a particular response.

EK: We were looking primarily for electrophysiological responses. We were among the early people who adopted a neurophysiological methodology in our department. It was a famous department; people came from all over the world to learn EEG and electrophysiology.

KK: During that time, we were also blessed with starting a family. Some of the research I had done with Eva, but I also did research with others at UCLA, for example James Olds, a psychologist, who made the observation that if you electrically stimulate a part of the chameleon brain, there would be a repetitive behavior associated with it. That part of the brain became known as the pleasure center, and we convinced Jim to do some drug studies in his lever pressing animals to get "pleasure."

EK: That was one of the great advantages of a mixed group working in a laboratory, that nowadays, with shortage of funding, you can't do. At that time, there were enough funds so it was possible for analysts, physiologists and psychologists to work together. It was Keith who introduced Jim to the idea of putting a drug into his preparation to measure how it altered lever pressing and in order to see what it would reveal about the site of action of the drug. If there had been no pharmacologists in the group, the research would have been much narrower.

KK: I'd like to reinforce something Eva referred to earlier, and that is the creativity of Magoun. He was able to amass a variety of scientists from all over the world and the United States, and have them work on a variety of projects. At lunch time, we were constantly apprising one another of what was going on and if a new idea occurred, it was implemented by the next afternoon.

EK: I think of the similarity between that and what we had at the early ACNP meetings. We were among the founders of the ACNP. As a pharmacologist when I went to the meetings of the American Psychological Association, or to Basic Science meetings, I was unable to find among the thousands of people anyone interested in drugs for mental disease, or interested in exchanging ideas. But we found that the ACNP was a place where we could talk and exchange ideas. The meetings were small with not too many people, and in those early days nobody was worrying that somebody was going to steal their ideas. Everybody came with a few slides to project or something they could show to others. It was similar to what we had at UCLA. That was a wonderful period in the history of this society.

KK: I could work with Jim Olds on the behavioral side, and with Reese Jones we could look at the way behavior was organized and how it could be manipulated by the psychotropic drugs available at the time. We used coded stimuli that could be tracked through the normal brain rhythms to see how various parts of the brain processed information. And, by interrupting behavior with drugs, we could see how the behavior de-coupled from electrical activity of the brain, and re-coupled as the effects of the drug wore off. That led us into the next aspect of our work, because it wasn't enough simply to say we saw something on the oscilloscope. So, we started to use computers for the analysis of spontaneous and evoked electrical activity. Prior to doing that we had done a lot of work with averaging techniques; I had been to MIT and worked with groups on the LINC program. The Air Force and NIH pooled money together and selected twenty-five groups around the country to establish computerized laboratories for more rapid and efficient conducting of experiments. And, as Eva mentioned, we had Jim Hance join us from Philip Bradley and Joel Elkes' laboratory in Birmingham; Jim was without a doubt a wizard with respect to the introduction of computers into science. He and I went to Boston to build one of those computers from scratch, while Eva stayed home and had our first child. The new computers also led us into programmed instruction in teaching pharmacology. Then we had a job switch. It was sparked by going on a sabbatical to Marseilles and the laboratories of Robert Naquet. Say something about our friend.

EK: Dr. Naquet is a very well known EEG specialist and also a specialist in epilepsy, who was trained by Gastaut. When we arrived at his laboratory we found he had animals that looked like little monkeys but were baboons. He obtained them through a friend in Africa. When we got there, Bobby told us that some of these baboons had seizures from flashing lights of a particular frequency, like humans. One or two percent of normal people who do not have epilepsy have seizures when exposed to a fifteen per second flashing light. These baboons had seizures when exposed to a twenty-five per second flashing light. So we started to work out a method of quantifying the seizures. When Gastaut came, he said, "there's no epilepsy in baboons," but when he saw ours he said, "Yes, it's epilepsy." We did a great deal of work with these baboons in Bobby's laboratory in Marseilles, and later we worked with them, trying to develop an understanding of the pathways involved in those seizures. Our particular interest was to find out whether we could use these baboons to test new anti-epileptic drugs. And we were able to develop a methodology to screen for and study antiepileptic drugs. Later on we worked with baboons raised in our own laboratory.

KK: This brings up the point that the trait for epileptic events was genetically determined in a strictly Mendelian pattern.

EK: While we were still interested in drugs for mental disease, the ways in which new drugs worked and what sites they worked at, we now started doing studies in parallel with anti-epileptic drugs to find out the site where they worked. We also developed methods for assessing their behavioral toxicity, a term that Joe Brady first brought up in some early conferences in Washington. When we talk about the toxicity of new drugs, we tend to talk about how much liver damage, loss of weight and so forth they cause, and say nothing about the behavioral toxicity they may have. So we developed methods to assess how an animal learns with and without being given a particular anticonvulsant drug. We used the adolescent baboon as a model of a child in school on chronic treatment with an anti-epileptic drug. When you work on animals to make inferences from it to humans you need to use matching doses in terms of effectiveness. Using our method we were able to assess the behavioral toxicity of anti-epileptic drugs and identify drugs for children who go to school which do not make them drowsy or interfere with learning.

KK: The switch in our research interest to studying anti-epileptic drugs occurred while we were at Stanford and was carried through when we moved to the University of California at Davis. The reason why we went specifically to Davis was the availability of a primate center where we could import animals from Africa. Some of the residue of the work we had been doing at UCLA and carried on while at Stanford was studying sleep mechanisms, looking at sedatives vs. major tranquilizers and minor tranquilizers and how various sleep patterns would be altered by these drugs. We were developing methodologies with respect to EEG quantification that made it possible to look more specifically at major differences between the benzodiazepine and barbiturate series.

   In addition to that, I, personally – since Eva was busy with our family – did some work for John F. Kennedy as part of his presidential science advisory committee, evaluating drug dependency as a problem in this United States. For a number of years, we spent summers at places where the problem of drug dependency was most prevalent and we became interested whether one could make predictions relevant to dependency by studying the effect of drugs on the brain. At Davis most of our research with baboons and learning, was done by Eva. We participated in a collaborative project sponsored by the DEA with Joe Brady and a group at Emory in Atlanta. We had a number of laboratories evaluating specific drugs of interest coming from the street. Each laboratory used a different methodology, and from that study we have EEG data on most benzodiazepines developed until the last five years, as well as a variety of other substances. At the same time, Brady and his group in the Chicago area, and a group at Emory were evaluating the strictly behavioral effects of these drugs. We were interested in how drugs affect the nervous system. We assumed that drug dependency is one type of learned behavior, regardless whether abnormal or normal. And that leads us to the end of our career.

EK: You might like to say something about the last switch.

KK: I have been fortunate to start working with two molecular biologists, Rhonda and Lynn Schwan; these two people are absolutely spectacular. We became very interested in the problem of why drug users were more susceptible to acquiring AIDS than people in the general population. We did not believe it was only because of needle sharing. So we developed a population of morphine-dependent animals, and then administered them a virus similar to the one that causes HIV.

EK: These were Rhesus monkeys.

KK: The most amazing finding was that the replication rate of viruses in morphine-dependent monkeys was three-fold higher than for monkeys not exposed to morphine. In addition, the rate of mutation of the virus was at least doubled and the generated mutants were AZT insensitive.

EK: These findings have important implications in terms of testing blood in blood banks, because if you have an increased rate of mutation with mutated viruses which are silent in current drug tests, lots of people can get infected.

KK: On the list of questions that they wish us to cover is the direction research is moving and research funding. It is very disturbing to both of us that many areas of research are not funded properly. Funds currently go almost completely to support molecular genetic studies. The number of grants funded for primate research, particularly in neuropsychopharmacology, is almost zero. We feel that primate research is an important bridge from preclinical to clinical studies. I sincerely believe that primate behavior and primate research in general is closer to research in humans than research in rodents despite the fact that it is easier to control the genetics of rodents. It is relevant in this context that anti-vivisectionists don't consider the rat an animal. We have been spending a considerable amount of time to marshal the efforts of the scientific community to recognize the challenge from the anti-vivisectionist groups. They claim that they are animal rights groups, but I believe to consider an animal has rights similar to a human is just an affront.

EK: We think the work we do and the kind of work we've always done has been very important to a rapidly growing field of medicine, and if animal research is cut from the curriculum of medical and veterinary students, we're going to have people who are unable to do anything but work with pencil and paper. And if you feed garbage into a computer it will be garbage that comes out of it.

KK: We have been very fortunate in our careers that we have worked with groups which, as Eva pointed out, have come from multiple directions; practicing psychiatrists could come and work in our laboratories and we could be educated by them concerning their problems and needs as well as the shortcomings of our models. We have been able to provide solid data regarding drug toxicity. With respect to the future, we believe that it looks dim, and not because we don't have bright students or bright people, but because of the problem of maintaining funding at levels where we can have an interplay between anatomists, molecular biologists, physiologists and psychologists. Is there anything else you'd like to add?

EK: No, except we didn't say very much about the history of ACNP, but other people will do that. We were among the people who joined the organization early and we strongly believe, despite the fact that we live on the other side of the continent, that the rule about coming to every meeting is right.

KK: We feel proud our colleagues elected each of us to be President of the organization. The amazing thing we've seen is the ability of people to pull together, work and accomplish things without any major reward other than that it was done for the College. That kind of spirit still exists in spite of expectations that external pressures on our field and on the college are more likely to increase than decrease. I wish we had twenty more years to help you all.

VINCENZO G. LONGO

Interviewed by Leonard Cook
San Juan, Puerto Rico, December 10, 1996

LC: We are at the annual meeting of the American College of Neuro-psychopharmacology in 1996. I am Leonard Cook and I will be interviewing a long time friend and associate, Professor Vincenzo Longo* from Rome. I have known him for perhaps thirty years.

VL: Exactly, I want to remind you when we met.

LC: I know: it was in Brussels.

VL: Yes.

LC: Dr Longo has played a very key and critical role in the evolution of modern CNS drugs over the past thirty-five years. He was one of the very few people, and certainly one of the early people, to integrate behavioral pharmacology – what we called neuropharmacology – with the recording of electrical activities of the brain. I'm going to ask Dr. Longo a few personal questions. Would you like to tell us where you were born and where you went to school?

VL: I was born in south Italy in Calabria. But, very soon I transferred to Rome where I completed my studies. I graduated in medicine in 1948. In my doctoral thesis, with the guidance of Professor Daniel Bovet, I discussed the effects of curare-like agents.

LC: So you were associated with Professor Bovet even in medical school?

VL: Even in medical school. One year later, in 1949, I joined the staff of the laboratory of therapeutic chemistry in the Istituto Superiore de Sanità, and stayed there all my life.

LC: Were you working with Professor Bovet when he did the pivotal work that led to his Nobel Prize?

VL: Well, the work for which he got the Nobel Prize was done in Paris before he came to Rome. It was research on sulfamides and antihistamines, and in general on structure-activity relationships. But Bovet, as you probably remember, was an exceptional researcher with what we call a "flare" for new lines of research.

LC: So, he had that knack.

VL: Yes, definitely. One time he called me and said we must move into new areas of research, and he used the word, "neuropharmacology," that sounded strange to me at the time. It meant pharmacology of the nervous system. We already had some signs that the central nervous system could be influenced by drugs in the late 1940s and early1950s. Before

---

* Vincenzo G. Longo was born in Reggio, Calabria, Italy in 1925.

that we had only a few drugs, like the barbiturates and bromides that could influence the central nervous system.

LC: So the new agents served as a very important tool.

VL: As tools and hints. For instance, in the late 1940s Parsidol (ethopropazine) and Parpanit (caramiphen) proved useful for tremors and Parkinsonian symptoms. Then it was discovered by chance that diphenhydramine, an antihistamine agent, has hypnotic properties. Later on, the first investigations started with chlorpromazine.

LC: Yes, of course.

VL: So, one day Bovet called me and said, "You must start searching for new laboratory methods which would help discover drugs acting on the central nervous system."

LC: What kind of methods did you think he meant?

VL: The first method we introduced in the laboratory was a test for antiparkinson drugs. We used tremor induced by nicotine in animals. It is suitable for studying drug effects because it is exactly the same as the tremor of Parkinsonian patients. As a matter of fact, we published an article on nicotine-induced tremor in the early 1950s in the *Journal of Pharmacology*. Later on, while searching for methods to study CNS drugs, I got interested in recording cerebral electrical activity of laboratory animals.

LC: I see.

VL: And I continued to do research in this field for a very long time. We also published our findings on the effect of chlorpromazine on the EEG of rabbits in the *Journal of Pharmacology*. In 1956 Bovet and I presented a paper in Brussels at the International Congress of Physiology, on the reticular formation, the meeting where we first met. Do you remember that magnificent dinner at the Grande Palace?

LC: I remember. You were one of the very early investigators who established criteria for the effects of drugs on EEG patterns.

VL: You might remember also that, in 1962, I published an Atlas of the effects of drugs on the EEG in the rabbit.

LC: At that time, you were alone working with that methodology. There weren't many colleagues around to discuss your findings.

VL: Very few people were interested in those days in the EEG effect of drugs

LC: Right.

VL: But I remember Bradley in England was interested in it. And Domino, here in the States, but very few others. The book was a good success; it was divided into chapters on convulsants and anticonvulsants, tranquilizers, opioids, adrenergic, cholinergic and anticholinergic drugs. I studied the effect of anticholinergic drugs for long time. As a matter of fact, I was promoted to become a member of a Cholinergic Club in Italy.

LC: A club?

VL: Yes, and in this club all the people interested in anticholinergic drugs gathered; I remember for instance that Pepeu was there.

LC: Of course. But he was very young at the time.

VL: He was. And when I visited Abe Wikler in Lexington he encouraged me to write an article about the effects of cholinergic drugs on the central nervous system. He liked it very much and later it was published in *Pharmacological Reviews*.

LC: Did you have any other interaction with Abe Wikler?

VL: I was interacting with him quite extensively on the effect of opioids on the EEG.

LC: And you were among the first to recognize the distinctive effect of neuroleptics, called tranquilizers at the time, on the EEG.

VL: Yes, we had our first report in that area of research published in 1954 in the *Journal of Pharmacology*.

LC: How did you end up at the Istituto Superiore di Sanità? Because of Bovet?

VL: Yes, because of Bovet.

LC: Besides running your laboratory, did you have any other tasks at the institute?

VL: Well, the institute is a mixture of your Food and Drug Administration and National Heart Institute.

   This is an advantage from one point of view and a disadvantage from another, because in addition to research, you have administrative duties. But let me tell you about another area of my research interests. At a certain point I became interested in the behavioral sciences and extended my research to study behavior. In the late 1960s and early 1970s people were interested in spontaneous and conditioned behavior and I became involved in studying the relationship between behavioral and EEG changes.

LC: The name of your collaborator at the time escapes me. He did the behavioral aspect of the studies in your laboratory.

VL: I had many collaborators. There was Scotti and Lipparini, but it was McGaugh's visit to the laboratory that had a great impact on moving our research into behavioral studies; he was interested in conditioned behavior.

LC: Yes.

VL: We published several papers with him. And even after he transferred to Irvine, California, we continued our collaboration.

LC: Your purpose in doing this was essentially descriptive; describing the effects of drugs on behavior and to find out how the behavioral effects correlated with the EEG changes.

VL: I was also interested in behavior; in 1972 I published a book entitled *Neuropharmacology and Behavior*. It dealt more with behavior than EEG. At that time I was visiting professor at Loyola in Chicago, working with Nicky Karczmar. Then, when neurotoxins like 5-hydroxydopamine became fashionable I switched to another area of research.

LC: How did you get to Chicago?

VL: When I was in Brussels in 1956, I met you and Dr. Unna.

LC: Yes, Dr. Unna.

VL: And Unna offered me a Smith, Kline & French Foundation fellowship to work in Chicago at the University Clinic. And there I did some work with Bill Martin. I also worked with Unna on the Renshaw cells.

LC: So at that time, Unna and Pfeiffer were around?

VL: Pfeiffer had already left for Atlanta. There was Unna, Cedric Smith, Bill Martin.

LC: Keith Killam had already left and came to work with me. What do you think was the most influential thing that happened to you in Chicago?

VL: My work in Chicago was strongly influenced by the personality of Unna; he came to see us every day to discuss the results of our experiments. But I was always under the influence of Bovet throughout my entire career. When I returned from Chicago to Rome, I continued to work on 6-hydroxydopamine. But, as you probably remember, in the early 1970s, there was an upsurge of interest in receptors. It was very difficult for neuro-pharmologists to keep up with the pace things were moving. I stayed with the dopamine receptor; and did a lot of work using biochemical methods that I added to my armamentarium. I published my findings in the early 1980s in the *Annual Review of Neurobiology*. It was a review paper on the effects of drugs on the various dopamine receptors. After that time, about ten years ago, I became head of the Laboratory of Pharmacology at the Institute and got more and more involved in tasks related to public health.

LC: They wanted to take advantage of your vast experience.

VL: Not of my experience in neuropharmacology, I must say.

LC: After you went back to Rome, if I recall, you started to go to the University of Sardinia.

VL: Yes, I was a professor in Sassari for two or three years. But, later on, it was forbidden for people working for the State to have other activities. So I had a choice, and I picked of course the Istituto. But by that time Bovet had already left. This was in 1968. He left for Sardinia and I stayed in the Institute.

LC: I remember going with you to Sardinia.

VL: Yes, of course, for a meeting at the University of Sassari.

LC: Very good memory. You have lived through and been involved in the evolution of modern neuropsychopharmacology by doing research in physiology and biochemistry. What do you think you have done that has had an impact on the development of the field? Don't be modest.

VL: I am not modest. I believe my EEG investigations contributed to knowledge on the effect of drugs in the central nervous system. I started by looking for the action of drugs on the reticular formation of the brain and formulated hypotheses that drugs have their central effect by acting on it. I remember that in 1967 I was invited to Puerto Rico, on the occasion of the tenth anniversary of the American College of Neuropsychopharmacology, and presented data on the effect of drugs on the central nervous system. My presentation shocked the audience because I said I was hesitant in accepting any longer that all CNS drugs act on the reticular formation.

I said my behavior was like Saturn's; I was eating my son, namely my theory the central effect of drugs was dependent on the reticular formation.

LC: The effect of drugs on the reticular formation wasn't the center of everything.

VL: Definitely not. I cast doubt on it.

LC: What do you think have been some of the critical things that happened during the past forty years in our field? We all see history from a different mountain top; from a different perspective.

VL: I hate to admit it, but I think the main contributions came from people who discovered new neurotransmitters, other than the ones I worked with.

LC: You hate to admit it?

VL: I hate to admit it because I had no means of discovering them, although I had hints of their presence; you couldn't explain everything with acetylcholine, noradrenaline, serotonin and dopamine. You had the feeling there was something else.

LC: If you were graduating now, having much more information than we had then and a broader perspective how would you start your career now?

VL: Molecular biology.

LC: Do you think that molecular biology is going to stand on its own?

VL: I think so. A couple of years ago I wouldn't have, but now I think molecular biology can go ahead

LC: You have been in a position at the Institute where you were able to learn about the new drugs entering the market, and even those submitted for review that didn't enter the market. With all that knowledge, where do you think we will be in the next 25 years; what kind of drugs are we going to have and what will they do?

VL: This field is very unpredictable, but I think that all the big pharmaceutical companies are oriented towards real innovation on one side, and having cheap generic drugs on the other side. Real innovation should give us novel drugs in every field. Every time I read the scientific journals, I see some very important contributions.

LC: One of the things that has always fascinated me is the fact that you and I have gone through an era of three to four decades working with drugs that selectively suppress behavior, selectively depress various electro-physiological phenomena. What I've been interested is the concept that drugs could selectively enhance cognitive effects. I saw enormous potential in developing such drugs. What is your perspective about drugs that enhance cognition and other functions?

VL: This is a very important trend in neuropharmacological research; enhancing instead of inhibiting. The latest drug introduced in the therapy of diabetes enhances the production of insulin. I don't remember the name of the drug, but this is something which struck me. There is already a tendency to enhance the functions of organs instead of inhibiting them. We have to go ahead along this line. Your latest research was dealing with drugs enhancing the production of acetylcholine.

LC: The name of the drug is phenoperidine, and I personally am very excited about its future. In your opinion, has the electrical activity of the brain continued to play an important role in research, or has its importance diminished in the last decade?

VL: Definitely diminished. We hoped for a lot in passing from gross recording with big electrodes to recording single cell activity, but even that didn't give us the expected results, because when you record the activity of one cell, you don't record the activity of nearby cells.

LC: Exactly.

VL: That's not very useful from the point of view of research.

LC: What other issues do you feel should be discussed? Is there anything you feel I haven't brought up that is important in your career?

VL: Well, now, I speak more as an administrator than a researcher. In the last years, since I retired from the Institute, I got interested in collaborative research between academia and industry. You have had it in America for some time, but in Italy this kind of collaboration was practically non-existent. So, in the last three years, I have been helping to develop such collaborations. We can see the first results of my efforts; a national program with funds from the Ministry of Research to encourage collaboration between industry and academia. This is important because as you know very well, even if industry has the money and the means, very often the ideas come from academia. Without such an, osmosis, research on drugs is hindered.

LC: One of the phenomena that I've observed in the last decade in industry– and I spent my whole career in industry – is that most big pharmaceutical operations and drug companies, have gone to focusing whereas years ago we had fifteen to twenty projects, and a lot of different programs. What happened was things evolved and we got results unexpectedly because we had a variety of studies. The industry is now focusing on one or two, or at the most three areas of research, and from my perspective this is going to limit discovery. I would be interested to hear your point of view. What do you think?

VL: I think you must have several lines, because this is a kind of evoked serendipity.

LC: Evoked serendipity?

VL: Evoked serendipity. You increase your chances of serendipity if you have fifteen projects instead of three. And serendipity, as we all know, plays an important role in the advancement of research.

LC: You have had many young people come through your laboratory. What are your views about training; how would you train young people today? Training in classical pharmacology and in vivo pharmacology is becoming increasingly neglected with the enormous shift to molecular biology. Do you feel that is okay? Or do you feel it should move to a more balanced type of training?

VL: I'm definitely for unbalanced training.

LC: Unbalanced?

VL: Yes, but this applies only to Italy. I'm not talking about any other country. Before retiring from the Institute I oriented some people towards pre-clinical pharmacology and others to molecular biology.

And there was one person interested in the relationship between data obtained in the laboratory and in man.

LC: Who were some of the important people that affected your career besides Bovet?

VL: I was strongly influenced by some people who visited our laboratory. I spoke already of Jim McGaugh, and I was also influenced by Maurice Rappaport. These were two people who influenced me. Of the Italians, Erspamer was a person I admired. Incidentally, he is still active in the field.

LC: Is he really?

VL: Yes, he is over eighty.

LC: Tell me something about your responsibilities at the Institute regarding matters that would be equivalent to activities of our Food and Drug Administration.

VL: In 1985 I practically left active research for administrative and organizing responsibilities. I was dealing mainly with drug approvals. Another important area I dealt with when I had the responsibility for the entire Institute was reimbursement by Social Security. For about one year, I was the head of the Institute.

LC: What is the main difference between processing of drugs for approval in Italy and the United States?

VL: Not many. The only differences I saw when I visited the Food and Drug Administration was the number of people doing the work. There are about ten to fifteen times more people involved here than in Italy.

LC: What are you doing now?

VL: Working for the Ministry of Research, trying to get together industry research people and university research people as much as possible. I'm a consultant.

LC: How about funding available for research today in Italy?

VL: Funds are available, not much, but they are available. The problem is that now we no longer have any Italian pharmaceutical firms. They were all bought by multinationals: Farmitalia Carlo Erba for instance, was bought by Pharmacia which has now merged with Upjohn.

LC: What about Milano?

VL: It was bought by Richardson and Merrell. The laboratory was dismantled; the main laboratory is now in France.

LC: What about employment possibilities for young scientists today in Italy?

VL: Our program covers this as well. The state is obliged to invest ten percent of the funds in the training of new people and the pharmaceutical companies must sign an agreement that they will employ the people trained.

LC: Where are the main training grounds for young scientists today?

VL: At the big universities. Milano, Rome, Naples, Bari, but the bulk are trained in Milano.

LC: And, the training is now focused on molecular biology?

VL: Yes.

LC: So, tell me what else is of interest to you?

VL: From which point of view? Hobbies?

LC: Yes, tell me about your hobbies.

VL: One of my hobbies is travel. I like to travel. Another of my hobbies is the theater. Everywhere I go, I go to the theater because I find that very stimulating. And my third hobby is playing bridge.

LC: In terms of CNS drugs, do you feel that research in the field is focused properly? Or do you think that we are missing certain opportunities?

VL: I think the CNS field is fertile enough; we have some new antipsychotics and some new antianxiety drugs.

LC: I feel that eventually the field finds its own balance.

VL: Yes, absolutely.

LC: Although we have already touched on it once or twice, I am going to ask again, what do you think are some of the critical things that will be done over the next two or three decades? How would you describe the future?

VL: We already spoke about molecular biology. But there is also another area of research that impressed me in the last few years, and that is the progress made with such techniques as PET and MRI. In some way these new technologies get back to the old investigations in anatomy. We are looking at the various nuclei in the brain in a more sophisticated way, and maybe these new anatomical methods can give us some new hints.

LC: Yes.

VL: And just one other thing I would like to say between me and you; we have to get oriented to perfection. I think that the National Institute of Aging has a beautiful motto, Aging to Perfection!

LC: Aging to Perfection. With that I thank you. It is always a delight to get together and hear your perspective on where we have been and where things are going in the future. Thank you very much.

VL: Thank you.

GEORGE K. AGHAJANIAN
Interviewed by Leo E. Hollister & Thomas A. Ban
Las Croabas, Puerto Rico, December 17, 1998

LH: We're in Las Croabas, Puerto Rico, where we are about to interview an old hand in the field, George Aghajanian.* I'm Leo Hollister, and I'm joined by Tom Ban for this interview with George. George, how did you get started in medicine and pharmacology? What persuaded you to make a career this way?

GA: I was interested in engineering first, and all through high school that was my leaning. There is one branch of my family, especially an uncle, who was involved in engineering in the early part of the century, pioneering the development of machine tools. So I had an interest there. But once I got to college, I started veering toward medicine, became a pre-med, and finally went to medical school.

LH: You went to Yale for both your undergraduate and postgraduate studies?

GA: No, I went to Cornell for my undergraduate studies. My postgraduate work was at Yale Medical School.

LH: And then, once at Yale, you stayed?

GA: Pretty much, except for a year of internship and a tour in the army. In those days, there was a doctor's draft, the Berry plan. I had to put in my two years' service in the army.

LH: Didn't you already start your training in psychiatry?

GA: Yes, I had postponed the army requirements until I finished not only residency but also two years of post-doctoral studies. I went in the army at thirty, when they finally caught up with me.

LH: But by that time you had a lot of training under your belt. Did the army make use of it?

GA: Yes, they did. I was trying to switch out of the Army into the Public Health Service and go to NIH. But when the Army heard I had experience in psychopharmacology research, and particularly with LSD, they said, "We want this guy." They sent me to Edgewood Arsenal, the Army Chemical Center, to work on incapacitating agents that might be used in warfare. That was their idea at the time but no longer is.

LH: I'm reminded of when I was first starting to work with reserpine, one of our staff in the hospital had the idea we could store the reserpine in Russian reservoirs and tranquilize them. So both sides were thinking the same thing.

GA: People had some pretty odd ideas about that at the time. First, the Army had the lethal agents program with the acetylcholinesterase (AchE)

---

* George K. Aghajanian was born in Beirut, Lebanon in 1932.

inhibitors. But later, they also had an "incapacitating agents" program that included very high potency antimuscarinic compounds.

LH: The BZ series.

GA: Yes. That was the code name for the most potent ones. They also had the LSD program.

LH: Outside of botulinum toxin, LSD is the most powerful biologically active substance known.

GA: Certainly at the time.

LH: One milligram a day is all you need and that's pretty good. Okay. What did you do after two years in the army?

GA: After I came out of the army in 1965 I returned to Yale and got an NIMH career development award. It made it possible for me to learn certain basic sciences. I started in electron microscopy and histochemistry, but in two or three years I shifted into electrophysiology.

LH: So you were preparing for a research career in neuropsychopharmacology.

GA.: In that regard, the person who had probably the biggest influence on me was one of the founders of ACNP, the late Daniel X. Freedman. Incidentally, I understand that he was the person who influenced ACNP to have their meetings in Puerto Rico. He was my thesis advisor when I was a medical student.

LH: So Danny was in the department of psychiatry at the time.

GA: Yes. When I was a medical student in the late 1950s, he was a young faculty member in a department that was predominantly psychoanalytically oriented.

LH: That was when Mort Reiser was chairman?

GA: Before that.

LH: When Fritz Redlich was chairman?

GA: Yes, Fritz Redlich was the chairman and his interests were quite eclectic, although he came from an analytic background. But there were Ted Lidz, Steve Fleck and many others in the department who had a dynamic, analytic orientation. It was a very interesting department; they were quite good in psychodynamics. It was Danny Freedman in the late 1950s who started the biological program in the department.

LH: He was working on it primarily with Nick Giarman.

GA: That's quite right. Your memory is very good. Nick Giarman was in the pharmacology department and it was through Nick Giarman that Dan Freedman was able to get a program going in neuropsychopharmacology. It was a joint program in pharmacology and psychiatry. So Dan was responsible for getting a number of people started in the field. I think that was one of the first training programs in neuropsychopharmacology.

LH: Who were some of the others in the program?

GA: Herb Meltzer and Jack Barchas were medical students like me at the time. Jack Barchas was in the class behind me.

LH: So the program was an incubator for neuropsychopharmacologists.

GA: Dan Freedman was a magnet for people who were interested in neuropharmacology and psychopharmacology.

LH: Was he always as nice a guy as I knew him?

GA: That was my entire experience with him. He was always very encouraging to young people.

LH: He was a fine gentleman.

GA: It was very important in the late 1950s and early 1960s for someone starting out in the field of neuropharmacology to have encouragement, because that was not the accepted way in psychiatry at that time. I was actually told that there would be no future for someone like me in academic psychiatry without getting analytic training. In fact, Dan did that even while bringing forth his neuropharmacology training program.

LH: He had a degree in psychology, as well, didn't he?

GA: Yes, I at a college level. I don't think he had a PhD in psychology.

LH: Do you suppose that Nick's interest got you into research?

GA: Yes, along with Danny. I did my medical school thesis on LSD. People, today wouldn't believe that LSD was not a controlled substance at that time.

LH: You could order it from the drug company.

GA: Sandoz would send it out to any physician who wrote in a request. There were ampoules of LSD lying around all over the place.

LH: I've still got 100 milligrams of LSD powder to make a solution. You could order it from biochemical supply houses without any control.

GA: Dan left a supply of LSD with me when I was a medical student, between my junior and senior years. I was doing a behavioral study on LSD when he went for sabbatical to NIH for a year. He just left with me a large supply of ampoules.

LH: What year was that?

GA: The summer of 1957.

LH: That was pretty early in the game, wasn't it?

GA: Yes, it was.

LH: It's pretty amazing that from 1943, or whenever the accidental discovery was made, how the number of papers on LSD started to escalate.

GA: It was only in 1953 and 1954 that the interaction between LSD and serotonin was discovered and the possible relevance of this interaction to the biochemistry of mental illness raised. The structure of serotonin had been discovered only a relatively short time before that. So it was only about three years later; Giarman had just come back from a sabbatical in

Gaddum's laboratory in England. Gaddum was one of the co-proponents of the serotonin hypothesis of LSD's mechanism of action.

LH: He developed a hypothesis about schizophrenia based on the antagonism between LSD and serotonin. Who was the other guy from New York who got the same idea?

GA: Woolley.

LH: Woolley and Shaw.

GA: They started with their research in New York about the same time as Gaddum was doing his work in England. Gaddum first published in 1953 and Woolley and Shaw in 1954.

LH: But they weren't using it as a neurotransmitter.

GA: They had no idea about its role as a neurotransmitter. The serotonergic systems were not discovered until 1965.

LH: It was probably all done in platelets.

GA: By 1953, it was known that serotonin was present in the brain. Nick Giarman thought of it as a neurohumoral substance. He referred to it as a substance that was present in the brain. There was no specific knowledge that it was actually within a specific set of neurons and might be a transmitter used by those neurons. That wasn't known until 1965.

LH: I suppose Brodie and his crew established prior to that, that serotonin has an important role in the action of reserpine.

GA: Certainly. Levels could go up and down; reserpine could deplete serotonin, but it wasn't known where the serotonin was in the brain. They were working with whole brain, with brain homogenates. At that time, nothing was known about the neurotransmitter role or localization of serotonin. All those classical studies of Brodie, Carlsson, Freedman, and others were done on brain homogenates. It was Freedman who found that LSD affected the levels of serotonin and its metabolites in the brain.

LH: I think it was also Danny Freedman and Nick Giarman who first came up with the idea that LSD produces a model psychosis by affecting serotonin.

GA: By the time they suggested that in the 1950s the model psychosis idea was around quite widely.

LH: I used to have friendly arguments with Danny about just how good the LSD model was for schizophrenia. But, regardless, he certainly started you out on the trail of neurotransmitters. You've studied them over the course of a lifetime.

GA: I started as assistant professor in the department when I got back from the army. It was at the time when the discoveries of the Swedish histochemists were published, showing for the first time that the origin of serotonin is in the raphé neurons of the brain stem and the fibers from those cells containing serotonin projected to all other parts of the brain. The information on the release of serotonin came just a little bit later. In one of my first studies I was showing an increase of serotonin metabolites in different parts of the brain after electrical stimulation of the raphé neurons in the brain stem. This was indicative that serotonin had been released.

LH: Did you measure it chemically or histochemically?

GA: I measured it chemically. That was about 1966–67.

LH: That was when fluorescence made the scene.

GA: Fluorescence measurements were already on the scene. That was when I switched to electrophysiology because I thought the activity of these neurons might be very important for determining what their function was. I had no background in electrophysiology, but I was able to interest a post-doc in the neighboring laboratory of the late John Flynn from Yale in starting some studies of this nature. We did our research at night. On the basis of Danny Freedman's findings that LSD raises the levels of serotonin but decreases its metabolites, I hypothesized that LSD might be inhibiting the firing of serotonergic neurons, and as a result the released neurotransmitter would back up but its metabolites would go down.

LH: Well, that's one of the possibilities, isn't it?

GA: We did the first experiment one night in the winter of 1967, and it did work. Nine out of ten, or ninety-five out of a hundred of my hypotheses do not pan out, but that one did. So I became a confirmed electrophysiologist from that time.

LH: Over the years, I noticed, you published papers with three ACNP presidents: Danny Freedman, Floyd Bloom, and more recently Steve Bunney.

GA: Yes. Floyd Bloom and I were in the same laboratory studying electron microscopy in the 1960s. Steve Bunney was one of the first post-doctoral students in my laboratory. He was a resident in our program in the early 1970s.

LH: And that's where he learned his electrophysiology?

GA: Yes. His older brother, William Bunney or Biff Bunney – whom I had known for some years because we overlapped in residency at Yale – steered Steve my way. Steve started with no experience whatsoever, as a post-doc in my laboratory.

LH: The first time I ever heard Steve Bunney give a paper it was at the ACNP meeting in Phoenix, I think. I was impressed and afterward I asked him, "Why don't you get your older brother to nominate you for membership of this organization?" And he did.

If you had to pick out of your many papers two or three you think represent your best work, which ones would you pick?

GA: The papers describing the recording of the electrophysiological properties of the monoaminergic neurons; it was made possible after the Swedish histochemists published maps showing where they were. The first recordings of this kind were of the effect of LSD on the firing of serotonergic neurons. Then, within the next two or three years in my lab, we went on to record from the dopaminergic neurons and neurons in the locus coeruleus. That series of studies and the ensuing papers represent my best work. They were the first recordings from monoaminergic neurons and described their basic electrophysiological properties and the effects of drugs on their firing rate. That started off many studies in this area of research, and as you know, became a major industry.

LH: Oh, yes.

GA: We did that early work in a period of five years starting in 1967 and running until about 1973. We did the LSD studies and described the electrophysiological properties of serotonergic neurons in 1967 and 1968, and published our findings in *Science*. We did the first studies on noradrenergic neurons in 1971 with a medical student working for the summer in the lab. Then, when Steve Bunney came along, his project was to record from dopaminergic neurons. That was in 1973.

LH: Was he doing it in a single neuron?

GA: Yes, in single neurons. Many of the properties of the monoaminergic neurons that are well known today were discovered in those studies. We learned that serotonergic neurons release serotonin in very slow tonic firing; that the tonic firing of noradrenergic neurons is very reactive to sensory stimuli; and that the firing of dopaminegic neurons is affected by amphetamines and antipsychotic drugs. One of the main principles derived from those studies is that monoaminergic neurons have autoreceptors in the somatodendritic region for their own transmitters and that these autoreceptors serve as a negative feedback regulating their activity.

LH: Well, that's an established principle now.

GA: Yes, that principle was derived from findings in these early studies.

LH: That's landmark work.

GA: It had a major impact for many years on the development in that field through the work of many, many investigators.

LH: Did you ever think that serotonin would be as versatile as it seems to be?

GA: I certainly did not.

LH: I don't think anybody did.

GA: I remember when Eli Lilly was developing fluoxetine in the early 1970s, they were not confident they were working on a drug that had any future. But there were a few people who did.

LH: More in Europe than in America.

GA: You're absolutely right. In Britain, there were those who were inclined toward thinking that serotonin would have a role in affective disorders. Also, in Sweden, Arvid Carlsson believed that serotonin might be important for depression. In fact, Arvid Carlsson was involved in the development of a serotonin reuptake inhibitor, zimelidine.

LH: That looked pretty good for some time, didn't it?

GA: Yes, but it had certain toxicities and was dropped. Meanwhile, Eli Lilly was developing fluoxetine, but because the developers were not confident about marketing of the drug, the basic science work went on for some years before fluoxetine got into clinical testing.

LH: If you look back though, both imipramine and amitriptyline were serotonin uptake inhibitors, but they also had an effect on norepinephrine. I used to joke that in this country we bought more norepinephrine than in Europe whereas in Europe they bought more serotonin.

GA: In recent years, because many atypical antipsychotic drugs block the 5-HT_{2A} receptor, interest in serotonin everywhere reawakened.

LH: Do you think that has anything to do with their antipsychotic action?

GA: The most critical test of this is currently ongoing. The atypical antipsychotic drugs that we had in the past also have other actions. Of course, it's difficult to sort out the 5-HT_{2A} blocking component in their action from the other components. Among the currently used drugs, risperidone comes the closest for testing the relationship between blocking 5-HT_{2A} and antipsychotic action. It has a very high potency in blocking 5-HT_{2A} receptors. It is about ten times more effective blocking 5-HT_{2A} receptors than D_2 receptors. Risperidone has now been clearly shown to be an effective antipsychotic, and it has antipsychotic effects in a dose range where primarily it occupies 5-HT_{2A} receptors without occupying D_2 receptors. In higher dose ranges risperidone will occupy D_2 receptors and produce extrapyramidal side effects. There is a drug which was originally called MDL 100907 and now M100907 because the new company couldn't get that many digits into their coding system. It has just gone through Phase-III clinical trials.

LH: Is M100907 solely a 5-HT_{2A} blocker?

GA: It doesn't touch D_2 receptors.

LH: Well, we shall see. I've been of the opinion that all of the atypical antipsychotics have in common a weak D_2 antagonism and that D_4 or D_1 antagonism doesn't mean a damn thing. Probably serotonin antagonism doesn't mean anything, but I may be completely wrong on that.

GA: That's why this new drug, MDL 100907 is so important.

LH: Wasn't ritanserin selectively blocking serotonin receptors?

GA: Ritanserin does block 5-HT$_{2A}$ receptors, but it also blocks 5-HT$_{2C}$ receptors, and it also interacts with a number of other receptors, so it is not quite as suitable for testing the relationship between blocking 5-HT$_{2A}$ and antipsychotic effects.

LH: It bombed out as an antipsychotic.

GA: It was said to be useful in improving negative symptoms, but maybe not the positive symptoms. It's quite interesting that ritanserin doesn't seem to do the trick, even in animal models.

LH: So it's not a true test of the idea?

GA: MDL will be the true test and the results are being analyzed now. But the question in my mind is being so selective as we believe, will it work, and if so would it be in just a subset of patients? Probably, all schizophrenias are not the same, and it might pick out a subset of schizophrenias where the 5-HT$_{2A}$ receptor is important in the pathophysiology; whereas it might not have an effect on other schizophrenias where the 5-HT$_{2A}$ receptor is not involved.

That brings me to the topic of recent research of mine. I'm inclined to think these days that it's really not the monoamine receptors that are primarily involved in antipsychotic effects, although they may have some impact. I don't think the existing antipsychotic drugs are so effective anyway. We know that schizophrenic patients are not going to pop back to normal living after they are given an antipsychotic drug. So, in our recent research we are studying whether an abnormality of glutamate release might also be involved. We were led to this hypothesis by studies on the mechanisms of 5-HT$_{2A}$ receptor activity, and the recognition that the 5-HT$_{2A}$ receptors are concentrated in the cerebral cortex. It makes a lot of sense they are concentrated in the cerebral cortex because psychedelic hallucinogens that work through the 5-HT$_{2A}$ receptor, and possibly to some degree through the 5-HT$_{2C}$ receptor, produce not only hallucinations and illusions but have an effect on all cortical functions, including cognitive and affective.

In recent years we've been studying, electrophysiologically, the role of 5-HT$_{2A}$ receptors in the psychoses induced by hallucinogens. We found that hallucinogens work as partial agonists of 5-HT$_{2A}$ receptors in that they don't have serotonin's full effect. What makes a hallucinogen, we believe, is that they lack the other actions of serotonin that counterbalance the dramatic increase in 5-HT$_{2A}$ receptor activity. In other words, they leave the increase of 5-HT$_{2A}$ activity unopposed. However, it is not necessarily the over-activity of 5-HT$_{2A}$ receptors that produces the hallucinogenic effect but rather, as our studies show, it is an abnormality of glutamate release that might be responsible for endogenous psychoses.

If overactivity of 5-HT$_{2A}$ receptors were responsible, then drugs that block 5-HT$_{2A}$ receptors should work right away. However, they don't. Even with MDL 100907, there seems to be a two, three or four week delay in the onset of therapeutic effects.

Currently there are also ongoing studies with the ketamine model of psychosis. Ketamine is an antagonist of one type of glutamate receptor, the NMDA receptor. The ketamine-model of psychosis at first glance seems to be a completely different model from the LSD, or psychedelic hallucinogen model of psychosis.

LH: I thought it was a much more realistic model.

GA: People have debated that because there's some overlap between the two models. One obvious difference is that NMDA receptors are blocked with ketamine but not by the psychedelic hallucinogens. Recently, however, Bita Moghaddam, a member of ACNP, found that ketamine induces an increase in glutamate release in the cortex, and since the effects of psychedelic hallucinogens have also been attributed to an increase of glutamate release, the two models seem to share a common mode of action. There are also findings in PET imaging studies in Europe that have shown hypofrontality, similar to that seen in schizophrenia, after the administration of mescaline, a psychedelic hallucinogen, and also after the administration of ketamine. During the past few years the so-called metabotropic glutamate autoreceptors have been discovered, and it has been shown that glutamate can act on these autoreceptors to suppress glutamate release by a negative feedback mechanism. In this respect the glutamatergic system is analogous to the monoaminergic system where monoamines can act on their autoreceptors to suppress monoamine release. At this time, agonists of these metabotropic autoreceptors have been developed that can block the effect of psychedelic hallucinogens. This fits with the idea that the effects of psychedelic hallucinogens are mediated through an excessive release of glutamate.

Furthermore, Bita Moghaddam has also shown that the same metabotropic receptor agonist that blocks the excessive release of glutamate induced by ketamine or PCP also blocks the behavioral effects of these substances. So we have at this time two glutamate models of psychosis, a psychedelic hallucinogen model and a ketamine/PCP model.

LH: I would have thought so, because clinically, the differences are substantial.

GA: That's quite true. One of the major differences is that there is blockade of NMDA receptors in the ketamine/PCP model.

LH: Then there's also a glutamatergic-dopaminergic link.

GA: Where that fits into the picture is a little unclear. Bita Moghaddam has shown in her studies, that PCP and ketamine increase dopamine release, but metabotropic receptor agonists don't interfere with that effect. So we've got a new ball game here.

LH: How exciting! I'd given up on hallucinogens.

GA: It's so exciting that Eli Lilly has become the leading developer of metabotropic receptor agonist drugs. These drugs are analogs of glutamate with different side groups. It had been believed that such drugs would not enter the brain, because they are too polar, but Lilly has succeeded in developing highly potent agonists, with nanomolar potency, that can be given systemically and enter the brain.

LH: Are they actually bioavailable or do they just overwhelm you with their potency?

GA: They have surprising bioavailability. They may actually be transported into the brain, but that has not been established yet.

LH: I think they are transported into the brain.

GA: They might be, through amino acid transporters, but that has not been shown yet. These drugs are effective in animals in very reasonable doses. They were originally developed for use in the treatment of anxiety disorders, and are being used currently in clinical trials in these disorders. But now, because of the new findings that implicate excessive glutamate release in both the ketamine/PCP and psychedelic hallucinogen models of psychosis, Eli Lilly, through Bita Moghaddam's and our efforts, is contemplating clinical trials in schizophrenia with these substances. We're anxiously awaiting the inception of those trials. I've just brought you right up to the present.

LH: This is exciting, because we've been desperately trying to get off the dopamine hypothesis.

GA: This even gets us off the serotonin hypothesis and gets us to the glutamate hypothesis, because all roads lead to either glutamate or GABA. One can think that monoamines are interacting with their G-protein coupled second messenger pathways influencing gene expression, but in terms of their immediate electrophysiological effects the main function of monoamines is the modulation of excitatory and inhibitory amino acid transmission.

LH: GABA and glutamate are far more abundant in the brain than monoamines, aren't they? We talk so much about the amines, but they are there in relatively small amounts.

GA: Right. So one can think of a defect downstream of the monoamines and a defect, let's say, in the glutamate release mechanisms. Monoamines through their action via monoamine pathways may have some influence on a defective glutamate release mechanism. Perhaps the influence will not be great enough and will be too slow to translate into optimal efficacy.

So, we are hypothesizing that the monoamines have a rather indirect and distant influence on what may be the core pathology, which would be downstream, involving glutamatergic or GABAergic transmission. What might provide specificity is that the metabotropic receptors which modulate glutamate release and transmission are expressed differentially in different parts of the nervous system. There's one type of metabotropic receptor that's very strongly expressed in the cerebral cortex in fibers that, we think, are involved in the action of the psychedelic hallucinogens.

LH: This isn't history. This is bringing us up to date. I didn't realize all these things are going on.

GA: I would say there are a good dozen posters on studies dealing with metabotropic glutamate receptors at this meeting.

LH: Well, out of five hundred posters it's hard to find a dozen.

GA: Eli Lilly has already shown that one can make highly selective drugs that hit predominantly one or another subtype of metabotropic receptor. So it's going to be very exciting in the coming years to see how these drugs, with an action on different subtypes of metabotropic receptors, will effect mental functioning, and ultimately what therapeutic benefit their use might have. The first of these drugs, LY354740, as I mentioned earlier, has already been tested in anxiety disorders and does seem to have anxiolytic properties. Moreover, these drugs should work very rapidly because they reach to the heart of the matter rather than influencing it indirectly as the monoamines have been doing.

LH: Well, there are lots of surprises. So, you come from monoamines all the way up to glutamate and the other transmitters.

GA: To me, the connection with glutamate was a surprise. We started only three years ago with these studies looking at the effect of 5-HT$_{2A}$ receptors on glutamate transmission, and at that time we had no idea how the metabotropic agonists might fit into that scheme. Nor did we have any idea that there were drug companies developing selective agonists of metabotropic receptors that would block the effects of hallucinogens.

LH: That's a novelty in itself.

GA: This has all happened in the last two or three years.

LH: Well, you've had a really exciting career.

GA: Yes, it's very exciting. One difference between the way things were in the 1960s, when I got started, and are now is that there was very little knowledge about brain systems at the time. It would take years to follow up any findings, but now things happen very quickly. The base of knowledge is expanding so much it makes one envious of the people who are starting out now. The knowledge basis is so much greater and the tools one has to work with are so much better than they were. The one way I would not be envious is that people starting out have a tougher road, because there's greater competition. There are so many more people in the field. When I was starting out, there was hardly anyone doing what I was. In fact, there was no one. But now, that's not the case. A young investigator comes up with some novel finding, and in no time at all, ten other labs will be doing it.

LH: One of the sad developments is that people are reluctant to share new information for fear it will be co-opted.

GA: When I started recording from monoaminergic neurons, no one else was doing it, and it actually took several years before other people started.

LH: Now, it would be several weeks.

GA: Yes, I think so.

LH: Well, thank you, George, for coming by and sharing parts of your most interesting career. I think we're going to have you back in another ten or fifteen years to bring the history up to date.

GA: I don't know about that because I've developed another interest, which might have a higher priority in the next ten or fifteen years. That's a game one plays with a funny looking stick and a little white ball you hit down a fairway. I've been corrupted!

LH: Thanks for spending time tracking the electrophysiology of neurotrans-mitters and I wish you a lot of luck with the golf. I'm sure Tom does, too, because, as clinicians, we feel deprived, not being in the forefront of things and not having as many drugs to offer patients as we would like.

FLOYD E. BLOOM

Interviewed by David J. Kupfer
San Juan, Puerto Rico, December 13, 1995

DK: I'm David Kupfer. I'm currently president of the College and it's my plea-sure to introduce and interview Floyd Bloom,* who is one of our illustrious past presidents. Floyd, the first thing would be if you could tell us about the kind of training you had that got you into neuropsychopharmacology.

FB: As a medical student I did neurophysiology research. On the basis of that research, I was going to secure my exemption from the military draft.

DK: This seemed one of the major motivating factors?

FB: Absolutely. That drove a lot of people into action in the good old days. When I was trying to get a place at the NIH the man I hoped to work with had left and Bob Berliner, the director of the intramural research program, was handling interviewees. He told me there was some "funny program" at St. Elizabeths Hospital that had to do with nerves, and maybe I should interview with them as they might have a place for me. That's where I met Joel Elkes for the first time and Nino Salmoiraghi. They accepted me, but I was told to come back after I completed my first year of residency in internal medicine.

DK: How many years was that before you started?

FB: Two years. I was a senior medical student at the time. I did an internship in medicine and my first year of residency and then went to the NIH to work at St. Elizabeths simply to establish an independent research record so I could compete for Chief Resident in Medicine at Barnes Hospital, which was the height of my aspirations.

DK: When was this?

FB: 1959. And, there was Joel Elkes, sitting behind what I thought was the world's largest desk, smoking what seemed to be the world's smallest pipe. He was fascinated by what I had done as a medical student and by what we could do in his Center at St. Elizabeths. Because he started his own research career studying the myelin X-ray diffraction pattern, he was interested in the peripheral nerves I had worked on. By the time I came back, in July 1962, Salmoiraghi had devised the technique of microiontophoresis, and that completely changed what I had thought I was going to be doing. Initially, I was going to look at how reserpine caused sedation in animals using the EEG and microelectrodes. But by then it was clear from the work of Costa and Brodie, that reserpine was able to deplete catecholamines and serotonin (and later also dopamine)

---

* Floyd E. Bloom was born in Minneapolis, Minnesota in 1936.

from the brain. Nobody knew what catecholamines in the brain did, so microiontophoresis seemed to be the ideal way to go.

DK: Was Mimo Costa at St. E's then?

FB: No, he was in the Heart Institute, but shortly after I started at St.E's he and I met at some seminar and struck up a conversation. After that he started coming over two and three days a week and most of the pharmacology I learned, I learned from Mimo during that time.

DK: So, that was in 1962? Were you still planning to return to St. Louis as Chief Resident in Medicine?

FB: The work went well and we were able to make headway in understanding the actions of norepinephrine in the olfactory bulb and later in the hypothalamus. And we did some of the first recordings on what dopamine would do to cells in the cortex and basal ganglia. As a result I had a lead article in *Science* with Salmoiraghi, and an *Annual Review of Pharmacology* paper with Salmoiraghi and Costa. It was a great time to be at the NIH, because Jacques Glowinski was there, Leslie Iversen, Dick Wurtman and Sol Snyder were all there, and the young kid seminars were truly exciting. We all were working on the same set of problems from different dimensions, so it was an exceptional time.

About the beginning of my second year, I went back to St. Louis and talked to my professor and said, "Dr. Moore, I don't think I'm coming back for the residency, this brain research stuff seems really pretty interesting." He puffed on his pipe for a while and said, "That's very good; I wish you well, but do you think you can make a living doing that kind of work?" I was aghast. That was the first time anybody had asked me to worry about making a living. I was free, innocent and scholarly and I thought that's the way you followed life. So while I was in St. Louis I talked to my other guiding lights, Oliver Lowry and Ed Dempsey, and both recommended I go to Yale to learn histochemistry with the electron microscope, because the question was not so much what norepinephrine does, but where is the norepinephrine synapse? It was at the time the Swedes were doing work in this area using histochemistry. And that's how I got to Yale.

DK: Before you got to Yale, you were busy as exemplified by your article in *Science*. Were you presenting this material at research meetings?

FB: The main places I presented were at FASEB meetings and summer ASPET meetings.

DK: After getting that interesting feedback in St. Louis what did you do?

FB: I continued to go to NIH. Electrophysiology is a pretty slow thing, so you do experiments three days a week. You've got two more days you can do something with, so I went over to the NIH main campus and learned elementary electron microscopy procedures from a classic electron microscopist, Professor Keith Richardson. He was willing to take me under his wing and teach me the manual skills required to take a huge sheet of glass and break it up into ultra-microtome knives.

DK: When did you start at Yale?

FB: Should have been July 1964. I applied for a special mental health fellowship and was able to go there with a rather ample fellowship stipend.

DK: You were showing the guys in St. Louis you were able to earn a living!

FB: Earn a living right away, yes. Almost the first week in New Haven while I was working in the lab of a man named Russell Barrnett, Daniel X. Freedman called me. He had heard what I was doing and he invited me to come to journal clubs he and Nick Giarman did. They had just written their *Pharmacological Reviews* paper on hallucinogenic drugs and the serotonin system. That was a different level of intellectual discussion, because this was now psychiatrists I was dealing with, as opposed to more or less basic neuropharmacologists. I very much enjoyed that conversation, but I also had this focus on trying to document electron dense reaction products by electron microscopy and that took a lot of time, too.

But by the middle of the first year the technology of autoradiography with the electron microscope emerged. At the NIH in Julie Axelrod's lab, Lincoln Potter and Axelrod had been able to show that if they injected animals with tritiated norepinephrine and fixed the pineal glands they could see where the radioactive norepinephrine accumulated. And Leslie Iversen and Jacques Glowinski had done the same thing, monitoring norepinephrine accumulation biochemically in the central nervous system. So it was a very fortunate moment. George Aghajanian had come back from the army, and having worked as a medical student with Danny, he and I teamed up in Russ Barrnett's laboratory. I went off to McGill for a long week to learn how to do EM autoradiography, and after I came back George and I did the first experiments; and lo and behold, we were able to see norepinephrine fibers in the brain with autoradiography.

DK: And then the two of you indirectly began influencing my career in medical school.

FB: Fred Elmadjian and his program. That would have been in 1966, when George and I moved over to the Connecticut Mental Health Center. I had no other place to go and it seemed like a very exciting place in neuropsychopharmacology. So when the Connecticut Mental Health Center opened, they gave George and me the first laboratories and we put an electron microscope in there. It seemed kind of ironic that the first instrument in a mental health center should be an electron microscope. In fact, we had a very good time in that place.

DK: So then you and George continued working together until when?

FB: Only two more years. In the early spring of 1968, Dr. Salmoiraghi had become the director of the Neuropharmacology Research Center at St. Elizabeths Hospital. He had taken over Joel Elkes' job when Joel left to take the Chair of Psychiatry at John Hopkins. The NIMH was growing. Groups that used to be Sections were now Laboratories and all that used to be Laboratories were now Divisions. So, Nino wanted me to come back to St. E's. And, since I worked on the histochemistry of the nervous system, I was recruited back from Yale in July of 1968. It was after the terrible series of riots that occurred in Washington. So, we started anew in the basement of St. Elizabeths Hospital. Mimmo Costa was also recruited back from Columbia University Medical School. We were now independent lab chiefs working side by side on two floors of a newly remodeled place. It was a big step up in what we were able to do. And of course, we didn't have to write grants.

DK: At this time are you regularly coming to ACNP? Do you remember?

FB: I was trying to think about that last night. I know I came once before the *First Generation of Progress* book. I had a chapter in that and I sat at dinner with Nate Kline, and he told me I had just been elected to the College. So, I think that must have been my second or third time. Nick Giarman brought me down all the times that I came. I got to know Danny and Mary Freedman very well through those meetings and I could also feel the kind of fellowship that was there. This was when we were still meeting at the Sheraton Hotel down the street in San Juan. The College was much smaller in those days and the sessions were much less planned, much less formal, lots more spontaneous discussion. I remember Joel Elkes discussing things at the end of what seemed like intense disagreements over psychiatric terms that I wasn't too clear on. But there was also a nice element of pre-clinical neuroscience work. So it was a strong precursor of the Society of Neuroscience, which didn't start for another four years.

DK: Then you were at St. E's between 1968 and when?

FB: From 1968 to 1975. We were able to build a pretty good laboratory system there. Several of the postdocs, who had been selected by Salmoiraghi, stayed on with me and have become famous in their own right; Roger Nicoll, Barry Hoffer, and George Siggins. We were able to do a very extensive analysis of "how does norepinephrine work," and surprisingly, because we were working next to Costa's lab where they were working on second messenger transduction, we were able to take their biochemical findings and immediately put them to the test with the electrophysiology. We were able to develop the Swedish method for fluorescence histochemistry, and combine electron microscopy with light microscopy. We started histochemistry in a major way with antibodies to cyclic AMP, which I was able to get from one of my previous teachers at Washington University, Charlie Parker. So it seemed like an ideal place to work. Then the government started becoming somewhat less pleasant, a lot of regulations, a lot of travel stipulations, a lot of pressure not to do things for money.

When I was at Yale, shortly before I came back to St. Elizabeths, Nick Giarman had been in a car accident, and died as a result of injuries. He had signed a contract to do a book for Oxford University Press, which was the course that Nick and Jack Cooper and Bob Roth and I taught to the first year graduate students in Pharmacology. So we finished the book to dedicate to his memory. I had to get special permission to leave Washington to Nick's funeral and work on the book. I couldn't work on the book on my own time, and every time there was a new edition, it was another series of hassles. I had been at NIMH seven years by that time. It just seemed to me there must be another way to do this.

DK: So, the popularity and success of the book was stimulating ?

FB: It was an important book; now in the eighth edition. We had no idea that writing a small irreverent paperback would become a lasting monument to our dear friend.

DK: So, then in 1975?

FB: In 1975, I started being open to invitations to look at other places. Normally, when someone would say, "What would it take to get you to do your stuff at our place?", I would say, "Oh, it'd probably take a million dollars," so they'd go on with their business and I would go on with mine. One day Frederic DeHoffman, who was the president of the Salk Institute, asked me that question and I gave him that answer, and he said, "I'll call you back next week." He called me back the next week and he had half the money. He said he felt sure that if I went with him to a couple of places we could get the rest of it. And he was true to his word. Jonas Salk was visiting Washington and I interviewed with Jonas and later looked at the place and gave my job seminar. They agreed to move a major part of my lab from NIMH there, set us up with the equipment we needed and build us a really splendid laboratory. And so we moved at the end of 1975, and the labs were up and running in the new location by July of 1976.

In that interval, my next-door neighbor at the Salk, Roger Guillemin, had discovered a couple of the endorphin peptides. In fact, while I was driving across the country, out came the paper by Hughes and Kosterlitz on the discovery of methionine enkephalin and leucine enkephalin. I read those papers when I got there, and Roger said to me, "We've just discovered another one of these peptides, but I don't know how to test them." And one of the things I was really good at was making intracisternal injections. So we had a ball in the first six months, without a lab, just working in Roger's space and around the Institute, injecting these newly synthesized peptides and watching what happened to the animals.

DK: What turned out to be, in retrospect, the most exciting work you did in the 1960s and 1970s?

FB: I'd always been obsessed with that initial question, what does norepinephrine do? We had a couple of insurmountable problems at the beginning. We didn't know where the cell bodies were that made the fibers, so it was very hard to envision the actions of norepinephrine in terms of circuitry. It was only possible to look at in terms of post-synaptic pharmacology, and show that a major part of its action could be mediated by cyclic AMP generation post-synaptically. It was just about the time when Earl Sutherland won the Nobel Prize for the discovery of cyclic AMP and second messengers. To be able to show that the nervous system exploited that same kind of thing was very exciting. But we spent a lot of time working with other postdocs devising methods.

Initially, Ed Evarts, another NIMH Lab Chief, started to record from the brains of freely moving cats to observe how cortical neurons changed during the stages of sleep. We thought that if we could determine where the norepinephrine cell bodies were located, we could do the same thing for them. By the early 1970s we knew where that was; we knew where the locus coeruleus was, and to record the serotonin cell body location from the locus coeruleus and the raphé nuclei during free spontaneous behavior. That series of experiments done at St. E's made very clear the regulatory role on cortical arousal that followed the origin and ending of the sleep stages. Putting those systems together, we began to get a kind of global view of how the pontine monoamine systems, projected to a lot of places, could modify their action in a way that might then lead to the enduring changes you could learn from. We ran a gamut of experiments with norepinephrine, just in studying its development, studying the origin of its synaptic inputs and outputs. So I would say that the characterization of the brain norepinephrine system and its actions stands out in my mind as what we wanted to do from the beginning, and only ten years later when the tools were there were we able to put it together. It became the paradigm for what we wanted to do with the peptide systems once we could see them. So when the neuropeptides became the focus of attention, then the same questions arose; Where are the cell bodies? What happens to the post-synaptic cells when you stimulate the pathways that have the peptides in them? And that's when we started with the opioid peptides; we tried to follow the same paradigm as before.

DK: Would that best characterize the era when you moved to California?

FB: Yes, it was very intensely focused on the neuropeptide systems, getting antibodies, using antibodies as early antagonists and then waiting for the chemist to synthesize new versions of them that we could use as agonists and antagonists, looking at processing, looking at the prohormones.

DK: Now, in your view, how was the College changing during this period?

FB: The main thing was the growth, bigger meetings, more formal presentations, taking advantage of the growth of the neurosciences; and there were lots of additional people, lots of guests who would be brought in for the meetings. I don't have a crystal clear memory of that interval.

DK: When did you become active on the administrative side of the ACNP?

FB: It was the year that I moved to California I missed the meeting, and when I got to California, Keith Killam called and told me, "Congratulations, you've just been elected to the council of the ACNP." I said, "I didn't even know I was running." So, I was on council for the first time in Keith's presidency in 1975–1976. And there were so many meetings, it was kind of onerous to keep up with all of them, especially when you are in California. There was one meeting in California, one meeting in Hawaii, and so that three year interval, went pretty fast. Then, I was gone for quite some time "doing my thing."

DK: How would you best epitomize "your thing" at that time?

FB: In 1979, a paper came out in *Nature* that completely revolutionized the way people were doing things in neuropeptide systems. The classic way that Roger Guillemin had done it, starting with 750,000 sheep hypothalamus, extracting the peptide from them and doing bioassays, was a major tour de force; it was the basis of his and Andrew Schally's Nobel Prize. But molecular biology was becoming a laboratory art, instead of something that people were afraid of, so cloning genes was now something people were investing in and the technology was moving along. In March 1979, Professor Numa's group from Kyoto published in *Nature* that with ten rat pituitaries they were able to extract enough messenger RNAs and clone them to identify the common precursor of ß-endorphin ACTH, later called "pro-opio-melanocortin" or "POMC." Moreover, they found buried in that molecule what looked to be yet a third hormone with ACTH and ß-endorphin. Within a week Dr. Guillemin's lab has synthesized that hormone and we were able to make antibodies to it and map it out.

It seemed like this technology would mean that if there are a lot more peptides – and that's what everybody thought – this would be the way to go at it. I went over to the Scripps Clinic, where I knew Richard Lerner, and he introduced me to his postdoc, Greg Sutcliffe, and I said, "How hard is what you do?" He said, "Oh, it's not hard at all." I said, "Well, why couldn't we just take the messenger RNAs from the brain and look for the ones that haven't been discovered yet? How hard would that be ?" And he said, "It's a lot of work, but it's not that hard." So we started a collaboration in mid-1979, and from that point on I was knee deep into the use of molecular biology for discovery. With the technical acquisition of in situ hybridization, you didn't have to wait for antibodies to map out where the cells were, and then to take those gene products and try to understand if they were really neuropeptides or some other kinds of substances. It led us to whole classes of molecules that had not been envisioned before. That kind of open ended mentally unconstrained attitude for discovery, with the use of molecular technology to probe the structure and function of the brain, is still very exciting to me.

DK: When did you move down the street?

FB: 1983. We had an alcohol center at the Salk, which allowed us to ask a lot of the fundamental questions of the catecholamine system. But it was my impression that some of the people at the Salk didn't think alcohol research was an honorable thing to do, and I still enjoyed doing research that examined people. We had a lot of projects that used event related potentials to study and predict who was vulnerable to alcoholism, so I was looking around at other jobs. I had been at The Salk for seven years, and seven years was a very long time for me to stay at any place. When it was clear that I was seriously looking at other job opportunities, Richard Lerner said to me, "Well, why don't you come here? We're expanding; whatever you want we'll get for you."

DK: This way, you didn't have to move.

FB: Well, five hundred yards. So we moved over a weekend into the new labs they had built for us and it's been a wonderful time ever since.

DK: It's been more than seven years.

FB: Twelve years now. The department has grown from 8,000 square feet, when we left the Salk Institute, to nearly 60,000 square feet and a faculty of 40 or so independent people doing their thing in neurobiology, neuro-immunology, a major commitment to CNS AIDS, the mechanisms of brain inflammation, actions of cytokines, transgenic animals and extensions of the molecular approach.

DK: It's interesting to me that the topics you're describing are somehow reflected in the topics of ACNP programs in that period. In other words, I suspect you're probably leading the curve so the topics wind up in our programs.

FB: Well, I think we got into molecular biology and neuropharmacology as early as anybody I remember, and we didn't do it, necessarily, for neuropharmacology per se, but with the idea that if you discovered new neurotransmitters, then you had some additional indices to use on measuring spinal fluids or brain tissues from people who died with mental illness, and maybe in some of the new indices we would find one that's really involved in these situations.

DK: It would be useful, especially, since our audience is to some extent the ACNP, if you could name people who spent time in your laboratories, who are members of the ACNP now.

FB: I have two former postdocs who are members here, and are chairmen of departments of psychiatry, and three who are chairs of basic science departments. I try to keep some of them with me, so we still have another four or five members of the College who are members of our department. It has been a productive relationship, promoting them to come here, getting them involved as independent people, so they are recognized for their own contributions. That allows me to be free and work on new subjects.

DK: What's your take on the way the College has changed over the last decade or so?

FB.: The problem now is that there is so much knowledge that just discussing the new discoveries crimps the amount of mental time you can devote to trying to put those together. And, I suppose, my view is a little biased because the political involvements and the time commitment to other things constrains how many sessions I can go to. But it's hard for clinicians to keep up with the pace of discovery in the basic sciences and hard for the basic scientists to keep up with the evolution of thinking about the kinds of mental illnesses that are distinct categories where you can look for unique mechanisms of prevention or treatment or diagnostics. If there's any regret I have, it's that the sheer weight of discovery has forced apart what was always the cohesive element, which was the intermingling between basic scientists and clinical scientists. As you and I have discussed many times, that's what we tried to achieve with the latest ACNP fourth Progress volume – to try to give them the hooks they could use if their scholarly interests awaken them to the opportunities that are out there.

DK: It still requires a lot of work to do that cross-talk.

FB: I guess anything important is going to require a lot of work.

DK: How do you balance everything you are doing nowadays?

FB: Well, there are still only so many hours in the day, so I make heavy use of computer-assisted communication. I do an awful lot of stuff by e-mail and by desktop video conferencing, so I can be in two places at the same time. I can e-mail; I can be in four places at the same time, but it has also cost me a lot of personal involvement in some of my research programs. I gave up a big grant in order to create time to devote to working as Editor-in-Chief at *Science*. It still takes an awful lot of time, and there's not a whole lot of free time left around.

DK: If you were to use your crystal ball, what's going to happen in the next ten to fifteen years?

FB: What's going to happen is our ability to image the human brain in action is going to improve with time and spatial resolution. The drugs that we work with to identify sensitive places in the brain will make markers that we can use on the living brain and test people sequentially.We'll be able to understand better the ability of experience to alter the structure and the function of the brain and the ways in which aging and other diseases may incapacitate those abilities to respond adaptively, constructively, to the events that we face with our brains. On the one hand, it'll be more of the same, but, on the other hand, we will know about the molecular events that take place from the moment that sensory events enter the brain until it modifies the association areas to take advantage of that information, store it and use it on another occasion.

DK: That's interesting. Despite everything going on in your life, you're still a regular attendee at the meeting. How's the meeting changed, the College in the last five or ten years? And what do you think is going to happen in the next ten years?

FB: Well, after I was president, we had another of our recurring crises on, "there's just too many good people out there for the number of people we admit," and we conceived that mechanism of bringing them in on associate memberships to start with, to kind of try out some of the talented people. But we have the problem that we are so popular and have such a good meeting that people want to join with us. At the same time, the more people who join with us, the further apart we are driven by the fact that there is only so much space for so many bodies. So, finding how to make an equilibrium out of that, how to maintain the vitality of the conversations and keep the young people coming in, but somehow turn us older ones out to pasture in some useful way, I think that's a real problem. This is not the biggest meeting we've had, but it's among the larger ones, and at last I've been able to get back into some of the sessions and listen to the science. And even with the science I know, I've learned from sitting in on those sessions, although only a month ago we had a neuroscience meeting, so things are really moving fast this time.

We have high quality people coming to the meeting, I would say, perhaps from broader areas than we used to be able to attract. There is a nice mix of the classic groups of people with European scientists coming to this meeting. I also think our global efforts in neuropsychopharmacology will allow us to maybe survive this period of suppressed funding, when we can work through cooperative consortium arrangements and not everybody has to do everything. To find trusted partners that you can work with and share your results in a way that you can each move forward with maybe not quite such an expansive attitude towards what you have to do.

DK: Anything else you'd like to say?

FB: Well, you know, when you were reading off the names of our dearly departed members, you sometimes recognize that you come here for people who aren't here any more physically, but who are really here mentally. And whatever we're doing with this videotape, it would be great if we could transmit through these videos some of the spirit of Nick Giarman and Danny Freedman and Nate Kline and the people who shaped this College at a time when they didn't know where it was going.

DK: And people who, I would say, independently influenced you and me in different ways.

FB: Absolutely. The heritage we indirectly inherited, which allows us a kind of instant rapport and a way of cross-checking our analytical insight into a particular situation, I think that's a remarkable feature of the College. Danny always used to call it a place where scholars came to share their information; that's what makes it different from an ordinary society.

DK: Good, thank you.

FB: Thank you. It was fun

JOSÉ M. R. DELGADO

Interviewed by Joel Braslow
Waikoloa, Hawaii, December 12, 2005

JB: I am Joel Braslow interviewing a distinguished colleague for the ACNP oral history series at our annual meeting in Hawaii on December 12. 2005. Please introduce yourself to our audience and the video camera.

JD: I'm José Manuel Rodriguez Delgado.* In Spain, you have a long, long name.

JB: Just tell me a little bit about your early childhood, where you grew up.

JD: I was born in Ronda in the south of Spain in Sevilla. Ronda was a beautiful town. We used to go there with my family for summer vacation in July and August. We had a really nice farm and I was born there. Then from there we went to Senegal in North Africa.

JB: Why were your parents in North Africa?

JD: My father was a major in the army and, we were fighting the Arabs, the Moors and the Muslims. We were in a beautiful place, in Helga. From there we went to Victoria in the Basque country and that's where I had my elementary schooling. Then I went to Madrid to get my MD degree and my doctorate in Science.

JB: When did you decide to become a physician and a scientist? And what made you decide to do that?

JD: I was in the third year of medical school when I started to do brain research with Professor Juan Negrin. Do you know Juan Negrin? He was the head of armaments during the time of the Republic. He was fighting Franco, and then the war was lost and he went to Mexico.

JB: After the Civil War?

JD: After the Civil War, in 1939, and he asked me to go with him to Mexico. I don't know whether I did right or wrong, but I wanted to stay in Spain. My problem was that Spain had no monkeys and I could not do my research without monkey brains. At that time, monkeys were not sold in Beijing or any of those countries.

JB: This was in 1939?

JD: No, I jumped in time. I am talking about 1940 or 1941. To solve my problem I went to Africa and brought about forty monkeys, two chimps and one gorilla back with me. At that time it was a long trip and took about two weeks. When I returned to Madrid, I asked myself, "what am I going to do? I'm going to do brain surgery on my gorilla? He's my best friend. I'm not going to do that."

JB: You became attached to the gorilla on the trip?

---

* José Manuel Rodriguez Delgado was born in Ronda, Spain in 1915. Delgado died in 2011.

JD: Yes, and I decided to give the gorilla to the Madrid Zoological Company. Then I continued doing research on the other monkeys. But it was after the war, and I had no instruments to do research in Spain. Then I found out that in the United States there was intensive brain research going on, so I decided to go there. And I met Professor John Friedman, Major John Lilly and many other people and began to do research at Yale University in New Haven, Connecticut.

JB: When was that?

JD: That was about 1942 or 1943, and I stayed at Yale for twenty-two years.

JB: Till 1974, is that right?

JD: From 1942 to 1973, something like that. Those were happy years. Those were the years when most of my research was performed.

JB: So, let's go back in time. Before you went to Yale, you had been doing what sort of work?

JD: I was in Madrid, at the Ramón y Cajal Center. At that time, the Center was in El Rápido, a beautiful park in Madrid. I started to develop electrodes for brain implantation.

JB: What motivated you to do electrical stimulation of the brain?

JD: I thought the most interesting field in medicine was the brain and I wanted to know what was going on inside the brain. Implanted electrodes were first used in 1932 by Professor Hess in Switzerland in cats. But he used a primitive technique. I should not say that, because he was a Nobel Prize winner.

JB: He got the Nobel Prize in 1949, is that right?

JD: I think later. I continued that line of research. I improved the electrodes. Instead of one I had seven electrodes, which were left in for weeks, months and even years. I did that, fifty-five years ago.

JB: So, you continued that work at Yale.

JD: I continued in monkeys for seven or eight years. I was able to induce yawning, multiple behaviors, pupillary dilation, so then I decided, if it works in monkeys why not implant electrodes in humans? Now we are in 1952, in Providence, Rhode Island, where in collaboration with Dr. Hannibal Hamlin, a surgeon, we began implanting electrodes in schizophrenic patients.

JB: Was this done for the first time in 1952?

JD: Yes; it was the first time that electrodes were implanted in human beings.

JB: What were your thoughts about that?

JD: Remember, 1952 was the age of lobotomy for which Egas Moniz won the Nobel Prize. I was not happy with lobotomy and wanted to see what we could do with implanted electrodes in schizophrenics, epileptics and depressed patients. John Fulton did not win the Nobel Prize, but he was the author of important work on the structure of the brain.

JB: You were in his department. Is that right?

JD: I had a joint appointment in physiology and psychiatry, a full professor in both.

JB: You were not happy with the results of lobotomy?

JD: I was asked whether I wanted to do lobotomies and I said no, let's wait until the methodology is improved. But, we had to treat epileptic, schizophrenic, and depressed patients.

JB: Treat them with what?

JD: With electrical stimulation, mainly frontal lobe stimulation.

JB: How did you do that? I mean, technically.

JD: It was necessary to make a little hole to place the electrodes steadfastly as possible into the brain, to stimulate it.

JB: How did you implant electrodes?

JD: The electrodes were implanted surgically.

JB: What did you find?

JD: In some patients it worked, in others it did not.

JD: Again, when did you do it for the first time?

JD: In Providence, Rhode Island in 1952.

JB: Was it done in a patient diagnosed with schizophrenia first?

JD: Yes, it was. And then, we did thirty-five or forty patients. In some of the cases we were very successful.

JB: Where did you implant the electrodes? Was it in the frontal lobes?

JD: In the frontal lobes and in the thalamus, mainly. We also implanted electrodes in the rostral part of the brain.

JB: Where in the rostral part of the brain?

JD: The septum and the head of the corpus callosum. These are the two areas with inhibitory functions, as demonstrated in monkeys, chimps, gorillas, sheep and many different varieties of animal. Then, I thought, if brain stimulation works so well with electricity we should try chemically. So I continued my research with chemoelectrodes. The chemoelectrodes were very small and had a very fine tubing that I used for injecting the chemicals. At that time we were working in monkeys, not in humans, and we were studying the effects of cocaine injected into the brain.

JB: And, this was in the mid 1950s?

JD: No, it was in the 1960s. I don't like to use pills. What happens when you take a pill? It will go through your brain but also the liver, kidneys and the whole body. I think it is better to inject the drug where the drug has its effect, inside of the brain.

JB: In your original research with implanted electrodes were you thinking of doing it for therapeutic purposes or for fundamental research?

JD: At the beginning it was only for fundamental research. In one of our experiments we were using computers and found we could establish communication between the brain and the computer and back. We did that at Holloman Air Force Base in the chimpanzee. It was really surprising. Through the computer, we established that each time an animal had electrical activity in the limbic system, the central gray matter was stimulated. And then, the chimp learned to inhibit electrical activity.

JB: It was like biofeedback.

JD: Exactly. I think we found something that could and should be used today.

JB: When was this work done?

JD: That was in the 1960s, quite a long time ago. We also used electromagnetic waves in chickens. That was extraordinary: It would modify the egg.

JB: What did it modify?

JD: The fertilized egg was modified. What happens with a pregnant woman? She has an embryo inside her tummy. The question was whether electromagnetic waves could modify the embryo in a woman? You cannot do experiments with embryos or pregnant women, but you could do it in chickens. We learned that by using electromagnetic waves the embryo could be affected. It could be damaged. This risk must be considered very seriously by legislators, by the government and by women themselves.

Then I moved from Yale back to Spain. I had a very nice invitation from the Minister of Education, Pilar del Castillo. She said, "You ought to come to Madrid. We're building a new Medical School at Autonoma University and we need your intelligence, your capacity to organize things." I responded, "I'm very happy at Yale. I don't want to go back to Spain now." But then, I thought, I owe some duty to Spain, after all I am from there. When I told Yale I was invited back to Spain, they said, "We'll give you anything you need, salary, instruments." That went on for several months. Then I asked my wife, "What do you think?" And she responded, "It would be interesting to go back, let's go back to Spain." So we went back and I became Director of the Department of Physiology at the Autonoma Medical School. Then after that, I moved to the Cajal Center. The Cajal Center was originally organized by Generalisimo Franco, and one of the professors at the Center was his son-in-law. That was a big problem because when the new government came after Franco, everybody at the Cajal Center was dismissed, even very good people, including myself.

JB: When was that?

JD: About ten or maybe, fifteen years ago. I said I have been productive in research for a long time, I should retire. But should I retire and do nothing? I decided I would continue doing something which is perhaps even more important than research, and that is thinking about research ethics, about the philosophical implications of implanting electrodes, injecting chemicals into the brain. What is the meaning of all this? What is the meaning of life? And what I'm doing now is even more important than what I have done in the past; I think about the ethical and philosophical implications of brain research, the implications of cloning.

JB: Did those thoughts enter your mind in the course of your career as well? You were obviously involved in some very fundamental work, looking at the relationship between the brain and behavior, and were using pretty invasive interventions over the last fifty years.

JD: That's right. But what is the meaning of all this? When you stimulate the brain, a nucleus of the brain, and get an inhibitory effect on behavior? Anything you do to the brain has behavioral implications, social implications, and philosophical implications. One needs to think about the implications of one's own research. What you're doing is modifying the chemistry of the brain. That's what all the pharmaceutical companies are trying to do, modify by chemicals brain functioning and behavior. All right, there's an anti-epileptic drug and it works. But should it not be possible to administer it more directly to a specific locus so that it would not have secondary effects? This should be the goal of the companies.

JB: Tell me about some of the philosophical and social implications.

JD: Take a terrorist. The terrorist could be a good father, a good person because his brain and behavior is normal in all but one aspect, destroying lives and property. Would it be ethical to modify the brain of a terrorist? Now, let us try to find out why the terrorist is a terrorist. He is a terrorist because he has been inculcated to become one. Could you be a terrorist? Sure you could, because you're a normal human being. We are dealing with a philosophical question. The brain is the material support of the mind. And what is the mind? Well, the mind is something that is supported by the brain. Take a computer or a videotape.

JG: The videotape is a nice analogy in that even understanding the mechanics, you're not likely to understand anything about the content on the videotape.

JD: Exactly.

JB: You've been in the press a lot over the course of your career, and as you were talking it made me think that perhaps you've been misunderstood in a certain way. Could we talk about that?

JD: It was not misunderstanding. It was a lack of understanding.

JB: Can you tell me how it affected your career?

JD: I was doing what most brain researchers are doing, just trying to see how the brain works.

JB: But not many researchers have ended up on the cover of the *New York Times*. On page one of the *New York Times*, is that right? What was that like, getting acclaim and notoriety for your research, and how did that affect your career?

JD: It affected it very little because I was totally concentrated on my work. I did not have time to think about the implications of brain research. I think the newer generation of investigators should do more thinking about the implications of their research.

JB: Am I correct when you say implications, you mean ethical, social and philosophical implications?

JD: I mean practical use of their research findings.

JB: You think that should shape what researchers do? I mean, in the sense of thinking about how the research is going to be used or not used?

JD: That's right. What is research? Research is to find out what is real, what is going on in the brain. The results of your thinking are limited by the functions of your neurons, the function of your amygdala. Neurons are very similar; in frogs, in cats, and in human beings. All species of animals have neurons. You modify cells and thinking becomes different. This is happening in mental illness. That's why we should investigate what is going on in the brain of schizophrenic and depressed patients.

JB: I'm thinking now as you're talking, and I'm wondering, in fifty years from now, what would you like people to remember about you? About your work?

JD: They should remember my discoveries, because it is in their discoveries that people are different.

JB: When you look over your career, what is the biggest discovery you think you've made?

JD: Probably the communication between the brain and the computer. Could we communicate with the brain without words? One of the great possibilities in the future is to communicate without words.

JB: I notice that your wife came along with you. She's been a part of your life for a long time. Can you tell me a little bit about her? I think she has been an important collaborator.

JD: My wife has been a very essential part of my life, not only personally, but scientifically.

JB: That's what I want to hear about.

JD: When I was writing a paper I thought was very good, and showed it to her, she would say, "It's a lousy paper." And then, without any scientific knowledge, she was able to correct it. So Caroline has played a great part not only in my personal life, but also in my scientific life. She has been a very powerful contributor intellectually to my research, and to some of my discoveries. I am very grateful to her. She has collaborated in my scientific accomplishments all through my life.

JB: How long have you been married?

JD: Forty, fifty, sixty years, don't ask me how long, because I'll give you the run around.

JB: We've covered a lot of ground. Is there any material you'd like to add?

JD: No, the main thing is the necessity of thinking about the dual possibilities of the brain.

JB: Are you working on a book?

JD: This is what I'm working on now.

JB: You wrote a very famous book in the late 1960s.

JD: It was on my research, but I think the ethical and philosophical aspects I'm involved with now are far more important.

JB: Is there anything you'd like to add? You were honored by Congress.

JD: Oh, yes.

JB: Can you tell me something about that?

JD: Well, that was very nice. A Senator from California, I can't recall his name now....

JB: It was Sam Farr.

JD: Thank you. Sam Farr. He was kind enough to propose me being honored for my research. Doing research is wonderful! But thinking about the implications of our findings is more important than anything else. And that is what we are missing today.

JB: Terrific. I really appreciate you taking the time. Obviously, you have done a lot to try to help us understand who we are.

JD: We hope we will learn even more about that.

PART TWO

Brain Imaging

SEYMOUR S. KETY

Interviewed by Irwin J. Kopin
San Juan, Puerto Rico, December 12, 1995

IK: I'm here to interview one of my major mentors in science, Dr. Seymour Kety.* Dr. Kety was born in Philadelphia, went to Central High School and to the University of Pennsylvania. He had training in Boston with Joseph Aub, went back to the University of Pennsylvania where he made some major contributions to studies of blood flow to the brain, then came to the National Institutes of Health (NIH), first as the scientific director of what was then precursor of two different institutes, called the National Institute of Mental Health (NIMH), which at that time included the National Institute of Neurological Diseases and Blindness (NINDB), among other things. Somewhere around 1956, he stepped down from his post as scientific director, to lead the Laboratory of Clinical Science. The Laboratory of Clinical Science has spawned some of the last century's greatest scientists, including Nobel Prize winner Julie Axelrod and many members of the National Academy of Sciences, and was the spawning ground of at least half the psychiatrists in the United States who were interested in biological psychiatry. I regard, and I think everyone else does, Dr. Seymour Kety as the father of biological psychiatry in this country, if not in the world, and it's indeed a pleasure to have an opportunity to elicit some of his early memories of his science and the major contributions he's made over these many years.

Seymour, can you tell us how you got started from your early years, during internship and research on lead poisoning; how did that lead to your later research? You went to Boston with this background, but soon you returned to the University of Pennsylvania; tell us about that.

SK: I got interested in lead poisoning because I had a summer job with a biochemist and toxicologist in Philadelphia who was doing a project for the lead industry, in which it was necessary to analyze the urine of men who worked with lead. I was given the job of analyzing the urine, and in the analysis one used sodium citrate to dissolve the insoluble lead compounds. It occurred to me that maybe sodium citrate would be useful in the treatment of lead poisoning. And when I was in medical school, I tested that possibility for a paper at a Student Research Day by feeding rats food contaminated with lead, and then giving them water with sodium citrate added. Then, analyzing their urine and comparing that to the urine before they had sodium citrate, we found that the urine lead content went way up with the sodium citrate.

---

* Seymour S. Kety was born in Philadelphia, Pennsylvania in 1915. Kety died in 2000.

Then, when I was an intern at Philadelphia General, I spent my evenings doing studies in the laboratory there and one of the studies I concentrated on was an examination of the lead citrate complex. I published my first paper in the *Journal of Biological Chemistry*, which was a characterization of the lead citrate complex. Later, Letonoff and I administered sodium citrate to patients at the hospital who were suffering from lead poisoning. Letonoff was measuring lead in the urine and lead blood levels and found that sodium citrate did have a therapeutic effect. That was the first treatment of lead poisoning with a chelating agent. Shortly after, much more powerful chelating agents were developed and lead poisoning has been treated with these ever since.

As a result of that lead study and my interest in lead poisoning, I applied for a National Research Council (NRC) fellowship to work with Dr. Joseph Aub, in Boston, who was the national expert on lead and lead poisoning. I won this fellowship and spent a year in Joseph Aub's laboratory at the Massachusetts General Hospital, which was a very interesting year. Dr. Aub was a great man. He was professor of research medicine at Harvard and at Mass General. We didn't do much on lead poisoning; however, because of World War II.

IK: This was about 1940?

SK: I went to Aub's laboratory from 1942 to 1943. That was before America got into the war, but the war was imminent, and I had attempted to enlist in the Medical Corps, but the army rejected me because of an old fracture I had with some infection of the bone. Dr. Aub's laboratory was working on shock, not on lead poisoning, so I participated in that. There was another postdoc in Dr. Aub's laboratory, Alfred Pope. He and I were the two low men on the totem pole and spent many evenings together taking care of dogs in shock, measuring their blood pressure regularly and so on.

IK: That must have been a rough year for you, because you were married and shuttling back and forth to see Josie in Philadelphia. Is that right?

SK: I married Josephine in 1940, just before my internship, and Josephine joined me in 1941, becoming an intern at Philadelphia General Hospital, as was I. Then she did her second year of internship while I was in Boston. Since that internship was a pretty rigorous period in which one spent a lot of evenings in the hospital, it really wasn't too bad, because I would come back to Philadelphia on weekends.

Pope and I became interested in the physiology of shock and we wrote a paper, which was published in the *American Heart Journal*, on the homeostatic reflexes involved in shock for the purpose of preserving blood flow to the brain. That got me interested in the importance of cerebral circulation. At the same time, I read a paper by Dumke and Schmidt. Schmidt was my old professor of pharmacology as a medical student, and this was a paper in which they were measuring cerebral blood flow in the rhesus monkey by using an ingenious bubble flow meter, which had been developed by Rachmael Levine. These were the first reliable quantitative measurements of cerebral blood flow, at least in lower animals.

I decided I would be returning to Philadelphia at the end of my fellowship. I had written to Carl Schmidt and asked whether I could work in his laboratory. He offered me a position, and I worked with him on the metabolism of the brain of the monkey, using the bubble flow meter. But we also measured arteriovenous (AV) oxygen differences and studied the metabolism in various states of wakefulness, anesthesia, convulsions and so forth. Around that time I began to think that although these studies in the monkey brain were interesting, they really didn't have the fascination the possibility of studying circulation in the human brain meant to me. This, I felt, would be a much more important thing to do, because it is the human brain which is heir to disorders that one cannot produce in lower animals, like schizophrenia and other mental illnesses; it is the human brain that experiences profound sorrow, laughter, jests and insights; it's the human brain that can speak and reveal its inner workings.

IK: At the time there were other people interested in similar problems. There was Himwich, and some of the people in Boston, who were measuring arteriovenous differences in oxygen. They were using the same data but came to different conclusions or interpretations.

SK: That's right. A Boston psychiatrist, Myerson, had developed a means of getting venous blood from the human brain by putting a needle into the internal jugular around the mastoid process. Since they were able to get cerebral venous blood and tap an artery to get arterial blood, they could measure the AV oxygen difference across the brain. And Lennox and Gibbs, working at the Boston Psychopathic Hospital, which is now the Massachusetts Mental Health Center, studied cerebral circulation by examining the AV oxygen difference and using the Fick equation, which states that blood flow through an organ is equal to the amount of oxygen taken up by that organ, divided by the AV oxygen difference. They weren't able to measure the oxygen consumption of the brain, but they were able to measure the AV difference. So, if you assume that the oxygen consumption is constant then the AV difference is inversely proportional to the blood flow. And, so, with that expedient, they would study cerebral blood flow under the influence of carbon dioxide, in epilepsy and a number of other conditions.

IK: They kept the numerator constant by fiat, by deciding that it was valid. And Himwich did just the opposite.

SK: Himwich was interested in metabolism rather than blood flow, because he was studying mental retardation and other mental disorders. He used the AV difference as a measure of the oxygen consumption with the assumption that the blood flow is constant. The difficulty with both these techniques is that the AV difference is the result of both oxygen consumption and blood flow to the brain.

IK: You've got one equation with two unknowns.

SK: Exactly. You have one equation with two unknowns, and that was a problem.

IK: Didn't this lead to some funny results, as for example with anesthetics?

SK: By and large, they guessed right. Although they weren't able to make absolute measurements, they would make qualitative measurements.

IK: What was the conclusion they reached with anesthetics?

SK: Well, they made some false assumptions. With anesthesia, the AV difference diminished. We know now the AV difference diminished because the oxygen consumption went down. But in their assumption that the oxygen consumption was normal, the AV difference diminished simply because the blood flow increased. So they assumed that there was an increase in blood flow with anesthesia.

IK: A huge increase.

SK: Yes, doubling. By and large, they guessed right. But they could never be sure, and the problem was that oxygen is a poor tracer to use in a situation like that, because oxygen is used by the brain, and used in different amounts under different states. In the very state one is studying, the oxygen consumption may vary. And so, I thought, why not use a gas that, unlike oxygen, isn't metabolized? The amount of gas that would be taken up would be the result of purely physical properties like the solubility of the gas in brain tissue, the principles of diffusion from capillary into tissue. These factors could be independent of whether the brain was thinking or sleeping or suffering from one or another disease that didn't seriously affect the solubility of a gas in the brain. When I was in Boston, I'd attended a number of "shock dinners" that people in Boston working on shock used to have, including all the staff of Dr. Aub's laboratory. We would invite outside speakers to the dinners, and these lectures were supported by the Macy Foundation.

On one of these occasions, André Cournand came to Boston to talk on his studies of cardiac output in human veins, using the Fick principle. He was measuring mixed venous blood by inserting the catheter through an antecubital vein to the right atrium. This was a very impressive lecture, because it was obvious he was studying physiological parameters in human veins, and measuring them more reliably and more accurately than had ever been done in animals by using an indirect technique which was minimally invasive; certainly not as invasive as the surgery that was required in most animal studies. That convinced me it was possible to study these physiological processes in human subjects, with indirect methods that were less invasive than one used in animals. The inert gas that I finally selected was nitrous oxide. Physiologists, before me, had used nitrous oxide as an inert gas for studies of cardiac output and for pulmonary function studies. I spoke to Dr. Stady at Penn, an expert in this area, and learned that nitrous oxide would be very nontoxic in human beings. At a concentration of fifteen percent, the subjects would not experience any anesthesia. That was the beginning of the nitrous oxide technique for measuring cerebral blood flow. I went to the Philadelphia General Hospital and practiced getting blood from the internal jugular using the Myerson technique on cadavers, and after I felt I was proficient, I approached a patient in the neurology building, who had been in that building for years and was happy to find a physician interested in talking to and studying her.

IK: At that time the Philadelphia General Hospital was part nursing home, wasn't it?

SK: No, the neurology building was more than a nursing home. It was a museum of neurological disorders, just full of patients who had all sorts of conditions and lived in the hospital most of their lives. This lady was very gracious and cooperative, and perfectly happy to have me study her cerebral circulation. So, I did the first nitrous oxide study with her cooperation. I got curves of the nitrous oxide concentration in femoral artery and internal jugular blood. And I published this pair of curves in my first paper.

IK: The pair being the arterial and the venous?

SK: Right. Now, with those two curves, it was simple enough to get the AV difference, but the difference was not constant as it would be with oxygen. It was a variable, because the brain eventually came to equilibrium with nitrous oxide at the tension in arterial blood. The AV difference started wide, and then gradually narrowed as it went along. So, one could integrate the AV difference and get the amount of nitrous oxide taken up by the brain. That was the area between the two curves, over a period of time. But how does one get the numerator of the Fick equation, the amount of nitrous oxide taken up by the brain? Well, if one waited until the brain was in equilibrium or close to equilibrium with the blood exiting it, which turned out to be about ten minutes on the basis of calculation and studies in dogs, the venous blood emerging from the brain was in practical equilibrium with the brain tissue itself.

IK: The same concentration as the arterial?

SK: No, it wasn't the same as the arterial in ten minutes. We saw a little AV difference, but all it had to be in equilibrium with was the venous blood, because someone could take the venous concentration and with a partition coefficient representing the difference in solubility could calculate, not the amount of nitrous oxide in the brain, but the concentration of nitrous oxide. That's why the blood flow emerged in milliliters per hundred grams per minute. I then explained this to Carl Schmidt, showed him the curve and told him I would like to apply this technique to studies in patients in the hospital at the university. Carl suggested that it would be a good idea to calibrate this technique against cerebral blood flow as measured with the bubble flow meter. I agreed, and together we did exactly that.

Carl set up monkeys with the bubble flow meter and I set them up to use the nitrous oxide technique, and we found that there was a good correlation between the values obtained by the nitrous oxide technique and those obtained with the bubble flow meter. And so, with that assurance, I published the first paper on the nitrous oxide technique with Carl Schmidt. That was in about 1943. Then we studied cerebral blood flow and cerebral oxygen consumption, because once one had the blood flow and the AV difference, one could calculate the oxygen consumption. I measured these functions in a series of normal volunteers. These were men who were conscientious objectors and who decided to volunteer for human medical biological studies as their way of contributing to the scientific community. It was also their social contribution in wartime. We published the values in these normal young men for cerebral blood flow and oxygen consumption.

IK: Did you do glucose utilization at this time also?

SK: We didn't do glucose utilization at first, but we did it shortly afterwards in normal controls. With the glucose utilization and oxygen utilization, we could calculate the energy release, and that turned out to be the equivalent of the energy utilized by a 20-Watt incandescent bulb, which was a remarkably small amount.

IK: It was a dim light.

SK: It was dim compared to the huge amount of energy necessary to feed computers at that time. Of course, since 1942 or 1943, computers have become miniaturized and the energy utilized by them is much less. I suppose it won't be very long before computers will be developed that utilize

20 Watts of energy and perform the kinds of functions that the human brain is capable of.

IK: How did you come to NIH? This was one phase of your career, a time when you were getting interested in mental disease, or at least how the brain worked. What stimulated the transition to the NIH?

SK: I moved from Carl Schmidt's department to join Julius Comroe, who was my true mentor in the period I spent at the University of Pennsylvania. Julius Comroe was a great physiologist of the pulmonary system, the lungs and respiration.

IK: Was he, in any way, the mathematician in the marvelous review you published on diffusion of gases, which has really been a classic?

SK: No, Julius didn't make any pretense of being a mathematician. As a matter of fact, I wasn't much of a mathematician until I got interested in working out the theory of the nitrous oxide technique, where I had to go back and brush up on calculus. I wrote that review because Goodman and Gilman, who were editors of *Pharmacologic Reviews*, asked me to write a review on the exchange of inert gas between blood and tissue, and I thought that was interesting, something I wanted to do anyhow.

I spent a year reviewing the literature and tracing the development of our knowledge of the exchange of inert tracers between blood and tissue. In the course of that, I made some original contributions; for example, I calculated, in a more extended fashion, the uptake of ether by the human lungs, circulation and brain, using a much more exact replica of the situation than Haggard, who was the first person to attempt to write an equation for the uptake of ether. The equation I came up with was more exact, and with that one could relate the speed of induction of inhaled anesthetics on the basis of their solubility in blood and of physiological parameters like ventilation and cardiac output. I also addressed the question of the exchange of inert gases or inert tracers between the capillaries of the brain and brain tissue itself, and derived an equation that would be of great importance to me in a few years time.

But you asked how I came to the NIH. Just about the same time I finished that review and sent it in for publication – it was published in 1951 – I had a visit from Bob Felix, who was the director of the National Institute of Mental Health, a new institute of the National Institutes of Health. He asked me if I would be interested in joining him as the scientific director of the mental health institute and we had a nice conversation. I thought he was a lovely man, and felt it was going to be difficult for me to turn him down because he was such a generous person, but I knew I wasn't going to work for the government. I was perfectly happy in academia, working at the university with Julius Comroe. But he urged me to visit the National

Institutes of Health, and so I went there with Josephine, and Bob Felix showed me the Clinical Center, which was still in the construction stage, walked me through the laboratories the mental health institute was going to have, and talked to me about the challenge of directing the greatest program for the study of brain and behavior the world had ever seen. Those were his words.

Well, it certainly was the largest program contemplated for the study of these functions that the world had ever seen. Whether it was going to be the greatest was to be seen later. In any case, I met with the people at the mental health institute, John Eberhart and others who were working with Bob Felix in the new institute, which hardly had a place where they could do administrative work, and I also met the scientific directors of the other institutes. I remember talking at great length with Jim Shannon, who was scientific director of the Heart Institute, with Harry Eagle and a number of the other scientific directors. Somehow I became convinced this was a challenge and an opportunity I couldn't turn down. So, I joined Bob Felix in 1951 as the scientific director of the mental health institute.

By that time, it was also decided to start another new institute, which was to be the Neurology Institute, and later became the National Institute for Neurological Disorders and Blindness. I was scientific director of both of those institutes at first, because the neurology institute was grown out of the mental health institute as Eve grew out of Adam's rib. Bob Felix became interested in talking to me because of the nitrous oxide technique and because I had collaborated on a study of schizophrenia, which was published in the *American Journal of Psychiatry*. Bob, with a little prompting by the directors of the NIH, decided it would be a good idea to have a scientist as Director of the NIMH and since the neurology institute was to be part of the affiliation it would also be good to get somebody interested in biology. And when he saw the paper on cerebral blood flow in schizophrenia, he thought I was his man. So I moved in 1951.

IK: That was a full four or five years before you ultimately stepped down from the position. At the time, you were recruiting people for the two Institutes.

SK: That was a very exciting period. I began to establish and organize the Intramural Program of the NIMH, and lay down its philosophy. I decided right off the bat that biology was going to be of considerable importance to psychiatry because I was convinced the brain had a great deal to do with mental illness. At the same time, I realized our knowledge of the biology of the brain was very rudimentary and there were a lot of half-baked studies on biological aspects of schizophrenia. People would come up with great new discoveries of chemical changes in the blood they found in patients with schizophrenia but these were all premature, very difficult to replicate and none were ever confirmed. They appeared in the Sunday supplement of newspapers and disappeared very quickly. It was obvious what we needed was a great deal of basic research. We needed much more information about the fundamental aspects of biological processes in the brain, before we could even think of attacking the practical problems. What we needed, if we were to build a bridge across the big chasm between basic knowledge of the brain and mental illness, was to firm up the foundations of the bridge on both sides. We had to firm up basic information about the brain and firm up knowledge of mental illnesses before we could upgrade the connection between them.

IK: Who were some of the people you brought in between1951 and 1956?

SK: That was a very exciting list. The first laboratory I set up – having said all this about biology – was the Laboratory of Socio-Environmental Studies. I set that up because that was the field I knew least about, and because I wanted to make sure we didn't forget about the extra-biological factors that determine mental illness. I sought a director for that laboratory and found we had an outstanding sociologist already working with Bob Felix at the NIMH, and that was John Clausen. So I made John director of Socio-Environmental Studies. Seeking a director for Neurophysiology, I discovered that working quietly in the mental health institute before I got there was an outstanding neurophysiologist, Wade Marshall. He laid the groundwork for studies of the motor and sensory cerebral cortex, which he eventually pursued with Rose and Bard at Johns Hopkins. Then Wade became seriously ill and left the project while Rose and Bard went on to pursue it. They made beautiful maps of the cortex of the cat and monkey, which was followed by studies of the human cortex by the neurosurgical group in Montreal. By the time I got to the NIMH, Wade Marshall had been discharged from hospital, had taken a job with Bob Felix in neurophysiology, and was also doing very nice work on the cerebral cortex.

IK: At this time, there was the beginning of a revolution in pharmacology and in psychiatry. Wasn't chlorpromazine being introduced as the first antipsychotic?

SK: Well chlorpromazine was introduced in the United States around 1952 or 1953.

IK: Right.

SK: In 1951 it was being studied in France. Wade Marshall turned out to be an excellent chief of neurophysiology and passing through his laboratory were some of outstanding neurobiologists.

IK: Evarts, Eric Kandel. . . .

SK: Evarts and Kandel, and also Bill Landau and Lewis Rowland, who became two of the outstanding professors of neurology in the country. I appointed

Giulio Cantoni as head of a Laboratory of Comparative Pharmacology, and he brought Seymour Kaufman into his laboratory. When I appointed these people, the understanding was they did not have to work on mental illness. They didn't have to promise to work on the brain. They were to work on what they felt would ultimately be of importance to an understanding of mental illness, but it was up to them to choose the direction in which they went. I also appointed Bill Wendell as head of a Neuroanatomy Laboratory and he recruited Sandy Palay as one of his section chiefs. Palay became an outstanding electron microscopist of the brain.

Alex Rich came from Linus Pauling's laboratory to see me about a position at the NIMH, and Alex impressed talking about the macromolecules of the brain, how protein synthesis might be taking place and how the proteins might be responsible for encoding memory. And I had a long conversation with Linus Pauling on one of his trips to Washington; I remember sitting on a park bench outside the hotel where Linus was staying, and getting his generous recommendation of Alex. So Alex came in as chief of a Laboratory of Physical Chemistry and brought into that laboratory a number of outstanding molecular biologists, who pursued their own careers in a very imaginative way.

Julie Axelrod came to see me from Steve Brodie's laboratory in the Heart Institute. He asked if there was an opportunity to join the mental mealth institute, and thought that he would like to work in Dr. Cantoni's laboratory, because Cantoni was head of the Laboratory of Comparative Pharmacology. I didn't think that was such a good idea because Axelrod was interested more in the applied side of pharmacology, the development of drugs and their metabolism but these were not areas Cantoni was particularly concerned with. But by that time, I had also appointed the head of clinical research in the Institute. This was Bob Cohen, a psychiatrist and psychoanalyst from Chestnut Lodge, who was developing the clinical program, which was largely non-biological. I thought it would be a good idea if Bob were to have a laboratory on the clinical side, interested in biology. Bob had already started such a laboratory with Marion Keyes and Ed Evarts, and was also working with Wade Marshall at the time. So I called Steve Brodie to make sure he knew I was thinking of offering Axelrod a position. We didn't want to rob another institute without letting them know.

IK: Julie had just obtained his PhD hadn't he?

SK: No, he hadn't. I referred Julie, then, to Bob Cohen saying he looked like an extremely attractive individual and it would be good if he gave him an appointment in the laboratory he was developing on the clinical side. So Julie joined the NIMH working in that program.

By that time, I had asked Lou Sokoloff, who had been working with me at Penn, to join me at NIH. I set up a Laboratory of Cerebral Metabolism and made Sokoloff chief of a Section in that Laboratory. That was the laboratory where I hoped to do some research in addition to organizing the Intramural Program. In 1956, I felt I had done my share. I'd spent five years organizing the Intramural Program, recruiting an outstanding group of people, and I spoke to Bob Felix about the possibility of stepping down from the position of scientific director to become a laboratory chief. Bob was very generous; he saw the possibilities, and permitted me to step down. I became chief of a new laboratory, which had already been started with Ed Evarts, Julie Axelrod, Marion Keyes and Roger McDonald, then nominally the chief. He had decided to call it the Laboratory of Clinical Science. They were all happy to have me as lab chief and shortly after that you turned up.

IK: Even before that you were interested in the adrenochrome hypothesis of schizophrenia.

SK: Was that before you came?

IK: That was about the time I came, because Julie was attracted to the path laid by you. This was around the time I came. I was your first research associate and we were talking about serotonin and tryptophan at that time. My first project was to make radioactive tryptophan, to follow along the serotonin line; but I think you also stimulated interest in the catecholamines because of the pink adrenaline story.

SK: Yes, I felt the function of this Laboratory of Clinical Science was to attempt to bridge the gap between basic science and the clinical program, and one thing we could start with was schizophrenia. Now, I definitely did not want to assign people to work on schizophrenia, but I thought it might be possible to stimulate interest in schizophrenia by having a series of seminars at which various members presented papers, reviews or whatever on the topic. Very early in that series, I talked about work I'd heard about in Saskatchewan by Hoffer and Osmond on adrenochrome. They claimed that oxidized adrenaline injected into human beings would produce symptoms like those of schizophrenia. That was a long story. First they became interested in pink adrenaline. During the war, people who got pink adrenaline – pink because it was oxidized to adrenochrome while sitting around – were claimed to have hallucinations. Hoffer and Osmond became interested in pink adrenaline and injected adrenochrome into themselves. They claimed they had hallucinations and that it produced all kinds of symptoms. In any case, it seemed it would be interesting to see what adrenochrome did in humans and study its metabolism. Their theory was that in the schizophrenic adrenaline was metabolized by an erroneous pathway to adrenochrome and that adrenochrome was hallu-cinogenic and produced the symptoms of schizophrenia. In order to test that, we were stuck, because we didn't even know the normal metabo-lism of adrenaline, let alone its metabolism in schizophrenia.

I thought the thing to do was study the metabolism of adrenaline under normal circumstances and in schizophrenics. But in order to do that I knew it would be necessary to get radioactive adrenaline of a very high specific activity, because adrenaline is such a powerful phar-macologic agent that one could only give traces of it. So it had to be loaded with enough radioactivity to measure. ^{14}C adrenaline, which was available, would not be suitable. I tried to get one or another of the laboratories working with radioactive materials to make some tritiated epinephrine. I finally got Seymour Rothschild at New England Nuclear to agree to a contract from the NIMH to make tritiated epinephrine and he worked on it for a while. Interestingly enough, by the time the tritiated epinephrine came to our laboratory Julie Axelrod had already worked out the normal metabolism of adrenaline.

IK: That was around 1957. I think it was at the Federation Meetings in Atlantic City in April of that year that Armstrong and Shaw found vanyllylmandelic acid (VMA), the major metabolite of adrenaline in the urine of patients with pheochromocytoma. Julie was in the audience and after he came back from the meeting he started to become interested in adrenaline metabolism and discovered catechol-O-methyltransferase. But I think the metabolism of adrenaline in animals or patients had not yet been worked out, and it was due to the tritium-labeled adrenaline produced under your prompting that made it possible for these other studies to begin.

SK: Well, Julie discovered catechol-O-methyltransferase and the metabolism by that route. In fact, he did the whole metabolic series and published before the radioactive adrenaline came.

IK: That's about the time that I arrived.

SK: What the radioactive adrenaline did was permit us to do the study in human brains. And using radioactive epinephrine, we did what I had hoped. We administered it to normal subjects and schizophrenics and studied what came out in the urine. Now, before Julie's contribution I thought that we would simply do chromatography of the urine and look for where the radioactivity was and see if the radioactivity appeared in spots in schizophrenics where it didn't appear in normals, and then try to track it down. But, when we started the work we knew what substances to look for and how to extract them.

IK: Roger McDonald set up these long columns for the assay of VMA.

SK: And LaBrosse and Mann did the analysis of the urine and studied the radioactive metabolites in schizophrenics and normals using Julie's methods for discriminating these substances and analyzing them. They eventually found they could not identify any adrenochrome in the urine of the schizophrenics and also that adrenaline disappeared in the blood of the schizophrenics at the same rate it disappeared in normals. So we were unable to confirm any of Hoffer and Osmond's hypotheses about adrenochrome. But Julie went on, and we also had Seymour Rothschild make radioactive noradrenaline. It was the radioactive noradrenaline that Julie used to make the discovery of reuptake, which I think was the discovery that won him the Nobel Prize.

IK: Right.

SK: He asked if he could have some of the radioactive noradrenaline, which I was only too happy to let him have, because that's why we made it, and he said he wanted to study its distribution in the body of cats, rats, or both. I said what do you want to do that for, it's sort of a half-baked idea to study the distribution of adrenaline in various organs. But, I gave him the stuff anyhow. He measured the distribution of radioactive norepinephrine and found it was highly concentrated in structures and tissues that had a high density of sympathetic nerve endings.

IK: Endogenous norepinephrine, right?

SK: From that he concluded that the radioactive noradrenaline he had injected, was being taken up by nerve endings and stored in the vesicles.

IK: George Hertting was with him at the time, and Fleckenstein from Vienna where George had come from in Austria, had described the potentiation of noradrenaline by cocaine. And there was also Bacq in Belgium, who reported that pyrogallol potentiated catecholamines. Those two findings, that pyrogallol was an inhibitor of catechol-O-methyltransferase, and cocaine inhibited uptake, led Julie to conclude that uptake is important and that perhaps drugs influence the uptake. And that's what started the story of transporters, because cocaine was the first drug to be shown to inhibit the uptake of noradrenaline. This was a paper published with George Hertting. It started an avalanche of research in the catecholamine area, and you played a very important role in stimulating the hypotheses of catecholamines in relation to depression. Joe Schildkraut had come into the lab somewhat later, but all the connections of biological substances with psychiatric illness grew out of the ideas you were fostering at the time and encouraged in the people who came into our lab.

SK: I didn't have much to do with the direct studies on catecholamines and mental illness. Joe Schildkraut developed the catecholamine hypothesis entirely on his own.

IK: I don't think that would have happened if he were not in the environment you created.

SK: He published a paper and put my name on it because we had many discussions together.

IK: He was right in doing that, because I don't think the theory would have developed without many of the concepts in biological psychiatry that were the basis of future studies, or without conversations with you. You helped generate the general concepts of the importance of biological interactions with drugs in brain as clues to mechanisms of mental illness. You may not take responsibility for these ideas, but if they had been bad you would have been blamed anyway, so you may as well take the credit you deserve.

SK: I remember making a big point about chemical neurotransmitters. I was fascinated by these chemical synaptic transmissions, which was a new concept then.

IK: We skipped one thing chronologically. Somewhere around 1960, largely in recognition of the importance of biological psychiatry and your critical role in it, you were offered and accepted, at least for a short time, the position of chairman of the department of psychiatry at Johns Hopkins. This was really a departure from the traditional appointment because I don't think you were a psychiatrist, although I understood from Josie that there was a time when you underwent psychoanalysis. Can you tell us about that? I remember a very amusing conversation you had with her in regard to an offer by the NIH to pay for your psychoanalysis.

SK: Seymour Vestermark, of blessed memory, was head of training in the early mental health institute, and right after I was appointed a scientific director, he came to me and said, "Seymour, I think you ought to have an analysis and we'll pay for it, because the scientific director of the NIMH ought to know something about psychoanalysis." I came home and told Josephine that they wanted to give me a free psychoanalysis, and she said, "If they offered to take your appendix out for nothing, would you let them do it?" That was enough for me to tell Seymour I wasn't interested. He didn't come back again until about 1960, when again he broached the subject, and this time I thought, well . . .

IK: Have your appendix out!

SK: I thought I'd have my appendix out for nothing. So they picked the dean of psychoanalysts in Washington, Edith Weigart, a lovely woman from Vienna, and I went through about a year of psychoanalysis, at which time . . .

IK: You qualified for chairman of the department.

SK: Yes, in the middle of that I was offered the chairmanship of psychia-
     try at Hopkins, which was the most distinguished chair of psychiatry in
     America; it was the chair Adolf Meyer established and he was the father
     of American psychiatry. I was struggling with whether to accept that posi-
     tion while I was in analysis, and I think I spent most of the time in analysis
     arguing with myself as to whether to take the job or not. I remember get-
     ting angry with Edith, because I would say, "You know more about me
     than anybody else. What do you think I ought to do? Why don't you ever
     give me any advice? Why do you let me struggle with these decisions
     entirely on my own?" Finally, I accepted, and the reason I was offered the
     position was that the search committee at Hopkins decided the time was
     ripe for a biologist to be chairman of psychiatry and didn't care whether I
     was a psychiatrist or not. In fact, I wasn't a psychiatrist. I was a physiolo-
     gist. And, so, I went to Hopkins for a year.
IK: About that time was when the American College of Neuropsychopharma-
     cology (ACNP) started.
SK: Yes.
IK: Can you tell us about your role in starting the ACNP?
SK: I was a charter member, Paul Hoch was a good friend of mine and also
     Fritz Freyhan. I had worked with Fritz; we had done studies of cerebral
     blood flow in schizophrenia. Paul Hoch was the one who started the
     ACNP, and he gathered around him a group of people, including me, and
     I was a member of the first Council. Joel Elkes, by that time, had come to
     the NIH. That was all I did with regard to the ACNP. I was a member of the
     Council.
IK: The time was ripe to have a College of this nature because of the interest
     in biological psychiatry and the discovery of the first psychopharmaco-
     logical agents. I think the founders of the College were following up on
     many of the ideas which you had a major role in developing; the impor-
     tance bridging the basic sciences of pharmacology and neurochemistry
     with brain function and mental disorders. That was probably why you
     were included in the group. I'm sure it was.
SK: I was one of the few people around doing biological studies in psychiatry
     or fostering that approach.
IK: What happened when you sat in Adolf Meyer's chair?
SK: The chair promptly fell down! We decided that Adolf's chair of psychiatry
     had to be repaired, so we called the maintenance department and had it
     repaired.
IK: I see. Did that repair entail your returning to NIH, because a year later you
     did?

SK: I discovered I really wasn't interested in being chairman of the department of psychiatry, because being chairman of any department is not a great pleasure nowadays. With psychiatry it's even worse, because you deal not only with administrative matters to do with medicine and research, but with administrative matters that have to do with nurses, police, social workers and a whole mélange of health professionals that I had very little interest in. I didn't mind administering research, but administering more than that was not of great interest. So, after a year, I screwed up my courage and went to the see the Dean at Hopkins and told him that I was sorry to say I would like to relinquish the position.

IK: You came back to NIH for a few years. Then you went to Paris for a year, and then we didn't see you again for a long time.

SK: I didn't go to Paris until 1967.

IK: That's right that was a number of years later. But you did not come back to NIH from Paris. You went to Harvard, and developed the Mailman Research Center at McLean Hospital. Later, we were fortunate enough to attract you back to NIH. I'm not sure how that happened, but it was certainly a good thing for us. You've continued as a senior scientist, influencing research and that seems sort of full circle, because people are doing a lot of the things you set out to do when you were doing your early cerebral blood flow research, studying the metabolism of the brain and how it changes. Now we use the new imaging techniques that Sokoloff developed out of much of the work you did. He attends many of the ACNP meetings, and we see imaging as part of understanding how the brain works. All that is really an outgrowth of work back when you started studies of cerebral metabolism, and the biological psychiatry you fostered has grown.

      I think that we've used up about our allotted time. There's so much more we could talk about because you've had such a distinguished career and influenced so many people. Fully one half of the College is descended from people you've trained, either directly or indirectly as grandchildren and great grandchildren of the trainees that came through the Laboratory of Clinical Science.

SK: Well, we've spent a lot of time talking about what you think my contributions were to biological psychiatry and to pharmacology; but we haven't talked about the studies that really had little to do with pharmacology, namely the use of the adoption strategy, the study of the genetics of schizophrenia, and also the regional blood flow studies which I did shortly after I came to NIH. While I was still scientific director, Bill Landau came to see me from Wade Marshall's laboratory, thought it would be nice to measure regional cerebral blood flow and asked if he could work with me doing that.

IK: You had all those equations worked out already.

SK: I said, "You came to the right person, because I have the equations that I've been dying to try out but haven't had the chance; if you're interested, we can try to apply them to our study. Bill Landau got Walter Freygang to join him, and Lou Sokoloff by that time had come to NIH so I asked him to join us. Bud Rowland who was a postdoc in Wade Marshall's lab also joined us, and the four of us spent a good year or two developing the regional blood flow studies using those equations and a band-saw to cut up the frozen brains of cats, which were loaded with a radioactive inert gas, trifluoroiodomethane, to make autoradiograms. These were the first studies of the regional circulation of the brain. Bill Landau then published a paper with all of us, measuring the cerebral blood flow in twenty eight regions of the brain. That was the technique which was eventually picked up by Marcus Raichle in positron emission tomography, using radioactive water in studies of regional blood flow in the human brain. Lou Sokoloff took off from that and went further. It had been my hope that, eventually, once we measured regional blood flow it would be possible to measure regional oxygen consumption. But Lou decided that regional glucose metabolism was going to be easier to measure and developed, with Martin Reivich, the deoxyglucose technique. It was the deoxyglucose technique that first established a raison d'être for the positron emission tomography (PET) scanners, which then became the first instrument for measuring blood flow and metabolism in the human brain.

IK: I don't think we have too much time left, but tell us a little bit about the genetics of schizophrenia, because that was a landmark study, and the beginning of the genetics of mental disorders.

SK: In 1959, I wrote a review for *Science*, on the biochemical theories of schizophrenia, in which I reviewed research purporting to show a biochemical lesion or a biochemical fault in schizophrenia. I discovered, to my disappointment, that most of these theories did not hold water, and were based on poor techniques and poor controls, with a lack of replication. But the one area that seemed the most promising was the evidence that genetic factors play a role in schizophrenia. What was the evidence? Well, schizophrenia runs in families, but that had not really disturbed psychiatrists very much because they agreed the reason it ran in families was because parents taught it to their children. And so, the schizophrenogenic mother and schizophrenogenic parent hypothesis flourished to explian the familial distribution of schizophrenia. Then there were the twin studies, and there were a number of twin studies in which high concordance rates were found in monozygotic twins with lower concordance equal to that found in fraternal twins. But even that didn't shake the psychogenic theories of schizophrenia, because they argued that monozygotic twins share their environment much more than dizygotic twins, and one couldn't be sure it was genetic rather than environmental factors.

It was then I thought there was a better way of separating the environmental from the genetic factors and that would be the study of adopted individuals who developed schizophrenia. In order to do this, I decided that one would need a national study and I suggested this in the review I published in 1959. I laid out the strategy one could use for studying the distribution of schizophrenia in the biological and the adoptive families of adopted schizophrenics, and pointed out it would require a national sample and that effort would have to be made to minimize subjective bias. I then discovered that David Rosenthal at NIMH was interested in doing an adoption study of the children of schizophrenic parents and how they developed schizophrenia. Paul Wender was not only interested in doing an adoption study, but actually started to collect a sample population. His interest was in the adoptive parents of schizophrenics to see to what extent the schizophrenia in these people could possibly be attributed to the adoptive parents. He was pulling together a sample of adoptive parents but he was not having a great deal of luck doing this in America.

We learned about Denmark, which had wonderful population records and psychiatric records, and a national psychiatric register, and so in 1963, I flew over to Copenhagen and met with Fini Schulsinger, who introduced me to the records they have. With our assurances of complete confidentiality, they made those records available to us and we set up a national register of all the adopted people in Denmark who had grown up. In that register, we found those who had developed schizophrenia. Then we were able to trace their biological relatives and their adopted relatives and find out if schizophrenia runs in families, and which family of an adopted schizophrenic it runs in, the biological family or the adopted family and we found that it ran in the biological families.

IK: Well, it's really been great for you to review with us some of the early history of your career and about the impact it has had on biological psychiatry, which is really what the ACNP is all about. So, thank you very much. It's been a real pleasure for me to be able to review these things, most of which I didn't know, some of which I did.

SK: You cut me off before I was going to talk about your coming into the laboratory.

IK: We're not here to talk about me. We're here to talk about you.

LOUIS SOKOLOFF

Interviewed by Thomas A. Ban
San Juan, Puerto Rico, December 8, 2003

TB: This will be an interview with Dr. Louis Sokoloff* for the Archives of the American College of Neuropsychopharmacology. We are at the annual meeting of the College in San Juan. It is December 8, 2003. I am Thomas Ban. I think we should start from the beginning. Please tell us where and when you were born, something about your education and so on.

LS: I was born in 1921 in Philadelphia, one of two sons of immigrant parents. We grew up in the 1920s and 1930s. It was the great depression, a very bad period. My father was a working man, and there was always a problem of finding a job. It was also a time of intensive union organization and there were frequent strikes during which he could not work. The depression years were very formative in establishing my attitudes and viewpoints. I think that its impact on me probably made me a liberal for life. We didn't have money for fun, and so I spent much of my time in reading. The public library system in Philadelphia was quite good, and I used it constantly to take out books.

My brother was six years older than I, and he had a big impact on my interests. He was academically inclined and had always wanted to be a physician, but we did not know if we would ever be able to afford the tuition for higher education. When he graduated high school in 1933, however, he won a scholarship to the University of Pennsylvania. While there he majored in zoology, and probably because of that I also developed an interest. My brother lived at home during his college years and had all his textbooks there. I would read them and learned a pretty fair amount of zoology before I even got to college myself.

The depression did have some beneficial effects on our educational system. The faculties in the Philadelphia public high school system were excellent, because many of the teachers had previously been on university faculties. Many universities, the University of Pennsylvania included, were closing down departments to save money, and so there were former faculty members who needed jobs. Some of them might have chosen to transfer from the universities because of higher salaries in the Philadelphia high schools. Therefore a number of the teachers, perhaps as many as half in my high school, were PhDs. They were excellent and very stimulating teachers. I knew that I would be unable to afford to go to college unless I also got a scholarship. Fortunately, I managed to do so by graduating first in my class in high school. At that time the person

---

* Louis Sokoloff was born in Philadelphia, Pennsylvania in 1921.

who graduated first was granted a four-year scholarship to the University of Pennsylvania.

TB: When did you start college?

LS: In September 1939, just a couple of weeks after World War II had begun in Europe. I began my studies at the University of Pennsylvania with the intention of majoring in zoology. The College of Arts and Science in the University had a liberal arts and sciences program in which the first two years were largely defined or prescribed. As I remember, the requirements included three semesters of English composition, one each on the history of the English language and English literature, and also choices of courses in the physical and social sciences. Majors were chosen at the end of the second year. In my first year the science courses I chose were General Zoology and General Inorganic Chemistry, and in my second year Qualitative and Quantitative Analytic Chemistry and Organic Chemistry. I found that I really liked chemistry, but my heart was still set on biology. Penn at that time had separate departments of Botany and Zoology, and although I was mainly interested in animal biology I also took a couple of courses in botany.

When the time came for me to choose a major, my brother, who by then had had six years of experience, advised me and convinced the family I should not major in zoology. Because we were still in a time of depression, he thought I should choose chemistry rather than zoology as my major because there were few jobs for zoologists but greater employment opportunities for chemists. At that time the Atlantic Refining Company and Sunoco Oil Company were located in Philadelphia, and these oil companies were still occasionally hiring chemists. I stubbornly resisted his advice, but compromised by choosing zoology as my major but also taking as electives all the courses required of chemistry majors.

By my third year, the United States was also in the war. Although I was eligible for the military draft, I was granted a deferment because I was a potential medical student, and premedical and medical students were being deferred. It was during this school year that I took a mixed graduate-undergraduate course called General Physiology, but it was really cell biology. This course was taught by an outstanding cell biologist, Louis Victor Heilbrunn. He was to my knowledge the first, certainly the most vociferous one, to propose a key role for calcium in a variety of physiological and cellular processes, such as blood clotting, muscle contraction, regulation of protoplasmic viscosity in cells, membrane integrity and permeability, and cellular excitability. He argued that excitation in cells was associated with increased intracellular free ionic calcium concentrations derived from increased membrane transport and/or release from bound stores. Much of this is now accepted as true, but he was ahead of his time and considered by many to be obsessed with calcium.

This was a two-semester course with both laboratory work and lectures. In the first half of each semester we had assigned laboratory experiments, essentially exercises, we had to do, and then in the second half of the semesters we were required to carry out an original research project. My research project in the first semester was to determine if the flow of protoplasm in the pseudopod of the amoeba obeyed Poiseuille's Law. I found that it did not. In the second semester my research project, mutually agreed upon by Heilbrunn, Dan Harris, one his senior graduate students and teaching assistants, and myself, was to fractionate cells into their subcellular components and identify enzymes localized in each of the fractions. For a variety of reasons, mainly because the project was part of a teaching course and not supported by any research grant, we had to choose a cell type that was cheap, readily available, and relatively pure. We chose the frog egg because it met all of the above criteria. By using differential centrifugation we separated from the homogenized cells cytosol (called plasmasol at that time), pigment granules, lipid fraction and yolk. We found lipases in the lipid fraction and dipeptidases in the cytosol. I don't recall what enzymes we looked for and found in the yolk. This was in 1942, a couple of years before Schneider and Hogeboom reported their fractionation of cells into much more interesting subcellular components, for example, mitochondria, microsomes, and cytosol. I guess you can say we missed the boat, but the project certainly stimulated my interests in biochemical and biophysical aspects of cell biology.

This experience led me to enroll during my last year in an elective course called Undergraduate Research in Zoology, which allowed me to carry out further research under Heilbrunn. Because the United States was at war, Heilbrunn had switched his research activities to a defense-related project supported by an army grant. This project was to study the effects of heat on tissues. The army was interested in this research because of the numerous heat-related casualties the British 8th Army in North Africa was suffering. Heilbrunn's entire staff, postdoctoral fellows and graduate and undergraduate students were all working on various aspects of the effects of heat on tissues. My assignment was to use the rat sciatic nerve/gastrocnemius preparation, to determine the relative sensitivities of nerve and muscle to heat. The preparation was dissected out, and either the nerve or the muscle was submersed in Ringer's solution at 42°C. The nerve and muscle were alternately stimulated electrically, and the muscle contractions were detected by means of a mechanical lever and smoked drum. The stimulations were continued until muscle contractions ceased, and the time for this to occur was recorded. We found that the nerve was quite resistant and could be heated for some time before it failed to transmit the stimulation signal to the muscle. In contrast, when the muscle was in the heated bath, muscle contraction elicited by nerve stimulation was rapidly lost but was maintained considerably longer in response to direct muscle stimulation. This indicated that the myoneural junction was the most vulnerable component of the preparation to heat.

Heilbrunn considered this observation sufficiently interesting to merit publication. I began to work on a manuscript at a desk located in an office I shared with Paul LeFevre, who was then a graduate student of Heilbrunn's and later became well known for his work on red cell permeability. One day, as I was working on the manuscript, he told me that he had run across a paper that might interest me. Indeed, it did. It was a chapter written in French in 1870 by Claude Bernard in a book, *Dictionnaire de Physiologie*, edited by Charles Richet. Claude Bernard had carried out almost the identical experiments that we had, except that he used oil instead of Ringer's solution, and he obtained the same results and drew the same conclusions as we did. I guess the culture of science was somewhat different then from today; it was a time when quality of publications rather than their number was what counted. Even though Bernard had done the work and published it more than 70 years previously, Heilbrunn acknowledged that we had been scooped and decided not to publish our results because someone else had already published the same findings and conclusions.

Because of my experience in Heilbrunn's laboratory, I became so fascinated with laboratory research that I asked him if he would accept me as a graduate student to work for a PhD in zoology. He said he would be willing to accept me but advised me not to do that. His reason was that because of the war he was having trouble keeping his graduate students from the military draft. He advised me instead to go to medical school which would allow me to be deferred until I finished. I also remember him saying that he generally did not care much for medical education, but added, "Medical school doesn't necessarily spoil everybody for scientific research." He also said, "I'll write you a strong letter of recommendation, and when I write a letter that strong, the student is always accepted." He did write such a letter, and I was accepted into medical school at Penn. Because of the war the medical school had adopted an accelerated program, and therefore my classes began at an odd time in March 1943. The accelerated program was designed to complete the four-year curriculum in three years to speed up the supply of physicians to meet the needs of the armed forces. The acceleration was achieved by having the courses immediately follow one another with no breaks or vacations.

TB: You started medical school in 1943.

LS: Our first course was anatomy, and it made me think of quitting medical school. The atmosphere and my experience was enormously different from what I had enjoyed so much while working in Heilbrunn's lab. There we had been treated with respect as though we were mature scholars, whereas in the anatomy classes we were treated like kindergarten children. Everything was presented as an absolute fact to be accepted and memorized. There were no dynamic processes to be analyzed and no room for questioning or argument. Because of the war I stuck it out, and subsequent courses in the first year turned out to be more interesting. They included physiology and biochemistry, both of which I enjoyed very much, as I also did pharmacology which followed.

About three months after starting my first year the military took over the medical school. We were given the choice of joining either the army or the navy, provided of course we could pass their physical examinations. We had the option of not joining either, and anyone who chose not to would be deferred from the draft until graduation. However, we were encouraged to join because the military would pay all the tuition and provide the necessary textbooks and equipment, while those not joining had to cover these expenses themselves. The tuition fee alone was $400 per year which does not seem very much today, but it was a great deal at that time. My family's resources had been stretched by the payment for my first year, and I doubt we could have afforded the costs till graduation. Joining the military was, therefore, a great opportunity for me. Because my myopia disqualified me for the navy, I joined the army in July 1943, and went through the remainder of my medical education while a private in the Army Specialized Training Program (ASTP).

All through medical school I found that I enjoyed the basic science courses most. These were physiology, biochemistry and pharmacology. I suppose that I also enjoyed bacteriology and pathology, but not nearly as much. Although I was less interested in the clinical courses, I managed to do all right and graduated second in my class in March 1946.

TB: What did you do after graduation?

LS: Immediately following graduation from medical school, the army released me into the inactive reserves. This was a temporary arrangement to allow me to complete an internship and obtain a license to practice medicine, after which they would recall me to active duty as a medical officer. I served my internship at the Philadelphia General Hospital (PGH), which doesn't exist anymore. It was a city hospital with 2,500 beds. The internship was a rotating one, which the state of Pennsylvania then required for licensing. My first rotation was in psychiatry. Subsequent rotations – not necessarily in this order – were in tuberculosis, obstetrics, gynecology, laboratory medicine, internal medicine, orthopedic surgery, general surgery, neurology, and clinical pathology. Some of these rotations, such as obstetrics, were mandated by the state. Because the internship was also an accelerated program during the war, it was compressed from its normal full year into nine months during which we met all the required rotations.

By that time the war had ended, and it was decided in the midst of my internship to return to one year. In order to return to the normal July 1 to June 30 schedule, my class was given an extra six months, all to be served on a single service. The service to which I was assigned was Psychiatry. The transition from the nine-month to the full year schedule resulted in several months of overlap of a new group of interns with our class, during which the members of our class assumed duties and activities more like those of a resident than an intern. During that period I gained a lot of experience that included insulin coma and electroshock therapy. It was also a time when many physicians were returning from military service and seeking advanced training in medical specialties supported by the GI Bill of Rights.

PGH had a very active psychiatric program with an almost unlimited supply of patients. It was housed in its own building which contained about 300 beds for inpatients and very active outpatient clinics. Furthermore, it was a teaching hospital with four psychiatric services, each chaired by a faculty member of the various medical schools in Philadelphia. Medical students from those schools served their rotations in psychiatry there. The PGH Division of Psychiatry, headed by John Stouffer, became a training center for physicians returning from the war, and our faculty included, among others, O. Spurgeon English from Temple University, Samuel Hadden from the University of Pennsylvania, and a Dr. Schlesinger, whose first name I cannot recall, from Jefferson Medical College. The training program included formal classes, lectures, and clinics, in which interns and residents were allowed to participate. This greatly expanded our learning and experience beyond practical experience in the wards and clinics which was also quite considerable. In addition to outpatient duties each intern was responsible for two wards of approximately forty beds each. The psychiatric services were very active with a large turnover, and we experienced and learned a great deal.

My internship ended in June, 1947, and we were allowed a couple of months to take our state board licensing examinations after which the army recalled us to active duty. I reentered the army as a medical officer in August, 1947, and was assigned to the Medical Field Service School in Fort Sam Houston, Texas, for basic training that included setting up and operating battlefield aid stations and field hospitals. After about a month of training we received permanent assignments. To encourage us to choose careers in the army, they sent a plane-load of brass from Washington to interview us about our preferences for specialty and place of assignment. We were allowed three choices for each. In keeping with my interest in the basic medical sciences, my first choice for specialty was physiology and specifically in the army's environmental physiology laboratory located at Fort Knox, Tennessee. My second and third choices for specialty were internal medicine and neuropsychiatry. My second and third choices for places of assignment were Europe and California, in that order. In typical army fashion, they gave me none of my top choices and assigned me to Camp Lee, Virginia as Chief of Neuropsychiatry in a 150-bed station hospital. My assignment to neuropsychiatry was undoubtedly due to my previous experience during internship and probably because of the army's shortage of psychiatrists at that time.

TB: So this was in some way your third encounter with psychiatry.

LS: When I reported to Camp Lee, I found that there had not been a psychiatrist there for about six months. Their last one had completed his term of service and been discharged, and the army had been unable to find a replacement. In the interval neuropsychiatry was covered by the medical service which was very happy to see me come. When I arrived, I was given the option of keeping neuropsychiatry within the medical service or restoring it to its previous independent status. I chose to keep it within the medical service so that I could maintain some contact with internal medicine in which I was still interested, particularly metabolic disorders.

Although I did participate in the care of patients in the medical service, most of my time was spent in neuropsychiatry. There were some neurological patients, but these were infrequent in subjects of the age group with which I was dealing. Most of the neurological conditions I saw were acute and most often due to injuries or sub-arachnoid hemorrhages, but I did see one case of a relatively rare and interesting condition, Thomsen's disease, myotonia congenita. I was also Chief of the so-called Psychiatric Consultation Service which was responsible for evaluating all soldiers considered for court martial and those with behavior problems who were under consideration for discharge due to inability, inaptitude, or undesirable traits of character. Many of the latter fell into the category called at that time "Constitutional Psychopathic Inferior," and now Sociopathic Personality. Most of my time was spent with psychiatric patients covering the whole range of disorders. These included psychoses such as schizophrenia, but we did not have to treat psychotics. They were rapidly transferred to an army general hospital, usually Walter Reed. Consequently, most of my patients were neurotic. We were responsible for the care not only of the military personnel but also their families. This was fortunate because it gave me the opportunity to acquire experience with a greater variety of conditions and types of patients that included soldiers' wives and children.

Patients voluntarily coming or referred to me obviously needed help. What kind of help could a psychiatrist give them? Neuropsychopharmacology had not yet evolved. Psychiatry in the US at that time was largely dominated by psychoanalytic thinking. I had never been trained as a psychoanalyst, but I had been extensively exposed to it during my internship and had read a great deal of the psychoanalytic literature. It seemed to me that it offered the best opportunity to provide effective psychotherapy to neurotic patients, so I adopted a sort of a modified or diluted psychoanalytic approach to psychotherapy. Most of my psychiatric patients were outpatients. I usually saw them for an hour twice a week during which they were allowed to freely associate and were interrupted only by an occasional question or comment. One of my patients, the wife of a sergeant, had been referred by the medical clinic. She had been a patient for a long time with a history of a variety of physical complaints, joint pains, headaches, gastrointestinal disturbances, chronic fatigue, etc., but they could never find any physical basis for them. They finally decided that she was a hypochondriac and referred her to me. I met with her twice weekly for an hour each time over a period of about six months. Generally, I would begin each session with the question, "How have you been feeling since I last saw you?" I vividly remember the occasion when, after about six months of psychotherapy, her response to the question was, "Wonderful. I haven't felt this well in 13 years." I was flabbergasted. Although I had provided her psychotherapy, I really didn't have much faith in it. How did it happen? How could having her do most of the talking twice weekly for six months relieve her of all her physical complaints? Being strongly oriented toward the physical sciences and biology, I was sure that it had something to do with physiological or biochemical changes and, most likely, in the brain. To psychoanalysts, I suppose, this didn't matter.

Leon Eisenberg, a medical school classmate of mine, has since became a prominent psychiatrist and is now at Harvard. You may know him.

TB: Yes, I do.

LS: This is a digression, but I believe an amusing one. Several years ago Leon was invited to present a lecture to the Royal Society of Psychiatry. This required a manuscript, and he sent me a draft of it. It was entitled "Mindlessness and Brainlessness in Psychiatry." In it he compared the state of psychiatry in earlier days, for example when I was in the army practicing psychiatry and it was strongly influenced by psychoanalysis, and its present state. To psychoanalysts the brain was irrelevant. They were concerned only with the mind, whatever it might be and wherever it resided. Today psychiatry is concerned mainly with physical elements within the brain, such as receptors, neurotransmitters, synapses, second messengers, genes, etc. Little thought is devoted to the mind per se.

At any rate, even in those days I had faith that psychiatric disorders, not only those associated with organic brain disease but also the psychoses and neuroses, were diseases of the brain and had a biological basis. Of the functional disorders this seemed to me to be particularly true of schizophrenia. I had several clinical experiences that tended to reinforce that belief. When I was at PGH, we saw many catatonic schizophrenics which are relatively rare today. They frequently exhibited signs that suggested abnormal physiology. For example, I remember one catatonic patient who wouldn't eat, and we had to feed him by nasogastric tube. We would insert the tube through his nose, and when the tip reached his pharynx, we would squirt a little water through it to stimulate his swallowing reflex. He did not appear to resist, except on one occasion he contracted his nares so firmly that we could hardly move the tube in or out. That indicated extraordinarily strong muscle contractions beyond the range of normal physiological function and suggested that there was some neurophysiological alteration. Therefore, although I used a psychoanalytic approach for the treatment of my psychiatric patients, I always believed in biochemical or biophysical abnormalities in the brain as the cause of mental diseases. As a result of my experiences in psychiatry at PGH and in the army and my long interests in physiology and biochemistry, I began to consider a career in which I might combine those interests in studies of the biology of mental disease, and that to me meant studying the brain.

The required duration of my army service, beginning in August, 1947, was two years, and toward the end of 1948, I began to give serious thought about what I would do when I was discharged in 1949. After my time and experience in neuropsychiatry an obvious choice would have been to serve a psychiatric residency and obtain board certification in psychiatry, and I gave this possibility serious consideration. I still, however, entertained thoughts of getting back to basic research, particularly on the brain. Sometime late in 1948 I ran across a series of papers by Seymour Kety and Carl Schmidt on the development and use of their nitrous oxide method for measuring cerebral blood flow and metabolism in man. I knew both of them from medical school. My class in medical school was Kety's first after he joined Schmidt's Department of Pharmacology. I remembered him as a very kind, considerate, and supportive person and an excellent teacher, not much older than we were. He was about six years older than I was, about the same age as my brother. In fact, Kety and my brother had attended Penn at the same time.

The nitrous oxide method measured the rates of the brain's blood flow, oxygen consumption, glucose utilization, and use or production of any other substrates and metabolic products that could be assayed in blood, and it did this in unanesthetized humans. A description of the method and a number of its applications were reported in a series of six papers published in 1948 in a single issue of the *Journal of Clinical Investigation*. There was another one in the *American Journal of Psychiatry* on its use in schizophrenics. When I first saw these papers, I was immediately impressed by the potential of this method as a powerful tool with which to study the human brain in health and disease, including psychiatric disorders, and that was something I really wanted to do. I wasn't entirely sure, however, and did not exclude the possibility of first serving a residency in psychiatry.

TB: What did you decide?

LS: My parents were still living in Philadelphia, and so when I was discharged from the army in August 1949, my wife (whom I had married during my internship) and I returned to Philadelphia and lived with them while I was deciding what to do. I did nothing for two weeks, except to think about visiting Kety at Penn and inquiring about the possibility of working with him. Finally, I screwed up my courage and did so without making any prior appointment. I went directly to the office of the Department of Pharmacology in the Medical School building, where he had been located when I was a student, and asked the secretary if I might be able to see him. She replied, "He's not here anymore. He's now in the Department of Physiology and Pharmacology in the Graduate School of Medicine, not in the School of Medicine." I knew that Penn had a Graduate School of Medicine, but I had never heard of its Department of Physiology and Pharmacology.

I later learned that large numbers of physicians returning from military service were taking advantage of their eligibility for further education supported by the GI Bill of Rights to obtain such education at the Graduate

School of Medicine. One of the School's programs led to a PhD in Medical Sciences, and this program required further education in the basic sciences. The University had therefore established or expanded its basic science departments in the Graduate School of Medicine. There had previously been a small Department of Physiology, but it had expanded into the much larger Department of Physiology and Pharmacology with Julius Comroe as Chairman and Seymour Kety as a full professor, both of whom had previously been in Schmidt's Department of Pharmacology in the School of Medicine. The offices of the Department in the Graduate School were in the basement of the Medical School building, and I found my way down to his office where I asked Mrs. Sullivan, the Department's secretary if I could see Dr. Kety. She told me that he was meeting with someone, but if I was willing to wait, she was sure he would be able to see me. After about a half-hour I was able to meet him. I explained the purpose of my visit, my interest in his work on cerebral blood flow and metabolism, and my desire to work with him. I admitted I was bringing no original research ideas of my own and that my goal was to learn and work in whatever projects he chose for me. He replied that he remembered me from medical school and would be willing to take a chance on me. He then added something which he later claimed not to remember, but which I do very clearly. It was that he had just been notified his grant had been approved and would be funded, and it included the salary for an unfilled position. The position and its salary, however, were for someone with much more experience than mine. Nevertheless, he was willing to take a chance on me but, in view of my inexperience, at a lower salary. He then added that with the money left over he could appoint another fellow like me. Very practical, I thought. His acceptance of me was conditional, however, on its approval by Dr. Comroe, the Department Chairman who of course, would have to interview me. I returned to Mrs. Sullivan to make an appointment and obtained one for two weeks later.

There was an amusing sidelight associated with this interview. While I was standing in the hall waiting to see Kety, Comroe had walked by and, seeing me, asked if I were waiting to see him. At that time I was not yet aware that he was the chairman of the department, and so I said no, I wanted to see Dr. Kety. When I arrived for the interview with him two weeks later, the first thing he said was, "So you thought you could get away without seeing me." What a way to begin! I thought that was the end, but when I explained to him why I was there, he replied that he also remembered me from medical school and would approve the appointment. He asked what my plans were for the future. I was surprised by the question and replied that I thought my plan was obvious. It was to work for Dr. Kety. He explained that he meant my long range plans. Was I coming with the intention to make a career in physiology, or since I had a medical degree, was I coming to spend a year or so in laboratory research before returning to clinical medicine?

My reply was I didn't know. I knew only that I always liked basic science, but since I was just about to begin doing research I did not know if I would prove suited for a research career in physiology. His response was that he remembered me from medical school, was confident I would do well in research, and hoped that I would decide to make a career in physiology. I was flattered and pleased to hear that, but then he added, "But not here." I was surprised and asked what had I said or done wrong for him to have already decided that. He explained there were between 20 and 30 members of the Department, but only three of them were on university salaries: himself, Seymour Kety, and Mrs. Sullivan. "I am 38 years old and in good health and not planning to leave," he continued, "Kety is 35 years old, and as far as I know, also in good health and not planning to leave, so you cannot replace either of us. And as for Mrs. Sullivan, the secretary, I don't think you could do her job." He then added, "You are coming here to help us do our research. In return we will teach you how to do research. If and when you learn enough to be able to do your own research, we'll help you find a place to do it, but somewhere else."

In those days NIH did not allow principal investigators any salary from their own grants. Maybe you remember those days. That was the basis of Comroe's statement that only three in the department were on university salaries. All the others were getting their salaries off Comroe's and Kety's grants. When any of those became independent enough to get their own grants and wished to remain in the department, their salaries would then have to come from the university, and such salaried positions were not readily available. When, I understood this, his statement seemed reasonable, not a criticism of me and I accepted the position.

TB: So, you accepted the position.

LS: It turned out to be a wonderful choice and a great experience. The department was outstanding, arguably the best physiology department in the country at that time. I learned a great deal from Kety and Comroe and from many of the others. One important and lasting lesson was to be completely rigorous and as critical of one's own work as that of others. We learned in our weekly seminars that every statement we made had to be backed up by relevant and substantive facts or reasoning, or else we were subjected to strenuous questioning and criticism. I was indeed very fortunate and happy to have trained there.

TB: When did you join the department?

LS: I joined the department in the fall of 1949. Sometime late in 1950 a couple of men in white uniforms who we thought were naval officers came to see Kety. His office had two doors, one in front opening to the hallway and the other a side door that opened into a large room where all the research fellows had desks. The latter door was almost always open, and we would often go into his office and bother him, or else he would come out and talk with us. He seemed to like to be interrupted and to interact with us. On this occasion that door was closed, and the two uniformed men spent nearly all day in his office. Finally they left, and the door opened. All of us were keenly interested because we knew if the navy wanted something from Kety, it was likely to impact us. We asked Kety what the navy wanted, and he told us they were Public Health Service officers. One was Bob Felix, Director of the newly established National Institute of Mental Health (NIMH). You know him I suppose.

TB: Yes, I do.

LS: The other one was Joe Bobbitt, the Executive Officer of the NIMH. We asked Kety what they wanted, and he informed us they came to offer him the position of Scientific Director of this new institute and also the newly created but smaller National Institute of Neurological Diseases and Blindness (NINDB). His responsibility would be to direct the intramural research programs of both institutes. When we expressed doubts that a full professor in a prestigious Ivy League university, in an excellent department with a very supportive Chairman, would be interested he surprised us by saying he had always been interested in mental health and considered the position a great challenge to do something worthwhile in the field. He would have almost unlimited space, budget, and positions with which to create a formidable research program in neuroscience. The challenge appealed to him, and he would not reject it out of hand. We then asked why they would want a physiologist with little if any training and experience in psychiatry, to develop and head a program in mental health research. He replied that was a good question he himself had asked. Their answer had been that was exactly why they had selected him. They thought a scientific director of a major research program on mental and neurological diseases should be a basic scientist and not a psychiatrist or neurologist.

TB: They wanted a basic scientist.

LS: Kety had received great acclaim and recognition for his development of the nitrous oxide method for measuring cerebral blood flow and metabolism in man and was at the top of his career. He was naturally reluctant to give this up and enter into essentially a new career, and he spent several months agonizing about the offer and consulting others for advice.

Finally, he decided against most advice to accept the offer, and moved from Penn to the NIH, late in the summer of 1951.

TB: What about you?

LS: I stayed at Penn. By then I had become his most senior postdoctoral fellow and continued the research for which Kety had received two NIH grants. Because NIH policy at that time would have prevented me from receiving any salary from those grants if I became principal investigator, Comroe assumed the role of principal investigator and allowed me to continue working on them. The department had two main areas of research directed by Kety and Comroe. Kety's domain was cerebral blood flow and metabolism and peripheral circulation. Comroe's was respiratory physiology. It was an outstanding department. The pulmonary physiology program under Comroe was arguably the finest in the world as was the cerebral blood flow and metabolism program under Kety. Richard Wechsler, who later went into internal medicine and gastroenterology, was Kety's first postdoctoral fellow, and I was his second. We were subsequently joined by Renward Mangold from Berne, Switzerland, who also became a gastroenterologist; Charles Kennedy, a pediatrician who became the first person to be boarded in both pediatrics and neurology; Benton King and Eugene Conners, anesthesiologists; Jerome Kleinerman, who also went into internal medicine; and Reuben Copperman, a graduate student in biophysics from whom I learned a great deal of mathematics. It was a smooth working and very collegial team while it lasted. Kety, of course, had been the magnet that attracted and could assemble such a team. After he left no one new came and the team disintegrated. I was left with Copperman and a technician. Those of us who remained were still happy with our own research, but the atmosphere became somewhat boring because we did not have a critical mass with whom to converse and exchange stimulating ideas. Comroe's pulmonary physiologists did not have much interest in cerebral circulation and metabolism, and we had little interest in their field.

The US Navy had the Naval Air Development Center in Johnsville, Pennsylvania, just outside of Philadelphia. They had established the Aviation Medical Acceleration Laboratory to study the physiological bases for blackout and red-out in pilots undergoing gravitational stresses during maneuvers. This facility was equipped with a centrifuge that had a 50-foot arm and a gondola at the end with which they could subject animals and people to gravitational forces comparable to those encountered by pilots. It was hypothesized but not proven that blackout was due to inadequate perfusion of the brain, and they appointed me as a consultant to assist in the development of a method to measure cerebral blood flow and metabolism during imposed gravitational stresses in the centrifuge. I went to Johnsville once or twice a week to participate in experiments designed to develop such a method. After a couple of years they offered me the position as head of their physiology laboratory.

Because of my feelings of isolation in the department at Penn, I decided to accept the offer and went to Comroe to tell him of my decision. He did not want me to leave, especially to work for the Navy, and asked me to remain in his department and join the group working in pulmonary physiology. I explained to him that lung function might be interesting to some, but I did not find it particularly stimulating and wanted to pursue my interests in cerebral blood flow and metabolism. He then called Kety at NIH to tell him that I wanted to leave the department and suggested he offer me a position rather than let me go to the Navy. Kety then called to offer me a position and explained he had not done so previously because he had not wanted to rob the department at Penn. Since I was leaving anyway, however, why not come to NIH? I accepted his offer.

TB: What year are we in?

LS: This was in 1953. I signed in sometime in December 1953, but did not really begin to work there until early in 1954 because the laboratories were not ready. In the interim I continued working at Penn. When I finally arrived, Kety was working on the development of a method for measuring blood flow in different parts of the brain. There was need for such a method. The nitrous oxide method, which measured only average rates of blood flow and metabolism in the brain as a whole, had shown only reductions in cerebral oxygen consumption in states in which consciousness was impaired. It had failed, however, to show increases in any conditions and did not detect changes in a variety of physiological, pharmacological, and pathophysiological conditions in which cerebral function must certainly have been altered. For example, it showed no changes in cerebral oxygen consumption in subjects during mental arithmetic, slow wave sleep, hyperthyroidism, sedation, inebriation, etc. Cerebral oxygen consumption was also found to be unchanged in schizophrenia, which led Kety to jest that perhaps it took just as much energy to think an irrational thought as a rational thought. These results led to speculations about why cerebral energy metabolism appeared to be unaltered during obvious changes in brain function.

A popular belief at the time was that cerebral metabolism was already operating at its maximal rate which could be reduced by conditions that impaired consciousness but could not be detectably raised by increased functional activity in the brain. The brain was compared to a radio in which most of the energy is used in the filaments to heat the cathodes of the vacuum tubes but is negligibly altered by the signals or information being transmitted, whether it is music, speech, or static. We, however, did not believe that. Our hypothesis was that the nitrous oxide method failed to show increases in energy metabolism during functional activation because it measured only the average in the whole brain while specific functional activities are localized to particular regions of the brain. What was needed was a method that measured energy metabolism in individual regions of the brain. Furthermore, it had to be a method that could be applied without the need for general anesthesia which itself was likely to alter brain functional activity. Kety initiated a project to develop such a method shortly after he arrived at NIH. He was assisted by William Landau and Walter Freygang, both Research Associates in the Laboratory of Neurophysiology, NIMH, and Lewis Rowland, a Clinical Associate in the NINDB, and I joined this group when I arrived.

At that time it was not obvious how one might measure local energy metabolism in the brains of un-anesthetized, behaving animals. Kety's previous research on the principles of inert gas exchange between blood and tissues had led, however, to a possible approach to the determination of local cerebral blood flow. Blood flow in the brain was thought to be adjusted to metabolic demand. This approach proved successful. We succeeded in developing the first method for determination of the rates of blood flow locally in every region of the brain of unanesthetized animals. The method was based on the uptake from blood to brain of a chemically inert, radioactive gas, ^{131}I-labeled trifluoroiodomethane ($[^{131}I]CF^3I$), and it took advantage of a unique quantitative autoradiographic technique that made possible the measurement of local concentrations of the tracer within brain tissues. With this method we were able to measure the rates of blood flow in all parts of the brain in conscious and thiopental-anesthetized cats and found that anesthesia reduced blood flow in all gray matter structures, but particularly in sensory cortical regions, which is the main purpose of general anesthesia.

We also used the method to demonstrate that local blood flow does change in brain regions with normal alterations in functional activity. For example, retinal stimulation with a photoflash was found to increase blood flow in all stations of the primary visual pathways in the cat, and these changes were clearly visualized in the autoradiograms. This was the first demonstration of functional brain imaging. It should be noted that although the blood flow technique was originally developed for use with the ^{131}I-labeled gas $[^{131}I]CF^3I$ and autoradiography, it was later adapted for use with the non-volatile ^{14}C-labeled tracer $[^{14}C]$iodoantipyrine and autoradiography in animals and with ^{15}O-labeled water and PET in man.

TB: Have you been involved in any other projects?

LS: There were other projects in which I was involved after my arrival. For example, I set up the nitrous oxide method for measuring cerebral blood flow and metabolism in man and used it in studies of the effects of LSD and normal aging. My main interests, however, were in metabolism, which required knowledge of biochemistry. Although I had learned a lot of biochemistry from textbooks and reading of the literature, I had relatively little biochemical laboratory experience. It turned out that NIH was a wonderful place to remedy this deficiency because we were all mixed together, biochemists, physiologists, pharmacologists, anatomists, etc. In fact, when I first arrived, I was in the Laboratory of Neurochemistry which contained, in addition to my Section on Cerebral Metabolism, the Section on Lipid Biochemistry and the Section on Physical Chemistry. I was surrounded by biochemists and joined a biochemical journal club. There I met Seymour Kaufman, an outstanding enzymologist who later distinguished himself by his work on the mechanisms of amino acid hydroxylation, for example, phenylalanine hydroxylation to tyrosine, dopamine hydroxylation to norepinephrine, and tryptophane hydroxylation to hydroxytryptophane, all reactions important to neurotransmitter syntheses.

In earlier studies at Penn with the nitrous oxide method we had found cerebral oxygen consumption to be entirely normal in adult patients with hyperthyroidism, in whom total body oxygen consumption was increased by 50–70%. I became interested in the question of what was different about brain energy metabolism compared to that of other tissues that made it unresponsive to thyroid hormones. It soon became obvious, however, that to answer that question one would have to know the mechanism by which thyroid hormones stimulated energy metabolism in responsive tissues. From exhaustive examination of the literature I arrived at the hypothesis that thyroid hormones primarily stimulated protein synthesis but had little if any effect in mature brain because its rate of protein turnover is very low compared to carbohydrate metabolism. I presented this hypothesis and the evidence in favor of it at a session of the biochemical journal club. It turned out that Seymour Kaufman had arrived at the same hypothesis but from a different direction. We decided to collaborate on a project to examine this. It was a fortunate collaboration for me because it was obvious that testing the hypothesis would require mainly biochemical experiments, and though I had always been interested in biochemistry and had acquired a pretty fair knowledge of it from books, I had relatively little experience in laboratory techniques. It turned out to be a very fruitful collaboration. We complemented each other. Kaufman was an outstanding biochemist and enzymologist who came from a background in organic chemistry while I came from a background in physiology and medicine. He was a stern and rigorous teacher who over a period of years trained me in practical as well as theoretical biochemistry and made me a biochemist. I became so intrigued by the power of biochemistry to arrive at definitive conclusions that I remained fully engaged in it for the next 20 years. Incidentally, we found that thyroid hormones do indeed stimulate protein synthesis in those tissues in which they stimulate oxygen consumption, and published this finding first as a preliminary note in *Science* in 1959 and then in more complete form in the *Journal of Biological Chemistry* in 1961.

Although my laboratory work during those years was largely in vitro biochemistry, I never lost my interest in cerebral metabolism and the possibility of using the quantitative autoradiographic technique developed for the local blood flow method to measure local cerebral energy metabolism. Autoradiography requires, of course, the use of a radioactive tracer. Of the two almost exclusive substrates of the brain's energy metabolism, oxygen and glucose, oxygen was impractical because the half-life of its radioactive isotope, ^{15}O, is only two minutes. Glucose labeled with ^{14}C was a possible alternative because its rate of utilization in brain is stochiometrically related to that of oxygen. I tried to develop such a method for use with [^{14}C] glucose shortly after the local blood flow method had been developed. My first step was to try to design a kinetic model for the behavior of [^{14}C]glucose in brain that would define the variables and parameters needed to compute the rate of glucose utilization from measurements of radioactivity in blood and/or plasma and cerebral tissues. I dropped this effort when I realized that [^{14}C]glucose metabolism to $^{14}CO_2$ in brain and the removal of the $^{14}CO_2$ from the brain by the cerebral circulation are so rapid that it was impossible to estimate the amount of product derived from [^{14}C]glucose utilization over a given interval of time.

In 1957 I was writing a chapter for the *Handbook of Physiology* on the metabolism of the central nervous system in vivo and working on the part in which I was arguing that glucose is not only the preferred substrate for the brain's energy metabolism but an essential one. The evidence was that insulin-induced hypoglycemia leads to loss of consciousness, slowing of the EEG, and markedly reduced cerebral oxygen consumption, and that when the blood glucose level is restored by glucose administration, all these changes are reversed. I was looking for additional evidence that the effects of insulin-induced hypoglycemia on brain functions were due to lack of glucose and not to the insulin per se. I was discussing this issue with Don Tower, a neurochemist in the NINDB. He told me about still unpublished studies being carried out by Bernie Landau in the National Cancer Institute in which he was finding that the administration of pharmacologic doses of 2-deoxyglucose, an analogue of glucose, produced a clinical state just like that of insulin-induced hypoglycemia, but in the presence of an elevated blood glucose concentration. The animals lost consciousness, just like in insulin-induced hypoglycemia. Apparently 2-deoxyglucose was interfering somehow with glucose metabolism in the brain. This was the kind of evidence I was looking for, and I cited Landau's work in my chapter as a personal communication. I remained curious, however, about the mechanism of its effects in brain. How did it produce coma? It was likely to be competing with glucose, but the dose that produced coma did not appear to be large enough for the 2-deoxyglucose to compete with the much higher blood glucose levels to the point that blood-brain transport of glucose was insufficient to maintain cerebral glucose utilization and consciousness.

It was known from the earlier studies of Sols and Crane that 2-deoxyglucose was a substrate for hexokinase and could compete with glucose for phosphorylation in the glycolytic pathway. Normally, however, there is plenty of glucose in the brain, and furthermore, hexokinase has a much greater affinity for glucose than for 2-deoxyglucose. It was therefore unlikely that competitive inhibition of glucose phosphorylation was sufficient to produce coma. There must have been some other explanation, but what was it? I didn't do anything about it except to follow the growing literature on the effects of 2-deoxyglucose. Finally, a publication by Wick, Drury, and others appeared which showed that it was not 2-deoxyglucose itself but its phosphorylated product, 2-deoxyglucose-6-phosphate that blocked glucose metabolism. The mechanism appeared to be as follows: Glucose-6-phosphate, the product of the hexokinase-catalyzed phosphorylation of glucose, is normally rapidly isomerized to fructose-6-phosphate which is then metabolized further down the glycolytic and eventually into the tricarboxylic acid pathway. In contrast, 2-deoxyglucose-6-phosphate lacks the oxygen on its 2-carbon position and cannot be converted to fructose-6-phosphate and metabolized further. Therefore, because the brain has very little if any hexose-6-phosphatase activity, 2-deoxyglucose-6-phosphate accumulates in brain to levels that exceed that of glucose-6 phosphate and inhibits glucose-6 phosphate conversion to fructose-6-phosphate. This effectively blocks glycolysis and glucose utilization in the brain and is responsible for the coma.

When I saw this paper, I immediately thought that this property of 2-deoxyglucose might offer a means to use the quantitative autoradiographic technique to determine local rates of glucose utilization in the brain. 2-Deoxyglucose is an analogue of glucose that crosses the blood-brain barrier and is metabolized in competition with glucose in the first step of glucose metabolism, but then its metabolic product, unlike those of glucose metabolism, is essentially trapped and accumulates in the brain. It seemed to me that this unique property should allow one to determine how much 2-deoxyglucose had been phosphorylated and from that one should be able to figure out some way to compute the rate of glucose utilization. To do so would, however, require some type of kinetic modeling and analysis that was not immediately obvious. I was at the time still deeply involved in studies of the action of thyroid hormones on protein synthesis, and so I set this idea aside as something to work on some day.

TB: When did you return to it?

LS: In 1964, Martin Reivich, who was serving his required two years of military service as a Research Associate in the US Public Health Service at NIH, joined our lab. He had previously been trained in neurology at the University of Pennsylvania, and came to work with Seymour Kety and me on cerebral blood flow. At that time, neither Kety nor I was working any longer on cerebral blood flow; Seymour had become involved in biochemical and genetic studies of schizophrenia, and I was working on the thyroid project. Both of us, however, had always had an interest in adapting the old autoradiographic [^{131}I]trifluoriodomethane gas method for use with a non-volatile, long-lived ^{14}C-labeled tracer because of the greater convenience and better autoradiographic resolution it offered. Reivich did just that while he was here. He succeeded in adapting the local blood flow method for use with [^{14}C]antipyrine, and in doing so he also modified the quantitative autoradiographic technique for use with ^{14}C instead of ^{131}I. Quantitative autoradiography with ^{14}C was, of course, an essential step toward the development of a method to measure local cerebral glucose utilization with 2-[^{14}C]deoxyglucose. We discussed this further application of ^{14}C autoradiography and agreed that some day we ought to do something about it, but not then.

In 1966 Reivich returned to the Neurology Department at Penn. Shortly thereafter he called me to ask if he could include in a grant application he was preparing a section on the development of the [^{14}C]deoxyglucose method, and if I would be willing to collaborate with him on such a project. I agreed on condition that the initial experimental work would be done in his lab because mine was totally occupied with biochemical studies of the action of thyroid hormones and the cerebral utilization of ketone bodies. The initial studies done in his lab showed that 2-[^{14}C]deoxyglucose and glucose were taken up from the medium by brain slices in vitro in almost exact proportion. This encouraged us to develop a model for their behavior in brain in vivo. The model was essentially the same as the one for the measurement of local cerebral blood flow with a chemically inert radioactive tracer, such as [^{131}I]trifluoroiodomethane or [^{14}C]antipyrine, except that it included a trapping step to account for deoxyglucose phosphorylation by hexokinase. The model was not wrong, but it led to a technically impractical if not impossible procedure that would have required simultaneous measurement of local blood flow and knowledge of some parameters that were extremely difficult to determine.

In 1968 I was presented with the opportunity to take a sabbatical year to work somewhere else. I realized that it might be my last chance to do that, so I decided to go to the Laboratory of General and Comparative Biochemistry at the Collège de France in Paris. This laboratory, headed by Jean Roche, was internationally renowned for its work on thyroid hormones. Professor Roche, who was also the Rector of the University of Paris, was fully occupied dealing with a student body in revolt, and the laboratory was being run by Jacques Nunez. I collaborated with him on the biosynthesis of thyroid hormones. A key step in the pathway of this synthesis is the iodination of tyrosine residues in the protein thyroglobulin in the thyroid gland. This reaction is normally catalyzed by the enzyme thyroid peroxidase. To study this peroxidase-catalyzed protein iodination reaction we used a model in which horseradish peroxidase was used to catalyze iodination of serum albumin.

The kinetics of this reaction turned out to be peculiar. It did not follow typical Michaelis-Menten kinetics which intrigued me. We did eventually find the explanation for the unusual kinetics. The action was a bimolecular one that required the sequential addition of two substrates, iodide and serum albumin, to the peroxidase enzyme. The order of addition was qualitatively random, but there were kinetic preferences in the orders of addition, and simulation studies showed that the observed aberrant kinetic pattern could be duplicated if appropriate rate constants in the various steps of the reaction sequence were used. One very fortunate outcome of working on this problem was that it taught me a great deal about enzyme kinetics. Furthermore, when the student revolt was over and they returned to the university, I was incorporated into teaching a graduate class in biochemistry. The subject of my lectures was the regulation of enzyme activities. This experience further prepared me for what was to come. I began to think about the 2-deoxyglucose method more as an enzyme kinetic problem rather than as a blood flow and transport problem.

When I returned to my own laboratory at NIMH in 1969 after spending my sabbatical year abroad, I found the thyroid project in shambles. I had the choice of trying to resurrect it or to take the opportunity to use the enzyme kinetics I had learned and switch my lab's focus to work on the development of the deoxyglucose method. I chose the latter. After initial biochemical experiments with brain homogenates in vitro, we carried out our first experiment in vivo in which we injected ^{14}C-labeled deoxyglucose into a rat and autoradiographed its brain. This was done in February 1971. The development of the 2 [^{14}C]deoxyglucose method for the measurement of local cerebral glucose utilization in rats was completed by 1974, and by 1976 we had completed its adaptation for use in monkeys. It was subsequently adapted by us and by others for use in cats, dogs, mice, and sheep and fetal lambs.

TB: When did you move from animal research to man?

LS: After the autoradiographic 2-[^{14}C]deoxyglucose method was developed, Reivich, a collaborator in its development and a neurologist who necessarily dealt with human subjects, raised the question about the possibility of adapting it for use in humans. I remember quipping, "Sure, maybe one of the countries that still uses beheading as a penalty would allow us to inject some [^{14}C]deoxyglucose into the subject before they behead him and then allow us to take the brain out for autoradiography. It's not very practical to do autoradiography on a human brain." He replied that maybe there was another way. He had met David Kuhl at the University of Pennsylvania, who was in nuclear medicine and had with colleagues developed a single photon scanner that could scan the brain for γ-ray radiation and localize its distribution. It had four scintillation counters arranged in a rectangle in a plane that rotated around the head and could measure the radioactive emissions from localized regions in slices of the brain, one plane at a time. I believe they had used it to measure local blood contents in different parts of the brain with radioactive carbon monoxide which bound to hemoglobin. I acknowledged that the scanner might solve one problem but raised another. It required an isotope that emitted γ-rays that could penetrate the brain and skull and be detected by the scanner outside the head. The problem was that deoxyglucose contains only carbon, hydrogen, and oxygen. There are no γ-emitting isotopes of hydrogen; oxygen has one, ^{15}O, but with only a two-minute half-life; and carbon has ^{11}C which has a 20-minute half-life. I didn't know how one could synthesize deoxyglucose labeled with any one of these short-lived isotopes fast enough. What was there to do?

Another possibility occurred to us. At the time I belonged to a wine-tasting group at NIH, composed mainly of biochemists who met once a month. One of its members was Peter Goldman, a biochemical pharmacologist, now at Harvard, who was then doing research on the biochemical properties of fluorinated analogues of natural compounds. Fortunately, I knew something about his work. He had, for example, shown that glutamate decarboxylase, the enzyme that makes GABA from glutamate, could also decarboxylate fluorinated glutamate to make fluoro-GABA. Fluorine is so small an atom that when it is inserted in place of a hydrogen in not too critical a position in a molecule, enzymes acting on the natural compound often act on the fluorinated compound, at least qualitatively, like on the natural compound. [18]Fluorine is a γ-emitting isotope with a 110 minute half-life, long enough perhaps to permit synthesis of practical quantities of 2 [^{18}F]fluorodeoxyglucose.

A further concern was where in the molecule to insert the fluorine atom to assure that the compound was still a substrate for the enzyme hexokinase. 2-Deoxyglucose has 6 carbon atoms, and it is phosphorylated by hexokinase on the carbon-6 position. The carbon furthest away from the phosphorylation site that could be fluorinated was carbon-2. It seemed, therefore, that the compound most likely to meet all the criteria was 2-[^{18}F]fluoro-2-deoxy–D-glucose ([18]FDG). We were not, of course, radiochemists, so Kuhl enlisted the aid of Alfred Wolf and Joanna Fowler from Brookhaven National Laboratories. Reivich, Kuhl, Wolf, Fowler and I, and some of their colleagues held a meeting in Philadelphia where we discussed our need for [18]FDG. Wolf and Fowler were sure they could synthesize it. I insisted they first synthesize a ^{14}C-labeled version of the species of fluorodeoxyglucose so that we could do the biochemical and in vivo animal studies needed to confirm the compound did indeed behave like 2-deoxyglucose. Kuhl and Fowler succeeded in doing that, and we used the ^{14}C-labeled FDG in enzyme assays and animal studies to show that the proposed [18]FDG would have the same biochemical properties as 2-deoxyglucose.

Wolf, Fowler, and several of their colleagues also developed a synthesis for the ^{18}F-labeled FDG, and studies with [18]FDG in human subjects were successfully carried out with Kuhl's Mark IV scanner at Penn in 1976–1977. These were the first determinations of regional glucose utilization in the human brain. The images, however, were not very good, nowhere near those obtained with the autoradiographic technique. This was because the spatial resolution possible with the single photon emission scanner was in the range of centimeters whereas that of the autoradiographic techniques was about 100-200 microns. Shortly thereafter, Kuhl left Penn to assume the role of Chief of Nuclear Medicine at UCLA. He took with him Michael Phelps and Edward Hoffman, who had been working with him at Penn but had previously been intimately involved in the design and development of the first positron-emission tomographic

(PET) scanners when they were at Washington University. At UCLA they acquired the first commercial PET scanner, the ECAT II. ^{18}F is a positron emitter, and its positron emissions are the source of the γ rays that were exploited by Kuhl's single photon scanner. The positron, which has the same mass as the electron, is emitted from the atomic nucleus. It is absorbed in the tissue by collision with an electron in its environment, and the masses of both the electron and the positron are converted into two so-called annihilation γ rays of equal energy. These γ rays leave the site of the collision in opposite directions at approximately 180 degrees. Because γ rays are less readily absorbed by tissue, they can be detected by radioactivity detectors outside the head. The γ rays move in opposite directions with the speed of light, and so by having two detectors lined up which can measure the γ rays arriving at them in coincidence, it is possible to localize the line in the tissue from which the rays originated. By having many such pairs of detectors around the head, it is possible to localize the region in the brain from which the two rays originated. Then, with the aid of computer images, the distribution of the radioactivity in slices of the brain can be constructed. This is, in brief, the principle of positron emission tomography. It provides much better resolution than single photon scanning, in the range of millimeters. This resolution is still far less than that of autoradiography, but PET does allow measurements to be made in humans. Phelps, Hoffman, Kuhl, and a number of associates then proceeded to adapt the ^{18}FDG technique for use with PET and applied it to humans in a variety of normal functional states and clinical conditions, among them normal aging, partial complex epilepsy, Huntington's disease, Alzheimer's disease, and, more recently, neoplasms. These studies established the usefulness of the ^{18}FDG method to study the human brain in health and disease.

TB: What was the time frame of these developments?

LS: The autoradiographic [^{14}C]deoxyglucose method was first presented in 1974 at the annual meeting of the American Society for Neurochemistry. In 1975 we published in *Science* the first report of how it could be used for the mapping and imaging of functional activity in neural pathways. This report in *Science* did not, however, include quantification; it showed only how changes in functional activity could be visualized and localized in the autoradiographic images that the method provided. In 1976 we published in *PNAS* its use to map functional activity in the primary binocular visual system in the monkey. This report included the visualization of the nature and extent of the ocular dominance columns in the primary visual cortex as well as the localization for the first time of the site of representation of the blind spots of the visual fields in the visual cortex. In 1977 we published the full details of the theory, procedure, and applications of the quantitative deoxyglucose method in the *Journal of Neurochemistry*, and later that year we published a short review of its many applications in the same journal.

The development of the [18]FDG method for use in humans with the single photon scanner was completed in 1977, but not published until 1979 because of the many coauthors in different institutions who had to be allowed to review and edit the manuscript. It was eventually published by Reivich and the rest of us in *Circulation Research* at least a couple of years after its completion. The adaptation of the [18]FDG method for use with PET, in which I also collaborated, was completed somewhat later but also published in 1979 by Phelps et al. in the *Annals of Neurology*.

You might find it amusing to know why the full paper on the [14C] deoxyglucose method was not published until 1977 even though it had first been reported in abstract form in 1974. At the time when we were working on the development of the method, I was the Chief Editor of the *Journal of Neurochemistry* and a very conscientious one. I had a rule that any submitted or revised paper received in the mail had to be sent out for review by the next day. Also, any reviews received from referees would also be acted on by me by the next day and forwarded to the authors with a decision that was not a form letter but one tailored specifically to the manuscript and its reviews. That was practically a full time job helping others to get their papers published, and it did not leave me much time to write my own. At that time I had my first Japanese fellow, Osamu Sakurada, who was part of the group working on the development of the deoxyglucose method. He had come from the Department of Neurosurgery of Juntendo University in Tokyo, and a friend of his from that same department was a fellow in Janet Passonneau's Laboratory of Neurochemistry in the NINDS. Sometime in 1976 Sakurada asked me if there was something wrong with the deoxyglucose method. I was surprised and asked him had he found something wrong with it? He said that he himself didn't see anything wrong with it, but his friend had told him that at a journal club meeting in Dr. Passonneau's lab she had remarked that there must be something wrong with the method because the abstract had been published in 1974, and yet the full paper had not yet come out. This alerted me to the possibility of a serious problem, and so I resigned as Chief Editor of the *Journal of Neurochemistry* and spent the next six months writing the paper. That is the story of why the full paper followed so long after the abstract.

TB: Now, in the 1980s, you continued . . . ?

LS: Yes, I continued working with the method, to a large extent on the effects of neuropharmacologic agents related to the various neurotransmitter systems. These included, for example, dopaminergic, serotonergic, adrenergic, and cholinergic systems. Some of the drugs we examined were amphetamine, apomorphine, haloperidol, LSD, phenoxybenzamine, propranolol, morphine, diazepam, phencyclidine, and ketamine.

We also worked on the sites and mechanisms of activation of energy metabolism by neuronal functional activation. These studies definitively demonstrated the surprising fact that functional activation of a neural pathway stimulates glucose utilization in the neuropil, specifically the regions of the synaptic terminals in the projection zones of the pathway, and not at all in the perikarya in the region of origin of the pathway. The perikarya do consume glucose, but it is probably used mainly for "housekeeping" functions, such as the synthesis of proteins, nucleic acids, and lipids, as well as axonal transport, etc. and is not altered by functional activity in the pathway. Furthermore, the increases in glucose utilization in the terminal zones of the activated pathway are linearly related to the spike frequency in the afferents to the synapses, and is used mainly to supply the energy for the increased Na+,K+-ATPase activity that is needed to restore the ion gradients across the membranes which are partially degraded by the action potentials. An interesting outcome of these findings was the explanation of why activating an inhibitory pathway stimulated glucose utilization in its terminal zones just the same as activation of an excitatory pathway. It was not because inhibition required energy just like excitation, as was often speculated. It was because it was the spike activity in the afferent terminals that was responsible for the change in energy metabolism, and this would be the same whether it resulted in release of an inhibitory or an excitatory neurotransmitter. To determine which neurotransmitter was being released, it would be necessary to look at the next synapses of the pathway.

TB: What about in the 1990s?

LS: In the 1990s we returned in part to working on local cerebral blood flow. We were particularly interested in the physiological and/or biochemical mechanisms responsible for the increases in blood flow associated with increased functional and metabolic activities. We never did succeed in defining them, but we did make some interesting findings in the course of these studies. For example, we found that pharmacologic doses of 2-deoxyglucose or insulin-induced hypoglycemia of sufficient degree markedly increased blood flow everywhere in the brain. The glucose concentration in the brain under normoglycemic conditions, for example, plasma glucose concentrations of about 7 millimolar, is between 2 and 3 millimolar, approximately 50 times the Km of hexokinase for glucose. With progressively deeper levels of hypoglycemia brain glucose concentration falls almost linearly with plasma glucose concentration, but cerebral glucose utilization remains more or less constant because hexokinase still remains relatively saturated over a wide range of cerebral glucose concentrations. In this range cerebral blood flow also remains more or less constant. Eventually, however, when plasma glucose concentration falls into the range of 2–3 millimolar, cerebral glucose levels fall to levels around the Km and hexokinase becomes unsaturated causing cerebral glucose utilization to fall.

Surprisingly, we found that despite the decrease in energy metabolism, cerebral blood flow was markedly increased, a complete dissociation between energy metabolism and blood flow in the brain. The question was: why? Normally, cerebral blood flow is expected to be adjusted to metabolic demand. What in this case causes the blood flow to go up when metabolic demand goes down? We spent a lot of time studying that. Our first thought was that nitric oxide might be involved, and that perhaps it was formed or released by the reduced glucose utilization and was dilating the blood vessels. We therefore administered inhibitors of nitric oxide synthase. These did lower baseline cerebral blood flow but did not prevent or even reduce the increase due to hypoglycemia. Our next thought was that, inasmuch as hypoglycemia is one of Cannon's four stress conditions, it was likely to cause the release of epinephrine and norepinephrine by the adrenals, and that their elevation in blood might be causing the increase in cerebral blood flow. To examine this possibility, we measured blood norepinephrine and epinephrine levels and found that they did indeed rise markedly in hypoglycemia. We then infused the catecholamines intravenously at rates that raised their blood levels to the same or even higher levels than those found in hypoglycemia, but that failed to alter either cerebral blood flow or glucose utilization. It could not, therefore, explain the blood flow response to hypoglycemia.

We then considered the following scenario. When the brain glucose concentration falls to a level close to its Km, hexokinase becomes partly desaturated, and the rates of glucose phosphorylation and utilization fall to rates insufficient to maintain normal rates of ATP synthesis. ATP levels then fall while those of ADP and AMP rise. AMP is the substrate for 5'-nucleotidase which dephosphorylates it, generating adenosine. Adenosine is known to be a potent vasodilator, probably via its action on the adenosine A_{2a} receptor, and has been shown to be involved in the regulation of the coronary and probably also the cerebral circulation. To test this hypothesis we measured brain adenosine levels during both insulin-induced hypoglycemia and after pharmacologic doses of 2-deoxyglucose at the levels that increased cerebral blood flow. In both cases brain adenosine concentrations were tremendously increased. We then reasoned that if indeed it was adenosine that mediated the increases in cerebral blood flow, then blocking adenosine receptors should also block the blood flow response. Since we had no idea which of the adenosine receptors might be involved, we used a relatively non-specific antagonist, caffeine. Sure enough, caffeine dose-dependently inhibited the blood flow response to hypoglycemia to the point of complete extinction. It was very gratifying to have a definitive answer to an interesting problem, and furthermore, it provided strong evidence that adenosine does indeed have a role in the control of the cerebral circulation.

TB: You are still active, right?

LS: I am still presently active, but my lab's personnel and resources have been reduced to the point where it has become very difficult to do the kind of work I used to be able to do. I am, therefore, planning to retire next summer.

TB: Next summer?

LS: Yes.

TB: What was your most important contribution?

LS: My most important research contributions were the development of the 2-deoxyglucose method and using it to show that local brain energy metabolism can not only be measured, but exploited to localize neural functional activity and even to image its distribution within the brain. In addition, we were able to use the method to define a number of the properties of metabolic response to functional activation. For example, we showed that the changes in energy metabolism evoked by alterations in functional activity occur in the synaptic regions in the neuropil and not at all in the neuronal cell bodies. Furthermore, the change in the metabolic activity found in these regions in the neuropil reflects mainly the change in spike frequency in the terminals of the afferent pathways to the region. I wish that those who use the [18]FDG version of the method with PET would pay more attention to this point. When they find a region in the brain with altered metabolic activity or blood flow, they should not, as they unfortunately often do, conclude that region is the site of the altered function. Altered metabolic activity in any given region may rather reflect altered function in regions upstream that project to it.

We also learned a great deal about the mechanisms that underly the functional activation of energy metabolism in the nervous system. These changes occur in the synaptic regions. Action potentials in the presynaptic axonal terminals and in the postsynaptic dendrites reflect sodium entry into and potassium exit from those cellular elements. These action potentials tend to degrade the ion gradients that generate the membrane potential and must be restored by pumping the sodium out of the cell and transporting potassium back into the cell. This is done by Na+, K+-ATPase which consumes ATP in the process, and this requires glucose utilization to provide the energy needed to regenerate the ATP.

There are, in addition, some other processes that are associated with neuronal functional activity and are also dependent on energy metabolism. The increases in energy metabolism associated with functional activation of a pathway are localized to the neuropil containing the synapses to which the pathway projects. Neuropil contains several subcellular elements, such as presynaptic axonal terminals, postsynaptic dendrites, and astrocytic processes. The deoxyglucose method is not yet capable of the fine resolution required to identify which of these subcellular elements contribute to the activated energy metabolism. Because action potentials in the axonal terminals and the dendrites degrade ion gradients, which must be restored, it is almost certain that these elements contribute to the increased energy metabolism.

There are, however, studies with cell cultures in vitro carried out by Magistretti's group as well as ours that indicate that astroglia may also contribute to the functional activation of glucose utilization. Astrocytic processes surround the synapses, and astroglia have the property of avidly taking up glutamate which is the most prevalent excitatory neurotransmitter in the brain and is released in the synapses of excitatory pathways. Glutamate uptake by astrocytes is associated with the co-transport into the cell of 2–3 sodium ions per glutamate molecule. This sodium must then be pumped out of the cell, and this is done by Na+,K+-ATPase which uses up one ATP molecule for every 3 sodium ions pumped out. The astroglia also convert glutamate to glutamine, a process that also uses one ATP molecule for each glutamate converted. The increase in energy metabolism observed with neuronal functional activation is, therefore, I believe, distributed among presynaptic axonal terminals, postsynaptic dendrites, and in glutamatergic synapses in the astrocytes with processes surrounding the synapses.

TB: So we should focus on the synaptic area to which the pathway projects, because this is where the activity is?

LS: Yes, and that is the reason I said that I wish those using the [18]FDG method with PET would appreciate this. If they find a region with a low metabolic rate, they should not conclude, as they often tend to do, that that is where the abnormality is. Not necessarily. It may be that the problem is somewhere else, for example, the origin of a pathway that is projecting to this area.

TB: How would this translate into the clinical interpretation of findings?

LS: I think the lesson is that in trying to localize the sites of abnormalities in disease or the actions of drugs, one should remember that what is observed in one area may well be a reflection of what happened somewhere else.

TB: Is there anything we did not cover?

LS: Well, there are probably a lot of things.

TB: But you think that we covered the important things.

LS: I think so. We got the most important things.

TB: When did you become a member of ACNP?

LS: I am not sure, but I believe it was some time in the nineteen seventies.

TB: Have you been attending the annual meetings regularly?

LS: Oh, yes, I usually come to the meetings, at least two of every three years, and have participated in many sessions.

TB: What would you like to see happen in your field in the future?

LS: I would like to see the biochemical abnormalities in schizophrenia identified. It won't, of course, be by me. I think that the imaging field is going to get better and better as the instrumentation improves. It should be remembered, however, that one should not derive a functional model from what is imaged with PET or fMRI. The model should be designed from what is already known about the processes involved, and the images serve only to localize the process. For example, in the case of the deoxyglucose method, we first designed the model on the basis of known principles of enzymology and the results of basic biochemical and physiological studies in animals and man. All this was independent of and preceded any imaging techniques that were later used. The imaging techniques, first autoradiography and then single photon emission tomography and PET, were added only to obtain localization of the metabolic process within the brain and played no part in the theoretical basis and design of the model. The fact that the imaging techniques allowed us to visualize the distribution and the levels of metabolic activities within the brain, and in colors of the rainbow too, was only a secondary gain. If, on the other hand, we had begun by injecting radioactive deoxyglucose and then examined the images, we wouldn't have had much of an idea about what was going on. If one were to inject radioactive shoe-polish and image the radioactivity in the brain, one would almost certainly find patterns of distribution of radioactivity in the brain which might change with functional activation. One would not, however, obtain from the images alone any worthwhile information or useful knowledge about the nature of the processes involved that would allow one to design a model. Just injecting a radioactive compound and getting an image is not enough. It must be combined with basic fundamental research beyond the imaging in order to get meaningful information.

TB: This is a reasonable note on which to end this interview.

LS: OK.

TB: Thank you very much for sharing all this information.

LS: Thank you. It's good to remind oneself of one's past.

NANCY C. ANDREASEN

Interviewed by Andrea Tone
Scottsdale, Arizona, December 11, 2003

AT: My name is Andrea Tone and we are at the forty-second annual meeting of the ACNP in San Juan, Puerto Rico. Today I am interviewing Dr. Nancy Andreasen.* Thank you for coming. Let me start with asking a question. Please tell me a little bit about your upbringing.

NA: I was born in Lincoln, Nebraska. My father had a degree in journalism. He originally wanted to be a dentist and started dental school, but couldn't afford to finish. Next, he married my mom. When I was a kid, the expectation was that my older brother would go into medicine or dentistry and I would do something else because I was a girl. And, as a kid, my brother got the chemistry sets and the radio sets and all those kinds of things. I was very clear, early on, that I wanted no dolls, and so I didn't get stuck with them. But I got a lot of books, which were the things guaranteed to make me happy. My father was an army officer in the Second World War, so we moved around. We were in New York City, Buffalo, Kansas City and Minneapolis. Some people don't respond well to going to a new place every two years but I loved the adventure of it. I had mostly a mid-western childhood, so I loved wildlife and being out in the country; I imagined I was an Indian or a scout. All those kinds of things. I was always a tomboy, loved sports, playing with my older brother and his friends. To some extent, my poor mother was in despair because she wanted a little girl who would be frilly and feminine, and I wasn't.

AT: Were there just two of you?

NA: Just two. From the time I was a little kid, I knew I was gifted with a good brain. I wouldn't have put it that way then, because I didn't understand the brain as much as I do now, but I did know I was, without any effort, the brightest kid in any crowd. Even my parents knew that and were proud of me. My older brother, who was plenty bright enough, didn't adapt as well. With things like math when you move every couple of years, you can get behind. But I could pick up. He didn't do it quite as well, so in that sense, the gap between being especially bright and being just bright was evident to everybody in the family. I have memories of my parents inviting the two of us into dinner parties with their friends when I was five or six years old, and people would say, "Nancy, what do you want to be when you grow up?" And I would reply, "I'm going to be the first woman president of the United States." I always had the sense that I was going to do something important.

---

* Nancy Andreasen was born in Lincoln, Nebraska in 1938.

As I grew older I skipped many grades. I finished high school at sixteen, college at nineteen and had my Masters at twenty. Had I stayed in graduate school, I would have had my PhD at twenty-two. I took a year out to go to Oxford on a Fulbright fellowship and after I came back I spent one more year teaching at a small college before I went back to grad school. So I was twenty-four when I got my PhD. The intellectual environment in our household was more oriented toward literature than science. My father had his degree in journalism and my mother was an elementary school teacher. She didn't actually teach but was a full time homemaker. That's the way they both wanted it; the conventional way with father as breadwinner and mother as the homemaker. So, when I was going through high school, whatever interest I had in science was discouraged. It wasn't suppressed, but when I would register for classes my parents would say, "Take history, English or foreign languages." They made me take Spanish instead of French, because they thought it was an easier language. It was a funny paradox, when I look back on it. They knew they had this very bright daughter but they were still giving her advice not to challenge herself.

The bottom line is I didn't have any math or science in high school. I had Latin and Spanish, and, then on through my Master's degree and PhD, French, German and Greek. I was deeply educated in the humanities. As a college student, I was a triple major; English, History and Philosophy. I started as a History major, and then I took additional classes for fun. Before I knew what was going on I had three majors. I learned a lot about classics and philosophy. When I went to graduate school, I ended up in renaissance work and did my dissertation on John Donne that later on I turned into a book. John Donne was a metaphysical poet who drew many of his images from science. Donne's father was a doctor. In one of his poems he talks about the way that a man loves a woman and says, "Our two loves, which are one as two stiff twin compasses are one and one soul in the center sits and the other rotates around." His beautiful metaphors come from geometry and physics and math. Another metaphysical poet, Andrew Marvell, writes: "our loves so truly parallel, though infinite will never meet." Of course, this is before Einstein's physics. We now know those two unrequited loves could meet in eternity as lines curve in space. Anyway, to do metaphysical poetry, especially Donne, my skill and knowledge of history and philosophy were really handy to understand the metaphors. I was married at twenty and my husband was a handsome, blue-eyed blonde; that's where my Danish name comes from. I acquired it when it was unthinkable that a woman keep her own name when married.

AT: How did you meet?

NA: People kept fixing us up. I recently married for the second time, and reflecting on that I told several people, "I was a pretty elusive cat." When I was in high school, I dated a boy who was a very fine man, and ended up being a very good surgeon. He wanted to marry me, not when we were in high school, but later and I kept saying, "No, I don't want to get married." In college I went with another fellow who also was a very fine person. He ended up being Dean of the college of education at the University of Nebraska. I just reunited with him last year, after many years.

AT: Did you keep in contact?

NA: He sent me e-mails off and on, tracking my career and congratulating me. But we only recently saw each other again. I think for both of us it evoked memories. We had been very fond of each other, but he wanted to get married and I didn't. I wanted a career, and you could have a husband or a career, but not both.

AT: What year was this?

NA: We're talking the 1950s and 1960s. When I insisted on going to graduate school, my parents were disappointed because they wanted me to marry. George, my first husband, was a friend of my brother's and that's how we got fixed up. My parents thought he was the perfect husband because he was very outgoing and spontaneous, with a lot of social skills, whereas I was quiet and intellectual. I wasn't a total nerd, but I wasn't Scarlet O'Hara, the little girl they wanted. I was a very serious little girl and very intense; always carrying a book, thinking, reading and writing. Anyway, we married, went to Oxford together and had a lovely early life. He brought me back to Nebraska, where he had gone to dental school and got his degree in orthodontics. That's where I got my PhD.

I had been at Harvard before. Some people, jokingly – or not even jokingly – say, "Here's Nancy Andreasen. She managed to do very well despite the fact that she got her degrees from lesser schools such as Nebraska and Iowa." Truly, I'd like to smack them when I hear that, because good people are good people, and it doesn't matter where they get their degrees. What matters is what they do with their abilities. We finished school in Nebraska with an agreement we would both take a job at the first place that offered us positions, his in a department of Orthodontics and mine in a department of English.

Back then, every university had rules against hiring two people married to each other. It was just forbidden. But we were okay, because I was in the college of arts and science and he was in the college of dentistry. Iowa was the first place that offered us both jobs. We had the University of Washington on the line, too. This was an achievement because they were both trade-ups from Nebraska. I had already, by twenty-three, published two papers, which is a huge achievement in a field like English literature, and George had done extremely well, too. He was a mechanical engineer before he went into dentistry, so we both had rich backgrounds; we were by no means a pair like Pasko Rakic and Pat Goldman, but we did have complimentary interests. I suppose, to some extent, his interest in mechanics and facial growth, and even brain growth, had a significant impact on my life. When we were at Oxford, he studied with Le Gros Clark, who was one of the really great neuroanatomists of the last century. He did many things; from studying optic nerves to discovering that the Piltdown man was a hoax by studying the teeth. For that reason, he was interested in taking George on as a student. George also studied with a fellow named Tanner, who established the Tanner Growth Curves that are still the standard by which normal growth is determined. The whole notion of understanding body and brain development was one of George's passions. So I listened and got to know people like Tanner and Clark.

AT: Was he supportive of your career?

NA: Very supportive. That was the reason I married him. When he asked me to marry him I said, "I want to have a career. I want to go to graduate school. I want to study in Europe." And he replied, "I'll go with you." When I said, "That could interfere with your career," he said, "That's okay." We still split up, but he pursued and finally I caved in. I thought if this guy wants to marry me that much, I'll go ahead and do it. We were a very happy couple and Oxford was a whole lot of fun. Then we came back to the US and got the next level of degrees and jobs at the University of Iowa. There I was in Iowa, twenty-four years old. I already had hree years teaching at the University of Nebraska and Nebraska Wesleyan. So it wasn't my first teaching job, but it was a different level. Iowa had never had a woman faculty member in the English department. I was a groundbreaker and there was a lot of debate as to whether they should hire me.

AT: You may have well been the youngest.

NA: I was easily the youngest. I still remember the first time I walked into my classroom at Nebraska Wesleyan; I was twenty-one years old and the students were eighteen or nineteen. When I got to Iowa I was assigned a graduate course in Elizabethan Drama, which wasn't my field. I was pretty good at Shakespeare, but we're talking about the lesser Elizabethans, Nash and Webster and so on. I had never taught the topic, so I had to teach myself the material for a graduate course where everybody was probably older than I was. It was really quite a challenge. The essence of this story is when we got there I discovered I was pregnant. This was when birth control pills were coming in, but I wasn't on them. So here I was with my first big time teaching job, expecting our first child. Not planned, although welcomed and I'm very proud of her now. I felt I had a responsibility to women to do a good job at this. It turned out, fortunately, that the due date was right around Spring break. I could have the baby over the Spring break week and be back teaching my class after a week. So I was teaching on Friday and she was born on Monday.

AT: Did you encounter any discrimination or hostility because you were so young and pregnant?

NA: No, but I was very self-conscious about it. Fortunately, I'm slender and had good muscle tone; I didn't look very pregnant. I didn't encounter discrimination for being pregnant, but I did for being a woman. The younger male assistant professors would take me out to lunch and we would discuss salaries. I was making something like $6,200 a year while they were making $8,000. Several times we had that discussion, and I said, "Why should I be making so much less than you guys, especially since I've published and you haven't? We're teaching the same classes." And they would flatly say, "Because we are men. Men should make more money than women. Everybody knows that."

Anyway, Susan was due to be born over Spring break. I was starting to get sick a month before she was born. My blood pressure was going up, and if it had been now, they wouldn't have let me continue to teach. I was in pre-eclampsia, so the delivery was extremely difficult. But we got through it and I was discharged from the hospital after five days, probably on a Friday. Over that weekend and on into the next week, I had severe postpartum hemorrhaging. I was really sick. I called my obstetrician a couple of times, and finally he said "you better come back into the hospital." I got to the hospital running a temperature of 104. I had puerperal sepsis, which has killed women in childbirth for centuries. I was put on IV antibiotics, and spent the next four or five days in the hospital with my arm stretched out, aching, while I was getting IV antibiotics. I realized that my life was being saved by medicine. I was also thinking I had the gift of a good intellect and wondered whether I was using it for the right purpose. I got out of the hospital and went back to teaching my classes the following Monday. I missed one week of class and was very exhausted at the end of that first week after my return. When I went home I fell into bed and slept almost the entire weekend. But I was determined to do my job, which was to help these kids learn to love English poetry as I did. I was teaching Elizabethan Drama, a freshman composition course, and a general literature course.

AT: You were teaching three courses?

NA: Yes. I did nine hours a week of class teaching. For something that you're not an expert in, like Elizabethan Drama, that requires a lot of preparation time. I noticed the kids wouldn't have minded if I'd been away for another week. I thought to myself, why am I pounding my head against the wall trying to teach these kids when it's not going to make an iota of difference in the history of mankind? So, I finished that second semester of my first year at Iowa, and then over the summer finished reworking my dissertation and submitted some of it to Princeton University Press, which was the most distinguished press for renaissance literature at the time. I learned very early on to submit my articles using my initials rather than my name. It was almost guaranteed if I said, "Nancy," it would be rejected. So, I used N. J. C., my first two names plus my maiden name, which was Coover. So the book was submitted as N. J. C. Andreasen, and within two or three months I had an acceptance. The title of the book was *Conservative Revolutionary*, and it was published by Princeton University Press in 1967.

AT: That was fast.

N.A: It was fast. I was twenty-five years old, a young woman professor and I had my first book published.

AT: And your first child.

NA: My first child, at the same time. Instead of feeling elated, I was reflective, and said to myself, "You know how much effort and energy goes into producing a book like this and what if you took that same amount of effort and energy and put it in a different field? Maybe I could do something like discover penicillin." This goes back to, "I'm going to be the first woman president of the US." I never set my sights low. I thought about it some more, and talked to George. I also talked to the couple who lived across the street who were our best friends; he was a physician, a pathologist. I decided I would change my field and go into science, probably to medical school. So I did, the next semester.

Somebody pointed out to me that to get into medical school I would have to take the MCAT and I would have to meet all the science requirements. I had all the biology required, but I hadn't had any math, physics or chemistry. Before I took physics, I should take advanced math. So that's what I did the second semester of that year. It was advanced college algebra, and having had only one year of high school algebra it was tough. It was also a different way of thinking from history or literature. But I absolutely loved it. I loved the pure symbolism of working through a problem at that high level of abstraction. There's just this elegant simplicity of it. I could intuitively see what the solution was before I worked out the answer.

I could also have the pleasure of writing down the steps to the answer. So I found I had a real aptitude for math, having been told by my parents that girls shouldn't take math. I found the same thing when I did chemistry and physics. I was much better in physics than chemistry, and much better in organic than inorganic chemistry, which was different from the average pre-med student. They were better at chemistry than physics and at inorganic than organic chemistry. Most pre-med students think organic chemistry is sheer torture. But I thought it was a blast, because it was problem solving at an abstract level; one had to figure how to synthesize compounds and had to know the basic principles of how they combine.

AT: Who looked after your daughter?

NA: We hunted around and found an older lady, who came to our home at eight in the morning and stayed until five in the evening every day. And she was healthy, so she was there every day. I didn't want my precious child to do anything except grow up in her own home just as she would if her mom had been there. You can't imagine the burden of guilt I had, because I was the only working mother known to mankind, certainly known to the neighborhood.

AT: What about day care?

NA: You have no idea what a silly question that is. Nobody would have ever thought the university should have day care. They didn't think women should be working, never mind there should be day care. There was no woman professor in history. I was the only one in English. Pick the department; there were no women faculty members. Nobody gave me a hard time for having a child, but it was still considered strange.

And, the story goes on. When I applied, my MCATs were outstanding. It was almost unheard of to have a prefect 4-point average. I was at the top of every class. When I took the MCATs I hadn't taken physics. Still, I got scores in the ninetieth percentiles in science. I still don't know how I managed to do so well, except I must have had intuitive sense to figure out what the answers were. The admissions committee had a huge discussion about whether they should admit a woman who had a child, because a woman with a child probably wasn't going to practice medicine. I heard they were going to turn me down, through my friend across the street, the pathologist, whose name was Mike Carnes. But Mike stuck up for me through a friend of his on the admissions committee. So they decided to admit me. But the associate dean for student affairs sat me down in his office and said, "I want you to know we're going to admit you, but I'm completely opposed to this. I think you're doing a disservice to medicine and you're doing a disservice to your family. Your obligation is to stay home with your child. You have no business going to medical school."

AT: I've heard they would not admit women to medical school on the basis they menstruated and attendance would be disrupted by the monthly cycle.

NA: I started medical school and it was much harder for me than physics, math or chemistry, because so much was absolute memorization. It was mindless. Most of my education to that point had been thinking, identifying fundamental principals, seeing how they applied in various kinds of situations. That didn't work for anatomy. Our first year was histology and gross anatomy. We had one hundred and fifty people in my med school class and we started with five women. One eventually dropped out. Then there were four of us. The guys were all in fraternities and had access to examinations passed on from one year to another, but women were implicitly excluded. At Iowa medical school, one of the first big events of your life is meeting your cadaver. You work with three other medical students around a tank dissecting the corpse. That's the main thing you do for the first semester of medical school. And the question is who are going to be your tank partners? It's like a little kid getting on the bus and wondering if anybody is going to sit with them. We got into the anatomy laboratory and I felt both honored and blessed because one of my former students came up to me and said, "Nancy, would you be willing to be our tank partner?" So I had three very nice guys as my tank partners through anatomy.

AT: How old were you when you started medical school?

NA: Twenty-six or twenty-seven.

AT: You had a PhD and a child; were you older than your classmates?

NA: A little older. I was significantly older in my view of the world. These were a bunch of rowdy boys. They would study hard all week and get drunk on weekends. Most were single. There were in our class one or two people who were married. I was odd person out with the women too, because they were not much younger chronologically, but mentally they were much younger. Every evening I would be home seeing Susan, cooking dinner, doing all the motherly things until nine or so at night, and then doing my reading. I would read until eleven. I'd set the alarm, get up at four or so and study from four until she woke up, then go to classes. This is why I sometimes get annoyed when people talk about all the special privileges women should have because they have children. Those of us who cut the path sure didn't have any special privileges.

The next piece of the saga is we decided to have another child and I scoped out that the sophomore year is the best in medical school to have a kid. So we decided to have Robin. Her due date was a month before the first board examinations. You take board examinations after your first two years in medical school in pre-clinical subjects, like anatomy, physiology, pharmacology, pathology, and then you take the second round of the boards after your two clinical years. My first round of the boards would have to be taken in March–April right around the time that Robin would have been a newborn. I thought, I don't want to take those examinations postpartum, especially given my previous postpartum experience. There was a Spring and a Fall sitting for taking the exams; the Fall sitting was largely for people who hadn't passed the previous Spring. So I said, "Heck, I'll take them in the Fall." Several people said, "You can't take them in the Fall because you wouldn't have finished your second year of medical school." And I said," I'll buy the books and study over the summer." I'd always taught myself. So I took the exams in the Fall, and passed them, in the ninetieth percentile.

AT: Did you find that year was easier because you had done so much?

NA: Probably. Medical school, as I perceived it, was a pretty mindless endeavor. There were a lot of things going on that kept you busy, but they weren't learning experiences. What I learned didn't help me with anything I had to do.

AT: Before you went to medical school did you have any inclination what specialty you would choose?

NA: Everybody tells you not to pick your specialty before medical school, to try a bit of everything. I knew I wanted to do something related to the mind/brain, ranging from neurophysiology through neurosurgery and neurology to psychiatry. Each summer, I did research that was brain-related. My first summer, I did a fellowship with a very nice man, Fredric Deeke. This was early in the era of doing single cell recordings, putting electrodes into individual cells and measuring their firing. This was a hot topic that had only been around for a couple of years. I worked in his laboratory looking at the effects of various drugs in animals, and I learned I didn't want to do animal research. I didn't like working with animals. I admire people who do animal research, but I realized I just wasn't cut out for it. I wanted to do human research.

So, the next summer I took an elective that involved a psychiatric rotation. That same sophomore year in medical school, when I was giving birth to Robin and taking the boards in the Fall, I spent hours and hours collecting articles on the effects of lithium on sodium and potassium transport and on the adrenocortical system. I found a psychiatrist, Russ Norris, who had an IND to use lithium before lithium was FDA approved. In my sophomore year in medical school I had a lot of physiology, studying kidney transport. The kidney has a major role in regulating sodium and potassium balances. Also the kidney plus the adrenals have a role in regulating cortisol function. I found that very interesting.

I also went to a renal physiologist in the Department of Internal Medicine, Walter Kirkendall. He was one of the most admired members of the medical school faculty. I was probably twenty-eight years old when I went to see him. I was 4'11", weighed a hundred pounds and looked far younger than I was. From his point of view I was a little girl with a stack of 3 x 5 cards full of notes on how lithium might affect both somatic and brain physiology. When I showed this to him, he said, "I'm so impressed that one of our students has put in so much original work into a problem like this." This was probably the first nice thing anybody had said to me in medical school. But he also told me, "I can't help you because I'm a renal physiologist, and you have to find somebody who knows about the brain, because that's where this is going to matter." He was the one who knew Russ was around. Now, Russ didn't really know anything about the brain, but he at least took me under his wing and we worked together on this project. That was my first project in psychiatry and became my first publication.

AT: Was this a time when many medical schools still favored psychoanalytic training? I don't know how psychiatry was presented at your school.

NA: I was very blessed that Iowa is a really good medical school. It's the only medical school in Iowa and it serves the entire State. So in our training we saw hundreds and hundreds of patients. And, because it's a mid-Western school, it's very practical. Although in a psychiatry department you are exposed a little to psychodynamic thinking, we were mostly in the medical model. The interest was in bipolar illness and nobody on the faculty at Iowa thought that mania was an illness that could be treated psychodynamically. Nobody thought that schizophrenia was an illness that could be treated psychodynamically.

AT: So, it was not psychoanalysis.

NA: That approach is just mind-boggling to me. It's hard to imagine not using drugs when one knows they will improve things. My education was an anomaly to the majority of psychiatrists. I went on to do my residency at Iowa and our training was geared to provide health services to people throughout the state. We were taught we were first doctors, and secondly whatever specialty we were in. You could be a psychiatrist, an ophthalmologist or an orthopedist out somewhere and have a patient who needed something other than orthopedics or psychiatry and you could be the only doctor for a hundred and twenty miles. So you'd better be able to take care of that person, because you're a doctor. If I'm the only doctor on an airplane and a medical emergency occurs I try to do whatever I can. I was once at a play in New York and somebody in the audience was having a grand mal seizure. That's pretty much in my territory, so it wasn't too hard to handle. I've forgotten who was on stage, I think it Jason Robards, but he stopped the play and said, "A person out there is very sick. Is there a doctor around?" I was there with one of my girls.

In contrast to the places where they wouldn't give medications or do a physical examination because they were psychodynamically oriented, in Iowa we were absolutely required to do a complete physical on every patient we took care of. That meant doing a rectal examination on male patients and a pelvic examination on females. We were trained to be general family doctors at the same time we were psychiatrists. Iowa is a square state with four state hospitals in each of the corners and another in the center, and if you are a doctor in one of those state hospitals and you're the only doctor, you're going to have to take care of a lot of general health problems for your patients or they're not going to get any health care. If it was something more complicated we would refer the patient to internal medicine or whatever specialty they needed. It was a completely different model from what existed up and down the East coast and West coasts but I didn't know that.

AT: Can you go back to your project with lithium, cortisol, and kidney functions?

NA: I was reading widely, as usual, and I found some papers written by Edward J. Sachar, who was at Einstein. So I wrote him a note asking about his serum cortisol assays, because things were just beginning to move from urinary assays to serum cortisol assays. He wrote back a long personal note about how he was doing these assays and gave me the procedures. He gave me his phone number, and encouraged me to call him any time. He also gave me the name of his co-investigator. I was still a humble medical student and it meant a lot that this obviously very intelligent man based on his articles would take time to write me a personal letter. I thought, this is the way I'm going to be if I ever get to that position. I wanted to do that kind of thing for young people who asked me questions. Ed, tragically, died young from a stroke and is no longer with us. But eventually I met him and we became very close friends.

Anyway I did the work on lithium, and in the process I met psychiatric patients for the first time. And that really hooked me on doing psychiatry. Jan Stevens was also interested in how the mind works, but went into neurology because she didn't think she could ask questions as a psychiatrist. I was spared that dichotomy because the psychiatry department at

Iowa talked all the time about the brain, how it worked and how it would produce symptoms and what its chemistry was.

The head of child psychiatry was probably the first person anywhere to treat Tourette's Disease with Haldol. I was a medical student and saw these videotapes of Tourette's before and after Haldol. There was a fellow named Bob Heath at Tulane who was putting electrodes in the septal region in the brain, studying limbic activity. We were taught all that and about a serotonin hypothesis of psychosis before Herb Meltzer ever talked about it. We had an active chemistry laboratory attached to our hospital, so it was a splendid environment psychometrics as well and we had a strong psychology division that taught us about cognitive tests. I was trained to administer electroshock and we had a strong electrophysiology laboratory where I spent six months doing an EEG rotation. So I got a really good general psychiatric education.

I eventually chose not to pursue the lithium research. It would have led me down the road of laboratory assays, and I didn't think we were going to find the mechanisms of major illnesses by measuring peripheral metabolites and cortisol. Even if they were the closest index to what's going on in the brain, I didn't think they would take us there. I could see all the different artifacts, like sleep disturbance and stress, so I decided not to do that. Eventually, I emphasized the use of experimental cognitive tests to assay the brain. And I also spent a good chunk of my time clarifying the descriptive psychopathology of mental illnesses. As I began to focus more and more on schizophrenia, I became deeply interested in the language and thought abnormalities. That was natural for me because I came from a background in language and literature. So I kept asking how we could accurately measure the disturbances of thought and language. I did a lot of work in descriptive psychopathology on classic thought-language-communication disorder scales.

At the same time, I was working on the inpatient wards. All of us carried about a thirty percent load of clinical work. The wards were specialized in terms of diagnosis and I chose to work on the ward that had the more severe psychotic patients. I was doing my best to help with the medications that we had available at various times. I could see we improved their symptoms. Interestingly, at Iowa our average stay in hospital back then was about two weeks for mood disorders and about four weeks for schizophrenia. We almost never kept anybody longer than six weeks. It was long enough to get to know the patient and treat them well but not so long that we interfered with their routine lives. We were always very conscious of the fact we wanted our patients to get back to their jobs or to school.

What I began to notice in my patients with schizophrenia was that their psychotic symptoms markedly improved and might even stay markedly improved. We told one another, "If we can arrest the psychosis, these people can recover and lead normal lives." This isn't 1950, it is late l960s, early 1970s. So we're still in the early neuroleptic era. Haloperidol was introduced when I was a medical student. We quickly used it for both mania and for schizophrenia in very low doses. It was recommended we start with 2 milligrams and work up very slowly with Haldol. That's what I did, and I don't think I ever had a patient up to 10 milligrams. Patients would remit and in contrast to what happened later on with these antipsychotics, they would remit on low doses. But they would show up, not infrequently, maybe two or three months later, brought back by family members. And we were told, "He got a job, went for a month or so and then stopped. We can't get him to do anything."

We readmitted the patients because they had what I came to call negative symptoms. I was not the inventor of that concept which I got from Hughlings Jackson who talked about it in the nineteenth century; Will Carpenter, in a paper a couple of years earlier, made reference to it. He had one sentence about psychotic symptoms which are florid responders to neuroleptics, and other symptoms, which are negative. An absence of activity as opposed to an excess; something that ought to be there isn't. There's no fluency of speech. There's no emotional expression. There's no drive and energy. There's no attention. I thought about that and put together scales to measure both psychotic and negative symptoms separately. That was a contribution to descriptive psychopathology.

AT: How were your scales received?

NA: Pretty much like many good ideas are received. It was noticed and caught on with a few people, and then became almost like a snowball rolling down hill. Everybody began to say, after about five to eight years, ah ha, this is really true. Negative symptoms are what we really need to be worrying about treating. It also caught on that this is an illness where cognitive impairment is extraordinary. I'd been measuring this with experimental psychology tools; I have a whole series of papers with various experimental psychology techniques, measuring memory and language in sophisticated ways, showing that people with schizophrenia have a serious and non-remitting cognitive impairment. All of that work was there through the 1970s.

The thing that changed my life as a scientist was that imaging came in. I hate to keep saying what a great place Iowa is, but we had the second CT scanner in the country. We've always been a cutting edge place. I remember sitting on the inpatient unit, still a resident. A Polaroid CT scan was passed around, and I said, "Oh, my God, you can see the brain." I had done electives in neurosurgery where we did pneumoencephalography and saw where the ventricles were, or arteriography and saw where the vessels were; these were our very distant ways of seeing the brain. But those are also invasive techniques so I was completely taken by this noninvasive way of being able to see the brain. Even a modern CT scan is crude and those old scans were really crude; still it was a picture of the brain.

AT: Do you think that brain imaging brought about a radical change?

NA: It represented a radical change, and Hounsfield who developed CT, got a Nobel Prize for it, so it wasn't a trivial achievement. And the people who invented MRI got the Nobel Prize last year. That wasn't trivial either. Those guys in Stockholm noticed that X-rays do not permit you to see the brain, it's not a tissue you can visualize with X-rays. You can see the heart, you can see the lungs, but you can't see the brain. The only two ways you could see anything; one was by draining out all the cerebral spinal fluid and injecting air, which is very painful, and then you could see the ventricles. The other technique was to inject a radiosensitive dye into arteries and see where it is. But this is invasive too because you don't stick needles in arteries if you can avoid it or you're going to have blood spurting all over with the heart pumping it out. So arteriography should not be done trivially; usually it's done only when one suspects a brain tumor. Arteriography injects radio-opaque dye to see where the arteries are, but that doesn't let you see the brain. Now with CT and MRI here are finally techniques that let you see the brain the way you could see the heart and the lungs with conventional X-ray.

It was in the early 1970s I saw the first CT scan. I finished my residency in 1973, so it could have been before or right after; anyway I said to myself, we've got something for the first time we can use to measure brain abnormalities in mental illnesses. Everybody else was measuring platelet MAO and cortisol from peripheral blood samples but nobody was able to measure the brain. We're all looking at distal measures; we're looking at metabolites. I'm looking at cognitive assays. I'm seeing how the brain responds when given a list of words to remember. There are more elegant and complicated paradigms but they're not seeing the functioning brain itself. Now, with the CT, in the early studies we looked at the size of the brain and the ventricles.

Eve Johnstone and Tim Crow did the first study and it was published in *Lancet* in 1976. It had to be about 1972 or 1973 that I saw my first CT scan and realized I could use the technique to measure the brain in schizophrenia. I applied to our institutional review board to do it and they said no, you will never find anything in the brain in schizophrenia. I was young and had no position or stature at all, so I was talked out of it. One of my indelible memories was sitting in my office when that article came out, I'm pretty sure it was the spring of 1976, and seeing someone else had done the study I wanted to do with positive results.

AT: You had to be very frustrated.

NA: It's even worse, because I tried again to do a study, and I still wasn't given permission. They still said, this is just one article, and it doesn't prove anything. It's flawed, as many first articles on a topic are, because they had a number of people in their sample who had leucotomies and already had brain injury. They were mostly older, it was a small sample and they'd been chronically ill; all reasons the ventriclescould have been enlarged that might have had nothing to do with schizophrenia.

The next studies were done by the NIMH group, principally by Dan Weinberger and his crowd back when he was a very young person. The IRB at NIH is nothing near as rigorous as the IRBs in the rest of the world, so they were able to get permission when none of the rest of us could. I was ultimately able to take the Crow (it's really the Johnstone) paper, and some of the Weinberger papers and get permission to study patients at Iowa with schizophrenia. The Johnstone paper was in 1976, the Weinberger papers were in 1979 and 1980, and because of the delay in getting permission I didn't have my first paper out until 1982. But that was a pivotal event in the history of biological psychiatry, the opportunity to use imaging technology to demonstrate that a major psychiatric illness like schizophrenia had measurable brain differences from normal controls. A lot of people misunderstand that, but what we found is that there are group differences between people who have a certain kind of brain pathology and healthy volunteers. So we can say, in general, something has gone wrong with the brain in schizophrenia, but we have to say it's not an individual diagnostic test for schizophrenia. These are group differences.

AT: Why is that important?

NA: People misunderstand what imaging can do, a lot think I can bring my son or daughter in and have an MRI or a PET scan and this will diagnose them as schizophrenic. But we are not at that stage yet. Imaging in psychiatry is not like imaging in cancer where you can do a PET scan and detect metastases, or you can do imaging procedures and see the tumor. We are not able to do that, and don't have perfect relationships between the amount of brain abnormality we can measure and choice of treatment or ability to predict outcome. Imaging tools in psychiatry are very important because they help us understand the ways the brain isn't working right in general, but they're not telling us it's a specific illness or this person should have a particular treatment. They're helping us understand the mechanisms, but they're not helping us predict outcome or choose treatment.

AT: It is potentially a technique for diagnosing?

NA: Potentially, yes. I think we have a ways to go though, before we get there. We probably need different and better tools, because I don't think we'll be able to do it with the ones we are using now. There are people who claim they can make a diagnosis from an imaging technique, but that just is not the case.

AT: Can imaging tell what can be attributed to genetics and what can be attributed to environment in the development of schizophrenia?

NA: No. Many of us are working very hard to answer those kinds of questions, but none of us has been able to come up with a perfect answer. It's not for lack of trying, but because the illness is so complex. Schizophrenia is not a disease of a single brain region. I come to this meeting and hear people present who believe schizophrenia is caused by something that went wrong in the temporal lobe at some particular moment in time or in the hippocampus or in the dorsal lateral prefrontal cortex. And it's not that those specific brain regions aren't important. They probably are, but schizophrenia is almost certainly a disease of what I call distributed circuits. A lot of us use that term. I sometimes say that in Alzheimer's disease you have a particular pathological lesion, which is plaques and tangles, but in schizophrenia there's no pathological lesion we can point to. We can go to one of our favorite regions like the frontal cortex or the temporal lobes, the thalamus or the cerebellum, to all these different regions and sometimes find things with neuropathology, but you will not find it in every patient with the illness. This is telling us is that schizophrenia is not located in a specific part of the brain. The essence of schizophrenia is it's a disease that affects many different parts of the brain which normally work together, in such a manner they are not communicating with each other. It's a disease of disconnections.

My frontal lobe is doing just fine now, hooking into my temporal lobe, my cerebellum, my thalamus and my motor sensory cortex while I'm talking to you. If I had schizophrenia, there'd be something going wrong with how my frontal lobe, temporal lobe, thalamus, cerebellum, and so on work together in helping each other to monitor what is going on. In people with schizophrenia, the different parts of the brain just aren't working in a coordinated way. And so, people subjectively feel disorganized and confused, they feel they can't think clearly and they sometimes feel bombarded by stimuli. I still see patients on a fairly regular basis, and am eternally impressed by how much they suffer because they know they are not able to think as clearly as they once did, or even feel as intensely as they once did. So, it's a disease of disconected thought.

AT: Did things change in your career after you started to publish your findings with imaging?

NA: People began to pay attention to my work. Some of the smarter people paid a lot of attention to the early discussion of negative symptoms and the link I made between negative symptoms and brain changes. Then again, Iowa was one of the first places to get an MRI scanner, and so I did the first MRI study of schizophrenia, which I published in the *Archives* in 1986. That showed decreased size of the frontal lobes in schizophrenia. When I started presenting it in 1984 or 1985 we had a trio that consisted of Pat Goldman-Rakic, me and Danny Weinberger, each of whom had his or her version of the story of the frontal cortex in schizophrenia. The 1980s was a big turning point in my career, because I had a number of good ideas that were published which were right, and I began to be recognized as a leader. I would say for most people to understand the value of imaging took years and it was not before the 1990s.

I remember being at one meeting of a collaborative depression study. It was a group that focused primarily on mood disorders, and the people in that group were some great names: Gerry Klerman, who is now dead; Marty Keller at Harvard; Jan Fawcett at Rush Presbyterian, who is still very active; Paula Clayton and Ted Reich from Washington University; and me from Iowa; as well as Bill Coryell and George Winokur. I remember people were saying that just looking at family studies in genetics and the clinical definitions of illness wasn't enough. I spoke up said that we have to introduce biological measures. Somebody looked at me and said, "why are biological measures so important?" And I replied, "Because they're critical independent validations." So someone else said, "Why aren't you doing some validation using biological measures?" Then I said, "Well, I am. I'm doing imaging." And they said, "That's not a biological measure." I thought how could measuring the volume of the brain or the frontal lobes and blood flow in the brain or frontal lobes not be a biological measure? Those are biological measures along with neurotransmitters.

AT: In addition to doing all those things, you picked up the editorship of the *American Journal of Psychiatry*, so could you say something about that?

NA: I was lucky there, too. I did have a very hard time, as a woman, early in my career, but as life has gone on I've been rewarded by people, like John Nemiah, who was editor of the *American Journal of Psychiatry*. He was a psychoanalyst, but he asked me to be on the editorial board, and then he asked me to be the book editor. Then when his deputy editor, Morrie

Lipton, died, he asked me to be his deputy editor, and I think he intentionally had me in training to be his successor. He was very good to me and I appreciate it enormously.

It is the most natural thing in the world for me, because I intended to get a degree in Journalism. My father's degree and my grandfather's degree was in Journalism, and my great grandfather was a newspaper editor in the Civil War era. So I'm the fourth generation in publishing in one way or other. I've grown up with books and writing and editing. When I was a little kid, the one gift my parents let me have that I loved was a little mimeograph machine I could use to publish my own newspaper; and then I was editor of the junior high yearbook, the senior high yearbook and the senior high newspaper. I started out in college as a copy editor. and even had a job on a newspaper for awhile. Writing is as easy for me as breathing, and reading is also very easy. I've been trained for years and years, thinking about page layouts and all the things you have to do when you edit a journal.

AT: Do you have any regrets you didn't pursue English literature?

NA: Not a single regret. I'm very grateful I learned so much about history, literature and philosophy, and I use it all the time, I mean, all the time. As I've gotten further away from it, I have less capacity to quote poetry from memory. But I have a reservoir of reference points most other people don't have I can draw on. I have ways to conceptualize what's happening in the world, and if you are trained in history, as I was, you're thinking about the way things were once upon a time, how you got to where you are, and about what's going to be happening in the future, and not just a year or two years, but in five years, ten years, or fifty years. If you want to be a good scientist you have to think that way. You can't always do that, because you don't know what kind of technologies are going to develop. But you still need to have a sense of what your trajectory is into the future. If there's a mistake young scientists make, it's learning something but not understanding new things are going to come along, and as they come along, having to figure out which the useful new things are, embrace them, learn them, incorporate them into their work and move on into the eternally changing future.

AT: I picked up on a comment you made earlier on, and I'm curious. You said women such as yourself really paved the way for others, and mentioned things you accomplished first as a woman. How important is it that one is the first woman to do this or that?

NA: I would almost never say that I'm the first woman to do this or that because it's bad taste. It implies that I got there because I'm a woman, rather than because of what I've done, and I'd like to think that most of what I've accomplished was because of sheer ability, rather than because I was a woman. I really believe that's true. Those of us in my generation who have succeeded when nobody was cutting women any slack, don't want to think of ourselves as getting where we are because we were women. We got there in spite rather than because of our gender. So, the question was?

AT: What do you think about the changes that have taken place, for example giving women special benefits at universities?

NA: Some things have changed and many of them are for the good. Men are helping their wives more in two-career families and I think that's a nice thing for both of them. I am glad that younger women have access to things like daycare centers and so on. There are things that bother me, though. For example, there was a young woman whom I went out on a limb to hire. She was very committed to doing work in imaging. Then she discovered she was pregnant. It was inconvenient, because I knew she was going to be taking some time off. It is a problem when women take time off, and men don't, because there can be bad feelings. That's one of the reasons I always made very sure I pulled my oar just as hard as the guy sitting next to me without special favors on call schedules and things like that. If somebody lost, it was going to be me, and not my kids or my male colleagues. I might get less sleep. There was a period in my life where I might as well have been living in a cave. I never went to a movie. I never read a book. I did nothing, because there was no time to do anything. I had no time to follow what was happening in music, in film, in theater, because there just wasn't time. There was only time for work.

Anyway, this young woman was pregnant, and came to me to work out her maternity leave. The standard in New Mexico as well as in Iowa is six weeks, which to me is a very generous amount of time. For each of my kids, I had one week. It's plenty of time for a woman to physically recover from childbirth. But she wanted six months, and I said that's just not possible. And then she started citing Federal law which gives women, I think, six months; a certain amount of time with pay, and then a good period without pay. It turned out the New Mexico organization she worked in was small enough so that law didn't apply so we struck a balance, it was two or three months, less than she wanted, but much more than I wanted. Then she decided she didn't want to come back to work. This is another thing that is not good for women in general. My younger daughter, Robin, who has a PhD in Philosophy of Science and a job at the University of Delaware as an Assistant Professor, had her first little boy about sixteen months ago, and she is now expecting her second. And she's going through agonies as to whether she should quit and stay home with Owen, or whether she should continue her career. I understand it. I would never say to her that if you do quit, you'd be fulfilling the prophecy that women can't be taken seriously, because they're going to have kids. That's the attitude I grew up with so I'm real sensitive to that issue.

AT: One final question. What would you say your key contribution has been to psychopharmacology?

NA: I've had two or three good ideas. We've already covered most of them. One was to focus on refined clinical descriptions, the definition of the phenotype, and do that really well. I just reread some of the papers I wrote twenty-five or thirty years ago on this topic and they were good. Another contribution was the emphasis on thought disorder in schizophrenia and developing ways to define it clinically, and measure it psychometrically with language tests. Another was the introduction of negative symptoms. I consider myself one of the pioneers in applying imaging tools, and particularly applying MRI technology in psychiatry.

Years ago, I edited a book called *Can Schizophrenia be Localized in the Brain?* I was one of the first people who took the approach of neurology by trying to localize symptoms, as in a stroke. Can we in psychiatry localize symptoms like hallucinations, delusions, negative symptoms, language abnormalities? I was one of the first people who said, let's try to localize symptoms in different brain regions. As I progressed I came to believe localization is in distributed circuits because that is the way the brain works; I was one of the first to emphasize that. That idea rests on my work with functional imaging and especially with PET. I think the cerebral cortex is of great importance, but I'm trying to get people to think about the importance of sub-cortical regions as well. We have been taught about the importance of basal ganglia for years, because that's a target for the antipsychotic drugs. But people have really not thought about two of my beloved brain regions, the thalamus and the cerebellum. The thalamus is just beginning to get emphasized and the cerebellum is going to be one of these days. Almost every good idea I've had has turned out to be true. I just have to wait to see them accepted.

Another thing we haven't talked about is that I've written a couple of books for lay people. I'm very proud of those. The first one, *The Broken Brain*, which had the subtitle, *The Biological Revolution in Psychiatry*, I wrote in 1982 and 1983. It was published in 1984 and it's often called "the first brain book." It was certainly the first book to articulate the notion that psychiatry was going to change from a psychodynamic to a biological model. That book also carried the message that mental illnesses could not and should not be stigmatized, because they're brain diseases.

AT: Wasn't it nominated for a National Book Award?

NA: It was. That book is still in print and most of it is almost up to date. It's a very readable, enjoyable book, and it has attracted a lot of medical students and postdocs, who read it and came to work with me. It's been translated into many languages.

AT: And psychiatrists recommend reading it.

NA: After I did *The Broken Brain*, my editor kept nagging me to write another book. People kept saying, "When are you going to update *The Broken Brain*?" But for me, that book was like Shakespeare writing Hamlet, and then somebody wanting Hamlet Part Two, which is fashionable now with Terminator and such things, but it wasn't for me. So it took close to twenty more years before I was ready to write another book on the brain that could say something new and different, and that's *Brave New Brain*, which talks about the fusion between what we learn at the system level with techniques like imaging, and what we learn at the molecular level with things like genomics; how those will merge so we begin to understand illnesses to develop better treatments and prevention.

That is another gift I have, the ability to write clearly. You don't know how your own brain comes across to other people. But by now, it's clear as a bell, because I hear it over and over; that I can take the most difficult concepts and explain them in a way that is totally lucid and makes people listening understand what I'm saying. That's a characteristic of these two books. Some people say they like the first one better, because it's a little easier and some people like the second one better, because it's a little more complicated. I regret that I don't have more time, because I really do enjoy writing books. My kids both say, "Mom, you're just a born teacher. You love to explain things to people," It could be psychiatry, it could be neurobiology; but it could be how roadrunners are part of the cuckoo family or it could be what Queen Elizabeth I was doing in 1603, or what John Donne was doing in 1611, or any of the interesting things in history or in nature. I was having dinner with somebody the other night and we were talking about the way the world is changing, for good and for bad. I feel I'm so lucky I was born when I was. Admittedly, it was a disadvantageous time for women, but a time when so much was happening in science. We have so much freedom to do whatever we want, whether it's traveling or career wise, endless possibilities, so we're privileged. I feel so lucky that I get to have fun in my work and actually get paid for it.

AT: Thank you so much.

ROBERT M. KESSLER

Interviewed by Andrea Tone
San Juan, Puerto Rico, December 15, 2004

AT: My name is Dr. Andrea Tone and we are at the 2004 Annual Meeting at the ACNP. I have the great pleasure of being able to interview Dr. Robert Kessler.* Let's start with your background, personal and professional. What did you want to be when you grew up and what did you end up being and why?

RK: I'm not sure what I wanted to be when I grew up. I always had an interest in biology, just fooling around with a microscope as a kid. I got the microscope as a present when I must have been about ten or twelve years old. My father had made a number of histology slides when he was an undergraduate and I used to look at those. These were slides made in the 1930s, but they were still perfectly clear, and so I developed an interest in tissues and microorganisms. So I had an interest in biology. Then in high school I had a biology teacher who was extremely influential to my future, a very nice man who had me go through a summer course he gave looking at blood cells and parasites. Parasitology was the main theme, and that got me more interested. At least two of us from that course went into academic medicine, one of whom became Vice-Chair of the Department of Microbiology at Emory.

AT: Who was that?

RK: Sharon Weiss. She and I shared a microscope in that course. So I became interested in biology, and then in high school, post-Sputnik, there was this craze for developing science in the US. I lived outside of Washington at that time, and the Montgomery County Heart Association had a series of lectures, given at NIH, to encourage kids to become interested in science. You took an exam at the end, and if you did well you were offered a chance to work a summer at NIH, which I did.

AT: What were the lectures on?

RK: They were just general biomedical lectures. We're talking ancient history but I did end up in the laboratory of a chemist by the name of Hank Fells, on the seventh floor of the Clinical Center. He was a delightful man and had a wonderful lab; the staff were very tolerant and supportive to an inquisitive, overly talkative adolescent. It was a great place to be at the time. Across the hallway was a fellow by the name of Bob Levy, and Frederickson's lab was there. Around the corner was Marshall Nierenberg who won a Nobel Prize; there were a whole bunch of interesting people I got to meet and they were extremely nice. It really piqued my interest

---

* Robert M. Kessler was born in Philadelphia, Pennsylvania in 1945.

in medical science, and I'd say that's where it started. When I went to college, I majored in chemistry, largely as a result of my exposure to Dr. Fells' lab. I also took a course in psychology.

AT: Where did you go to college?

RK: Yale. Physiological psychology was taught by a rather charismatic fellow, who was practically oriented. He wasn't so much animal-oriented. He kept coming back to the point that biological explanations for behavior were going to come at some point, and that made me think about the chemistry of behavior and motivated me to go to medical school. I thought about doing psychiatry but Yale Medical School at that point was very analytically oriented. It was a wonderful department with a lot of good people, but I gravitated more towards the pharmacology department. At Yale you had to do a thesis and I ended up working with Bob Roth, who's a member of the ACNP. I did work with catecholamines in his lab, and at NIH in the summers I worked in Brodie's lab, which was a great opportunity to meet a lot of wonderful people. I did studies on inbred strains of mice, looking at turnover of catecholamines in the heart. I was looking at the regulation of catecholamine turnover in the autonomic nervous system. A paper came out of that, which was fortunate. Then I began thinking that what we learn in animals has to be translated into humans and it's not going to be straightforward. If you look closely at the anatomy of rats and mice and at the anatomy of the human brain, that's a pretty long leap. Genetically it may not be so long, but in terms of the circuitry it might be bigger than people think. We were going to have to examine the human condition to make sure that it really applied. The question was how? I began thinking in terms of imaging but that was well ahead of its time and impractical. Had I submitted the idea to an NIH committee, it would have been rejected as ridiculous.

AT: What time period are we talking about?

RK: The early seventies, just before the advent of CT. So I went into a Radiology residency, thinking about visualizing brain function. What saved my neck was the advent of CT when I was a resident at Peter Bent Brigham and it became apparent we could now visualize the brain. Initially I thought about ways of using labelled neurotransmitter analogs, but that wasn't possible although using isotopes seemed practical and single-photon tomography had already been invented by Dave Kolipan.

AT: For those who may not have advanced training in radiology what are the things you are talking about?

RK: Single-photon tomography is a way of looking at cross-sections in the body or the brain after you inject isotopes and get a picture of isotope distribution topographically. This was a very crude technique initially. Then in the mid-seventies, positron emission tomography came along, where we used a different type of isotope that allowed for better sensitivity and spatial resolution. I'm sure many people have heard of fluorodeoxyglucose. This is a glucose analog developed by Lou Sokoloff at NIH, and subsequently applied by Marty Reivich at the University of Pennsylvania, and Al Wolf at Brookhaven National Laboratory. They attached fluorine so they could image the isotopes with the new tomographs. In conjunction with devices that localized isotope concentration, they used physiological tracers of energy metabolism. The brain uses glucose and oxygen to produce most of its energy; energy metabolism is tightly regulated in the brain, so where the brain is functioning it's using energy. If you can image energy metabolism, you have a way of imaging brain function. So, that was the first good functional technique for looking at three-dimensional brain metabolism. It was developed in 1977 the time I came to NIH.

AT: How fortuitous!

RK: Dumb luck wins again! It occurred to me this was something I'd been looking for, so I took it upon myself as naive junior person at NIH to team up with people in the Neurology Institute at the Clinical Center and obtain support from Psychiatry. We managed to get a positron tomograph at NIH in 1979 but since we didn't have a synchrotron to develop the isotopes we used the synchrotron at the Naval Research Laboratory. We thought we had reached an agreement with them but after we bought the tomograph, there was talk their lab was closing down. It was through the intervention of my Norwegian Elkhound puppy that we got the whole thing back on track; my neighbor was a hydro-nautical engineer and a great lover of my little dog, and one day he asked me, as I was walking the dog, why I looked so glum. I told him the story about the naval lab closing and the problem that would create for me. He said, "Let me take care of it." It turned out his best friend was the director of the lab! So because I got to this man through my dog the PET program at NIH was able to continue.

AT: A great story!

RK: Sometimes things turn out in quirky ways. Otherwise, the NIH PET program would not have happened until several years later. We got started with fluorodeoxyglucose and several investigators looked at issues such as aging and schizophrenia, Alzheimer's, brain tumors; those were the first studies. Subsequently, I moved to Vanderbilt in 1984, with the idea of setting up a program there. It took a few more years than I would have liked.

I began developing ligands for dopamine D_2 receptors with the idea of looking at cortical limbic dopamine systems. Dopamine is the neurotransmitter implicated in Parkinson's disease which is based on deficiency of dopamine in the basal ganglia, nuclei at the center of the brain. But there are also smaller quantities of dopamine in other areas, such as the cortex. Since the limbic system is responsible for emotions, mood may be affected, as well. There's also a long-standing history of studies showing that dopamine is involved in some aspects of schizophrenia, probably the dopamine that is in the cortex and limbic system. There was no good way to image those particular systems, so we developed and patented a number of ligands initially for single-photon tomography, and then went on, with the help of NIMH, to develop a number of ligands for PET. We have subsequently started studies in humans. Unfortunately, these projects take decades and not months. For developing those ligands we have had very strong support from chemists, especially from Thomas de Paulis, who had been at Astra pharmaceutical company prior to joining Vanderbilt.

We developed the ligands in animals, studied their behavior in monkeys and published several articles. We did binding studies in post-mortem human brain. Eventually, we did the toxicology studies necessary before human use and then the initial studies in humans. Now we are doing studies in which we manipulate the uptake, release or depletion of dopamine, so we can see different aspects of dopaminergic neurotransmission. We're also doing studies in disorders that may involve dopamine, for example, Attention Deficit Disorder, in which there is an increase in the amount of dopamine in the brain. It may be an overdiagnosed disorder, but it's very real when you see it. We also have plans to start studies in schizophrenia. Dopamine is a ubiquitous neurotransmitter that may play a role in depression, drug abuse, and many other conditions. We're thinking about moving on to study other neurotransmitter systems, with the idea of looking at the relationship between cerebral neurotransmission and higher cortical function. Psychiatric disorders have been the focus of most of what I've done for the last twenty years.

AT: How do you envision the impressive research you are doing will change clinical practice?

RK: I don't know. Science takes indirect paths to real life, but we've learned many things from the mode of action of antipsychotic drugs. We studied schizophrenic subjects who take antipsychotic drugs and we found that clozapine, one of the most effective drugs in schizophrenia, while it blocks dopamine receptors to some extent, also has unusual effects on dopamine cell bodies in the mid-brain. We think that has a lot to do with the cognitive enhancement seen with this drug. We hope to translate these findings into drug development. We're using imaging to find out where the changes occur with different drugs and by doing this we provide hints to design better new drugs.

AT: So there will be new drugs that would target specific areas of the brain instead of just flooding the brain?

RK: In a way you're right, they will have properties that produce specific effects in specific areas. This sort of thing is extremely important. And we always wonder how good the clinical diagnostic criteria we have are. Dementia is a good case to illustrate this; twenty-five or thirty years ago, in a pathology textbook dementia wasn't dementia; it was Alzheimer's disease, Pick's disease, etc. There are many kinds of dementia and we have thrown them into a wastebasket and treat them as if they are the same. Even if genetic therapies are developed, they will have to be targeted to specific disorders people have. Someone with a Lewy body dementia has a different brain dysfunction from someone who has Alzheimer's dementia, a β-amyloid disease. They're difficult to tell apart clinically. In mental illness, a lot of people wonder that even though we use a common rubric for depression, does everybody have the same abnormality? Does everybody really have the same abnormality in schizophrenia? Schizophrenia is a diagnostic entity; it was put together in the last century and not everybody agrees it is one entity. So, it would be very important that we individualize therapy for patients, based upon different etiologies and different kinds of illness. Imaging can tell us a great deal about whether our clinical diagnoses conform to a single entity, or maybe we're lumping together people who have a final common behavioral pathway from multiple etiologies.

AT: Do you find DSM sufficient, or if you had your druthers, how would you change it? A lot of people I've interviewed at this meeting have said quite a bit about DSM.

RK: I am not a psychiatrist, so I'm not the best person to say, but I've seen a lot of patients with schizophrenia and as a non-psychiatrist, there seems to be a wide range of life history, cognitive and behavioral differences among these subjects. And, while it's possible it's one entity, you begin to wonder whether this is an adequate description of reality. At some level they tend to share some features and people would argue they switch from one subtype to another, but I think there are huge differences. There are people who fell out of the womb as awkward kids; they may have been a little bit funny looking, didn't do well in school, are socially isolated, and then, as teenagers begin to hallucinate, and now they're suddenly called schizophrenics. Then we have people who are very social, do extremely well, who have high achievement, go to Ivy League schools, have very high IQ's, have lots of friends – you know, have a totally different behavioral trajectory – and then in their mid to late twenties or late thirties have a psychotic break and become schizophrenic. The one who was never right from the first may have a very different disease from the one who was a philosophy major. Those diseases may have very different etiologies. We just don't know; it's important to understand that.

AT: Do you think that imaging will have a role in diagnosing patients?

RK: "Perhaps" is the answer, but we are far from it. Psychiatric diseases are not like neurological disorders where you can look at an MRI scan and say, this person has multiple systems atrophy, changes which are typical of Parkinsonism. We don't have that, but I do think, as we get more specific in our biochemical concepts of where these idiosyncratic diseases come from, it will play a role in diagnosis. I also think it's going to be very important in determining and monitoring therapies.

AT: Can you say a bit more about that?

RK: I think people respond very differently to different drugs and if we have a profile of what their biochemistry is, we may be better able to treat their particular abnormality from what we consider normal. If people have, let's say too little of receptor Y – whatever receptor Y is – then maybe we need to provide in treatment receptor Y supplements, or augment receptor Y activity. Or if someone else has too much of neurotransmitter Q we need to block receptor Q activity. We need to be able to get into the real chemistry to know what to do. Right now we're treating everybody with a diagnostic entity pretty much the same. Again, I'm not a psychiatrist, but I see this all the time. Someone comes in and they're diagnosed as schizophrenic, so the patient is put on a second generation atypical neuroleptic, and if the psychiatrist is not happy with the response, the psychiatrist tries another drug. And you find these funny responses, some respond beautifully to risperidone but they may not respond to olanzapine or vice versa.

AT: It seems that the ideal way to treat psychiatric patients is inherently interdisciplinary; that involves geneticists, radiologists and others. I wonder if that ideal is at odds with the economic reality of healthcare delivery. Have you any thoughts about that? Imaging is very expensive.

RK: When CT scans first came out in the mid-seventies there was huge resistance because it was too expensive; the machines were a few hundred thousand dollars then. But then a body of knowledge was built up and CT came into its own after an NIH consensus forum was held on imaging and they used CT as an example which showed the benefits so outweighed cost that it was criminal not to use it in certain cases. On the flip side, these technologies tend to be overused. When properly used there is no question that in many disorders you're way ahead. And the cost of not doing it can be much greater than doing it. Take brain abscesses for example. The morbidity and mortality of brain abscesses were very high prior to CT, maybe fifty percent. Using CT, you can see a developing abscess and operate in time; mortality for brain abscess went way down. You have a test that costs a few hundred dollars telling you how to save lives and preserve function. On the other hand medicine has become so oversold people are demanding absolute knowledge and these tests are overused. That creates problems; you have an anxious patient wanting to have it, so the physician feels compelled to do it, and as a result, you get tremendous overuse. I think society will swing back by necessity to a more rational use of these technologies. There are lots of gray areas; for example, we can diagnose Alzheimer's disease very well with PET today.

AT: Even at an early stage?

RK: Even at an early stage. ApoE4 is a protein that has a variant associated with a very high incidence of Alzheimer's disease. Eric Reiman showed that if you look at people in their fifties, who have that genetic variance, even if they are cognitively normal and functioning fine, they have a genetic time bomb ticking and it's probably going to make them demented by the time they're seventy-five. You can do a fluorodeoxyglucose PET scan and compare them statistically to normal subjects. The scan is significant twenty-five years before they have the clinical illness. When people have cognitive impairment and memory failure, and you don't know whether it's a benign memory failure with age or Alzheimer's disease, predictive accuracy is very important. The question can you going to do anything about it? Well, maybe, maybe not. Maybe there will be neuroprotective therapies. Drug trials are now looking at neuroprotective agents and glucose metabolism. Or maybe it is worth the family knowing what's going to happen, so they can take care of things. It's surprising to me how many families, a spouse, a father or a grandfather, want to know what's going to happen. They're actually willing to pay without insurance, if they have the resources. That's a one-time investment. There may be big reasons for doing this, if only for peace of mind. It is unfortunate that once they become mainstream there'll be a reaction to overuse, until we get to something reasonable. At the heart of the matter is proper use.

AT: I was thinking of how ultrasound technology has fundamentally changed pre-natal care. There was a time when people said it's unnecessary, it's too expensive, but now, it's bedrock technology for diagnostic care. Everyone who has been pregnant in the last ten years, has had an ultrasound.

      I'm going to ask a couple of questions related to the popularization of imaging technology. I was in Atlanta until a few months ago, and I remember listening to radio stations on my way to the university that would say, you are at risk for all sorts of illnesses and won't know if you are susceptible unless you have full body imaging; you can have it this week at a discount, for $120.

RK: That's abuse and where the free market is going a little too far, preying on people's fears. The former Chairman of Radiology at Emory had one of those full body scans and they had some suspicious findings, which resulted in unnecessary surgery and complications. So it's a double edged sword. You can find things that aren't as abnormal as they appear and the complications of trying to treat those non-life threatening, probably normal variances, can be worse than not knowing. I think that's horrible, that's greed. It's not a good use of technology.

AT: As all this literature is being published on what the brain looks like, do we need to have someone like you at the other end of the technology, making sense of what's being seen?

RK: I think there are two layers here. It's healthy and good that people in psychiatry, neurology and psychology learn how to read scans. The problem is that somebody trying to explain a specific symptom by looking at the scan might not recognize something totally unrelated but more significant. Many times a highly significant incidental finding is missed by someone who is overly focused on explaining a particular finding by a scan. You may have a psychiatrist looking at a CT scan of the head they think they know a lot about, but they miss the fact the person has a cancer of the nasopharynx, which they're untrained to look at. That's the expertise issue.

The other issue is in terms of the acquisition of images, making sure that they're of optimal quality. Experts get a lot of training in quality control. And, a third point; people who order and interpret their own X-rays, order and interpret more than if they order and interpret them from somebody else. So at the clinical level, it fuels over-utilization. At the research level, I think it's important to have the interplay of psychologists, neuroanatomists, radiologists, psychiatrists and radiochemists, because that's the way things go forward. In one of our recent projects for example we have a psychiatrist, who evaluates the patients and screens them for behavioral issues; there's myself, who oversees the imaging; we have PhDs handling the data; we have physicists and mathematicians, who look at the tracer to make sure everything is going well; we have psychologists, who do behavioral testing and statisticians, who help with the interpretation of huge data sets. So there's a big team. I'm just one person and everybody makes an important contribution. I happen to coordinate it, but all of these people together are what's needed to progress in multidisciplinary, multidimensional fields. The problem with many imaging enterprises is that you need so much expertise in so many places that not all groups have equal strength, and as a result the data can be criticized from ten different points of view. If you don't have the strength in every area, the whole enterprise may fail over a very simple issue. From a research point of view, it's important to have everybody involved and to make sure that everything gets done in a careful way. There are a lot of simple issues to a physicist that are not so simple to a psychologist.

AT: You're a radiologist in the ACNP.

RK: Yes.

AT: How welcoming has it been for your field?

RK: Because of my background in pharmacology and interest in behavior, I think I speak the language reasonably well, and it's very transparent and very open and very welcoming.

AT: What do you feel you give to people here and what do you take home from the other side of the fence?

RK: What I've given is development of pharmaceuticals, radiopharmaceutical enriching that has helped imaging in psychiatry. I've helped people get started at a number of institutions on imaging in psychiatry. I tend to serve as a facilitator and in return I get a lot of biological and pharmacological insights. They're hard to get anywhere else, and this organization promotes a multidisciplinary approach. There are basic scientists, clinicians, people like myself from different disciplines. That cross-fertilization is incredibly beneficial for everyone. My principal benefit from being here is from accessing the minds of creative people in many different areas. It gets you thinking in a different way. It jolts you out of your complacency.

AT: Final question. How do you see the relationship of imaging and radiology with psychiatry twenty to fifty years from now?

RK: Psychiatry does not have a clear blood test, at this point. The question is whether this can be resolved by genetics. It remains to be seen why there are so many people with susceptibility genes who don't become ill. Maybe we'll come down to genetic screening, but I seriously doubt it. I think psychiatry needs help in evaluating patients and their therapeutic responses with objective measures they currently don't have. The idea 20 or 25 years ago that schizophrenia was characterized by loss of brain substance was not in the minds of most psychiatrists. It wasn't well accepted. There was some very old literature from the 1930s using pneumoencephalography that suggested bigger ventricles in schizophrenia, but everybody said it was an artifact. Now, with CT, we see that differences between normal subjects and schizophrenic patients are real and think they are probably developmental. Imaging fostered the neurodevelopmental hypothesis of schizophrenia. The dopamine hypothesis of schizophrenia was supported by post-mortem studies. Then, in imaging studies, the corresponding changes with the dopamine hypothesis were not seen and it was necessary to reevaluate the role of dopamine. So, it's an iterative process where findings from testing a hypothesi in psychiatry feeds back to pharmacology, and may go back to testing in animals and then back to humans. Imaging has become part of that process.

AT: Thank you. Is there anything you want to add?

RK: Not really. I feel I've gone on too long.

AT: You haven't at all. It's been really interesting.

RK: Well, good. Thank you so much.

AT: Thank you.

DANIEL R. WEINBERGER

Interviewed by Stephen Potkin
Boca Raton, Florida, December 12, 2007

SP: Hello, my name is Stephen Potkin and we are at the 48th annual meeting of the ACNP. I have the pleasure today to interview Daniel R Weinberger.* Daniel R. Weinberger is Director of the Genes, Cognition and Psychosis program at NIMH. We are going to cover Danny's early training and his latest research ideas. Danny you can tell us from where you started and where you were born and where you went to school?

DW: I was born outside of New York City in 1947 and grew up in Great Neck, New York; I went to public school and Great Neck South High School. Then I went to Johns Hopkins University and was a liberal arts major but interested, from early in life, in becoming a pediatrician. I thought that was what my life was going to be. While a liberal arts major I did the requisite courses for medical school admission; it was a lot easier to get into medical school in those days than it is today. In 1969, I went to the University of Pennsylvania Medical School, where I decided that pediatrics was not really what I was interested in; instead I got very interested in Neuroscience and thought about being a neurosurgeon, but was not too happy with the neurosurgical lifestyle.

SP: The early morning scheduling?

DW: I had a lot of trouble with the 4:30 am rounds. Then I was thinking about neurology versus psychiatry from a neuroscience prospective. That was at the end of the Vietnam War. I was in a very humanistic state of mind and felt there was a humanity issue in general medicine, and that moved me into thinking about psychiatry. I did a medical internship from 1973 to 1974 at UCLA in Harbor General Hospital outside Los Angeles, mainly because I wanted to experience the west coast for a year.

SP: I would like to recommend it.

DW: I hated it until about March and then I became very fond of it. I remember having a change of mind about March when I realized it was seventy two degrees and the sun was out. Then I realized that I really liked it out there, but by then I committed to do a residency at the Massachusetts Mental Health Center. It was at that time the premier-Harvard program and very psychoanalytically oriented. It was very humanistic, trying to understand mental illness from the perspective of mind mechanisms. By the second year of my residency, which was intellectually challenging, I became aware I was learning a lot about humanity, human behavior and psychology, but I was not learning much about mental illness. And, then, two

_____
* Daniel Weinberger was born in New York City, New York in 1947.

friends from my residency, David Shiling and Joel Kleinman, who were at NIMH, kept saying, you can learn a great deal of science here and understand mental illness from a whole different perspective. I followed them and joined the laboratory of Richard Wyatt in 1977 while you were there, Steve. I was extremely unsophisticated about clinical or basic research but since I was thinking of an academic career in psychiatry I tried to get a basic understanding of its challenges.

I had become very interested in schizophrenia as a resident; I thought it was a great challenge for neuroscience to understand how a brain could malfunction in this unapproachable way. I was very conscious of how profoundly debilitating it was. One of the unusual things about the Mass Mental Health Center in those days was that in my entire first year of residency I had only 28 admissions, which was probably two orders of magnitude less than any other resident or intern in the country. When you admitted a patient, it was your patient for the duration of your residency. So you got to know these people extremely well. One of the things I found to my amazement was that the hallucinations and delusions which were the most obvious florid characteristics, was not what was wrong with them. I became very conscious after three years of residency that what was wrong was they could not function. It was the hallucinations and delusions we tried to analyze and find meaning in, but I was convinced the reason these people were not back at work or at school was they could not seem to function. So I became focused on what I thought from my early clinical days was really the core problem of schizophrenia, which was how the brain manages complex environmental information. So I followed my friends to NIMH and worked in Richard Wyatt's lab and that was the beginning of my research career.

SP: What was the first project you did? Do you recall it?

DW: I recall it very vividly, because it was a project with Carleton Gajdusek in the neurology institute. I obtained ten samples of brains from Joel Kleinman, because I was interested in the viral hypothesis of schizophrenia. When I was a resident, I read papers by Fuller Torrey and became very neurologically minded.

SP: When were those articles published?

DW: In 1972. I liked his articles about temporal lobe epilepsy, his ideas about the temporal lobe, encephalitis, viruses and herpes, and, of course about viruses that affect the temporal lobe and can induce psychosis. So, I took Joel's ten samples and worked in Gajdusek's lab, for two days a week for about a year. During this time we injected about 55 monkeys and six chimpanzees for the slow viral dementia studies they were doing. This was before he got the Nobel Prize. That was the first project I was

involved with. We followed them for over eight years and nothing happened. They did not develop Spongiform Encephalopathy; they did not
develop Schizophrenia; it was a negative study. We submitted a paper
that was rejected by the *Archives of General Psychiatry*! They felt the
method was not proven. So I wrote a letter to Danny Freedman, and said,
excuse me, this method won a Nobel Prize, there is nothing wrong with
the method, it is just there is no slow virus in the brains of schizophrenics.

Then I ran one of the research wards at St. Elizabeths Hospital. At the
time that was a terrific environment. It was an opportunity to experience
things hard to imagine one would ever experience. We had patients off
medication; this was an opportunity to see schizophrenia in an untreated
state. We did a lot of medical procedures that would be hard to do these
days, although we did them with full consent. We got to know patients
very well, because sometimes we had them on the research ward for over
a year or two. So it was an intimate experience. We were a bit of an outpost; sort of like the French Foreign Legion. We had a cadre of scientists,
physicians and basic scientists working in the same place and the same
building.

SP: Are there any people that stand out, who were important in moving your
research career forward?

DW: Well, I think the environment was conducive to trying new things and
thinking out of the box. I was basically preoccupied with the brain and
was a good neuroscience student at medical school. When I left Mass
Mental Health Center to go to NIMH I was conscious I had lost my connection with the neuroscience of mental illness. I always thought mental illness was the ultimate challenge for understanding how the brain
worked. There were two things that were critical: one which was what
Joel Kleinman at St. Elizabeths was doing, basically grind and bind studies of D_2 receptors and measuring enzymes in the brain.

SP: Was the other, the post-mortem studies?

DW: The other was the CT scan that had just come out. I think the first CT
scanner in the USA was delivered to Georgetown University in 1975, and
the first CT scanner at NIH arrived in about 1977. So when I got there,
they had the EMI CT scanner. EMI was a music corporation which produced all the Beatles music, but EMI was also making CT scanners. They
had an EMI Mark III CT scanner. So, I thought here I am at NIH and if
schizophrenia is a brain disease, then maybe we should look at these
people's brains. I started sending all the patients from the ward up to
NIH to get CT scans and they would always would come back normal.
Richard Wyatt, who ran the lab, had the biggest influence on me at that
time; he provided an environment that allowed people to do things they

were curious about without discouraging them. That was something that was very rare anywhere in the world. It was also a time when the NIMH Intramural Research Program had extraordinary resources, so it was possible to do virtually anything that was reasonable scientific research. We did a lot of drug trials; a lot of experimental therapeutics. I remember giving apomorphine, thinking it would cause presynaptic inhibition of dopamine release. We also did a lot of analytical chemistry, measuring all kinds of body fluids. We used to have patients lined up outside the treatment room for arterial punctures to look at some methylated indol compound.

SP: Also CSF studies?

DW: We did tons of CSF studies and the patients were pretty good about these things. We had very good relationships with the patients, so they were not opposed to these procedures and it wasn't just that they were intimidated and couldn't say no. We actually had patients who would volunteer for procedures. There is an old saying that many very sick individuals are reassured by medical procedures, and there was a certain relationship that existed between the doctors and patients that made this kind of thing possible. So I started doing CT scans and Jan Stevens was very helpful. She was a neurologist from the University of Oregon who spent a lot of time with Richard Wyatt. Jan had written several seminal papers on temporal lobe epilepsy and psychosis including one on the "Neuroanatomy of Psychosis" that was published in the *Archives*, I think in 1973. It highlighted the role of the nucleus acumbens something nobody knew anything about at the time. Jan made a comment to me which was very important. She said, "Even though the scans may be normal, there may be more quantitative things that were not normal." This led to the idea that maybe we could make quantitative measures of cerebral spinal fluid spaces, which were the ventricles, cortical fissures and sulci, the only anatomical details on a CT scan at that time. We did that, and it was the first study in which I learned how to use a manual planimeter. I became this "gnomish" guy in the basement measuring all the CT scans.

We reproduced data from the 1920s, done with pneumoencephalography (PEG). There was only one prior study with CT scanning from England by Eve Johnstone and Tim Crow. It was a very small study of an elderly sample. We did a large study, probably about two hundred patients, in first-break schizophrenia, middle episode, and normal controls; we confirmed that patients had bigger ventricles. That led to a series of studies to try to understand what the finding meant. Another person who was very influential in my thinking at that time was Norman Geschwind, who I had brought down from Boston for a visit; I had been a student of his at Harvard. Geschwind was the father of behavioral neurology and he wasn't really interested in psychosis; he was interested in aphasia, apraxia, anoxia, the classic cornerstones of behavioral neurology related to stroke. When I showed him all these CT scans, he thought that the patients in their twenties tended to have more CSF than he expected. He made a great comment, saying "People who have these findings should be different in some way from people who don't have them; that is what we call clinical pathological correlation." That's the classic way a neurologist looks for a lesion and relates it to the clinical state.

That led to studies showing that treatment response was quantitatively worse the bigger the ventricles. It also showed that cognitive variables were quantitatively worse, and that led to our pre-morbid studies where we collaborated with you and Cannon-Spoor who had developed a pre-morbid adjustment scale. We showed that adult patients with bigger ventricles were a little bit more delayed in reaching various social and educational milestones than people who didn't have them. And that led to the idea which was one of the major conceptual developments that emerged from the work, namely that whatever these changes in the brain were, they seemed to have clinical manifestations long before the illness emerged. When I wrote a paper in 1985 about implications of brain development, I cited this comment by Bleuler that many patients with schizophrenia have a childhood marked by social and educational difficulties. His argument was this was either a cause of schizophrenia or "a manifestation at a different time of life of the morbid pathology" which pre-dated the emergence of clinical phenomenology. So my assumption was that these early developmental problems and enlarged ventricles were related. That was in many ways the initiation of thinking about schizophrenia in a much more neurodevelopment way than people had previously.

Then I got very focused on imaging because we could study the brain of real people with more opportunity for experiment than we could with brain tissue. CT scans translated into more functional studies, because the problem with the CT is that it doesn't tell you why the brain is not working right or what the nature of the problem is. CT scans identify that the brain may not be absolutely normal in its structure, but it doesn't go beyond that. So we started doing early PET scans with glucose, and developed our own regional cerebral blood flow system. I was very interested in the early work being done in London by Richard Frackowiak on C-11 water and I couldn't get anybody at the NIH interested in cerebral blood flow because they were so stuck on the 2-deoxyglucose method discovered by Lou Sokoloff at the NIMH and its evolution into the FDG PET technique. And they didn't have capacity to make the postitron emiting water at the time. So we developed our own cerebral blood flow system at St. Elizabeths, which was a radioactive xenon based system. It was not topographic. It was cortical only, and it was like the most Rube Goldbergesque contraption you ever saw. I don't know if you ever saw it, Steve, the old blood flow system. It was bizarre. I had thirty two Geiger counters on top of the head that were basically sodium iodide crystals which recorded the emission of photons. And we had people breathe radioactive xenon gas, which is a great blood flow radio tracer because it's completely inert and totally diffusible. It is a true tracer of blood flow and you get highly quantitative measurements despite its low resolution. The most remarkable thing which I still don't believe completely to this day, is that it worked! And it produced topographical maps of cortical activity, so you could have regional resolution better than an EEG and it was much more quantifiable as a pure metabolic signal.

The other seminal thing that happened to my thinking occurred after reading Joaquin's Fuster's book. It was in 1984, my parents lived in Fort Lauderdale at the time, and I was lying on a beach in Fort Lauderdale reading *The Prefrontal Cortex*; published in 1982. I can't remember how I got interested in the frontal lobe but it was probably because of David Ingvar's findings in his original rCBF study. I started reading this book and I thought this is highly relevant to schizophrenia. The problem I was preoccupied with even as a resident was these patients don't function and can't think ahead. The problem was they have poor judgment, don't have insight, can't anticipate their actions, can't put sequences together, so they can't plan adequately and can't respond when things don't go well, which are characteristics related to frontal lobe function. Now, with Ingvar's data about hypofrontality in schizophrenia from cerebral blood flow studies I went to Allen Mirsky, who was head of neuropsychology at NIMH, and asked him for help in how to target frontal lobe function. I was thinking about the Starling heart experiments. I thought we could put a load on the pre-frontal cortex, because at the time people were only doing resting studies which seemed absurd to me because there was no way of knowing what a patient with schizophrenia and what someone who is not schizophrenic is doing during rest. It's not that the resting data might not be meaningful, but you have no idea what it is telling you, because you really don't know what their experience was at that time. I thought we had to do something to influence what they were doing during the procedure.

I asked Allan Mirsky what we can do to turn on the frontal lobe, and he said there is the Wisconsin Card Sorting Test. I recruited Karen Berman, who was a Fellow under me at the time to help me work on this, and we automated the test. It was a slide show, because there were no computers then. We had a slide show using a sensory motor control task by pressing a button. This was four years before anybody in Saint Louis or anywhere else had done an activation study of cognitive processing using the subtraction method. We did not consider this approach a great neuroscience advance, but it seemed appropriate for seeing how the frontal lobe was doing when it was working. So we administered the Wisconsin Card Sorting Test and it lit up the frontal lobe, which blew my mind. It was another fact that our machine actually worked, which was inconceivable. The machine was made by Harshaw Chemicals, who also made all those sodium iodine crystals. I remember flying out to Harshaw Chemicals in Ohio. I was very close to the salesman, because they had sold only two or three of these instruments before in their whole lifetime. Anyway, it worked, and we did patients with schizophrenia and confirmed Ingvar's studies, which was that the frontal lobe did not show normal engagement during the Wisconsin Card Sorting Test. Ultimately we moved into other areas of imaging as MRI came around. With MRI the image got much more sophisticated, although I have to say that while we have much more sophisticated paradigms and we can now, with fMRI, dissect at a much more elementary level the cognitive components of functional deficits in patients, we are basically finding much the same story as back in the mid-1980s, namely that patients with schizophrenia have problems engaging certain critical cognitive neurocircuits related to frontal lobe function.

SP: When did the ideas of involving the genetic aspects come about?

DW: That happened when Harold Varmus came to NIH as director; his tenure let to fundamental changes in my thinking about genetics. I was always phobic about genetics because I couldn't understand it. I couldn't get it when Ken Kendler would show those "path" diagrams from family segregation studies. I could read the literature about what structural equation modeling was and I understood the principle of it, but I couldn't really buy collecting the frequency of illness data in extended families. By creating paths you haven't proven anything, and I never bought it, because it was too abstract, too statistically dependent, and I am basically a biologist. I didn't like reaching all these conclusions based only on statistics. At that point in time psychiatric and behavioral genetics, and most genetics other than Mendelian disorders, were about statistics and epidemiology and I was a more hands-on doctor who couldn't relate to that kind of stuff. So I liked imaging; I mean it was like doing an exam. I just couldn't relate and was very intimidated by the math of genetics. It was all probabilistic and you couldn't get your hands around it. But I accepted the twin studies as a method, and I don't know if you were there when we had the Genain Quadruplets on our wards?

SP: Yes.

DW: These famous monozygotic quadruplets, all with schizophrenia, taught us that whatever was genetic about them – they were identical quadruplets – it wasn't their symptoms but something else, because their symptoms varied across the whole spectrum of schizophrenia. One was a hebephrenic and severely ill, another was only minimally symptomatic, and the other two were in the middle. So it was obvious, even though they had the identical genetic sequence, there was a lot of variability in penetrance and expression. If you look at Kety's original adoption studies, it was very clear that it was not the diagnostic symptoms which were genetic.

In this context, I was deeply affected by the occasion of Harold Varmus' visit, when he became NIH director. He came to visit St. Elizabeths and everyone was really stoked. We were going to show him around and show him all of the great stuff we have. Richard had this dog and pony show and I showed him imaging. Richard was always trying to do something he thought was earth shattering science, and Varmus laughed at it. He just looked at us and said, "What are you people, doing?" And then he said, "You are not doing anything that is going to crack this illness. You are telling me about all these great achievements, I see nothing you are doing now that is going to make any headway beyond what you have already done." This floored me.

Then about a year later, I was at an NAS sponsored meeting with Varmus, Zach Hall and all the schizophrenia heavyweights; I had recently become a branch chief at NIMH. Pat Goldman-Rakic and everyone was there and everybody did their dog and pony shows. This was a two day meeting at the National Academy of Sciences. And at the meeting, Zach Hall stood up and said, "You people have been studying this disease for thirty years, and from where I sit, you have accomplished virtually nothing." It was incredible. I was flattered to be there, and didn't take anything personally, but of course other people got incensed. And then, Varmus said, "You people don't get it; the human genome is going to be sequenced within the next decade. And all the genes related to mental illness are going to be found. So whatever you are doing, if you are not dealing with those findings, then you are going to be dinosaurs." In effect he said, if you people are not dealing with the genetic basis of mental illness, then you have no clues for what these illnesses are. I had been doing imaging for fifteen years, and we had become increasingly sophisticated as we had just started doing MRIs. But I had to admit, in my own heart of hearts, that what he said was we were doing phenomenology. We were getting more sophisticated with it and we were showing associations, but it was still phenomenology. We weren't creating pathways to new treatments and we weren't identifying the cause of illness. As I thought about it I realized I knew almost nothing about the genome and modern genetics. It became clear to me I couldn't say that he was not right; he probably was right and investigators were going to find the genes and understand the cause of these diseases. It was obviously not going to be us, because we were not even looking for them.

I came back and literally said to every person in my lab, "We are changing; this whole lab is going to change. We are going to become a molecular biology lab and we are going to learn genetics." I took courses; all of us took lab courses. I spent four weeks in a lab at Catholic University. I had asked Ian Creese, who was doing D_2 molecular genetics at that time, and he said the best lab courses in the country are at Catholic University because they immerse you for sixty hours a week and you learn all the basic technologies of recombinant DNA in four weeks. We cloned genes and did sequencing; we did everything you could do in that period. I didn't become a molecular biologist, but I came to understand the procedures, what it meant to do these things, and I could read the literature. Then, I spent the next five years working with David Goldman, Michael Dean, and others to get a better understanding of the clinical genetic aspects. I slowly but surely immersed myself in how we would use genes to understand the biology of the illness we have been studying.

The other big change in my thinking came when we started doing fMRI in 1992 after it became clear we could do high resolution functional imaging without radioactivity. I had always thought the Holy Grail in neuroimaging research was that we could study the same person multiple times. I actually wrote a paper with Joe Frank called the fMRI interview. My fantasy was, just as you do an interview with a patient to make a diagnosis, you would do an interview during fMRI. You would do multiple scans; the principle was that you could use the fMRI to develop a phenotype. I wrote a paper about how fMRI was going to be a genetic tool, in *NeuroImage*, in 1996. It was on new developments and the paper was about fMRI becoming a genetic tool. It was published in a supplement to the journal. I gave a talk in 1994 to all my colleagues in the NIH NMR center, saying I think we are going to be able to do phenotypes of how the brain works and relate this to variations in genes. It seemed very logical to me because I though as I was beginning to understand genetics, that genes can't make you hallucinate but genes make your brain behave, develop and function in a particular way. Genes will impact on brain physiology which can be assayed with fRMI. When I said that, they laughed at me and the radiologists went wild: "Are you out of your mind?" Everybody thought I was an idiot. I thought, however silly all this may sound, why shouldn't it be right; genes are related to behavior because they are about the biology of the brain. It is a tool we can use to study many different facets of how a brain works. One has to look closer at how genes work. That's how my involvement in imaging genetics started.

Julie Axelrod said that doing good science is not about brilliance; it's about persistence and asking the right question at the right time. NIMH was a very unusual place. It would have been impossible to get funded for this in the real world; if you talked like this they would probably have you committed, let alone give you a grant. So that is where we started. We had to get into genetics, because we wanted to do genetics based on intermediate phenotypes. I got very excited about this in the mid-90s because after five years of not getting it I was finally understanding genetics; I was reading and working in the lab and I started to get it. I wanted to collect a clinical sample that would allow us to understand how genes played out in the brain. In 1996 I started what we called "the sibling study." I recruited Michael Egan to help get the study going, and he became its "boots on the ground" manager. It was a huge project to do at St. Elizabeths; it was unheard of that we would be able to collect families to do it. We were focused on unaffected siblings, because the concept was genes were about your brain and not whether you halluci-nate. So siblings who share fifty percent of the genes should have some of the same characteristics. We had done studies with Fuller Torrey in the late 1980s and early 1990s on twins, where we showed that even though discordant healthy co-twins of schizophrenics had no diagnostic symp-toms, they had cognitive deficits and blood flow changes which were the only things we could measure at that time. That led us to do the sibling study, and because of my work with David Goldman and Michael Dean in the Cancer Institute – who I used to call my personal trainers – we were very focused on adequate controls. I would rather err on the side of a type II error than not controlling for a type I error. I felt we needed to not fall into the trap of findings artifacts, so we opted to do family-based stud-ies, focusing on triplets and quads. We would have two affected offspring and one or two unaffected offspring. We would use the unaffected off-spring to find heritable characteristics of brain function and cognition, which would be the targets of susceptibility genes. And so, we started collecting these trios and quads. We hired a social worker named Mary Weirick, who is priceless. She found every patient who had been studied at St. Elizabeths for thirty years and tried to get them and their families to come back for our study. This got a lot of people, because they had already been here and we had a very good relationship with them. We collected probably one hundred and fifty trios in those first four years.

We studied them very extensively over four days. We picked COMT as the first gene to study, because it contained a common functional variant and we knew a lot about its biology. I had the hypothesis about the role of frontal dopamine and there was evidence that COMT affected frontal dopamine. We came up with an association of COMT and schizophrenia, but more dramatically, the imaging findings showed that the COMT genotype predicted frontal lobe physiology even in small samples. This was based on thirty subjects, which completely blew our mind. We replicated the finding in this original study in three separate groups, and then started a series of studies using specific genes; targeting specific neuropathways we believed the gene might impact. We focused primarily on snips or variants in genes we knew affected the function of the gene, so that we had lawful predictions of the gene being affected biologically. In our early big profile studies we worked with the serotonin transporter, COMT and BDNF, and our findings confirmed the strategy we used by showing the results we expected. I think our findings have been a boon to understanding how genes affect the brain and how genes relate to behavior. It has made the behavioral genetic business a lot more biological.

SP: When you think back, what were your most important contributions?

DW: Before answering your question I would like to mention that after two years at NIMH, I decided I knew very little about the brain. So because I was doing imaging work without understanding the brain very well, I felt rather lost and that I didn't have any credibility with the other people in neuroscience. So I went back and did a neurology residency, which was very helpful to me, and gave me a lot of understanding and confidence in myself as a clinical neuroscientist. It also made it possible for me to put the psychiatric brain discipline in the broader context of biological brain science. That was a very important experience for me. Because of that background I thought cognition was a quantifiable, much more stable, aspect of the problems patients with schizophrenia have than the diagnostic symptoms. As I look back on my career, I was probably as much a proponent as anybody, of making cognition a centerpiece of psychiatric research in imaging and clinical follow up, and ultimately a target for treatments. That was one of the big contributions I made. I was also important by orienting thinking in imaging toward specific cognitive probes and a variety of image strategies. The notion of thinking about schizophrenia in a neuro-developmental context is something I think my voice was a major factor in. The other big advance that came out of work from my lab is the opportunity to make sense of genes related to behavior by linking them to aspects of human cognition and image based phenotypes.

SP: What honors and awards have you received?

DW: The awards that matters the most to me was the Lieber Prize from NARSAD. I won a number of prizes from the American Psychiatric Association, and I have been elected to the Institute of Medicine of the National Academy of Sciences. I have also won most of the general psychiatry prizes. I was awarded the first Roche *Nature Medicine* Translational Neuroscience Prize. Last year, I was given the first NAMI research prize.

SP: Are you happy with the way things have turned out professionally for you?

DW: I am probably much happier than I ever expected, and it's all because of the genes. Out of all of the things I have done, I have always been proud of recognizing that cognition is what we had to study. I felt the neurodevelopment hypothesis was a real contribution, and I thought that most of the imaging work we did was good because it almost always was replicable and stood the test of time. But I never thought any of that was fundamentally profound. I do think that genetics is profound. That's why I think we all – I know you feel this way – get very stirred up by it. To make sense out of gene-related variations in human temperament, in human cognition, in human brain function and in psychiatric disorders, is a major development. I think that focusing on the brain-based phenotypes and image genetics is going to change the way we think about behavioral genetics.

SP: So where is this going to lead?

DW: Ultimately, this will lead to rethinking psychiatric illness. We will use genes because genes tell us what the illnesses are on a very basic level. As we have a better understanding of how these genes influence the way different brain systems operate and how they develop, how they process environmental information, we will have a different way of thinking about mental illness. I don't think we will be as stuck any longer on arbitrary diagnostic schemes that have hijacked the freedom to ask questions that generate new data. I used to say to Francis Collins in the early days that the modern age of the human genome sequence will do more to change our understanding of mental illness than they will in any other field of medicine.

SP: I want to thank you very much for such a candid and personal view of your research and your career.

DW: Thank you for taking the time.

INDEX

Note: The page numbers for each interviewee's entry appear in boldface type.

www.ingramcontent.com/pod-product-compliance
Lightning Source LLC
Chambersburg PA
CBHW081104170526
45165CB00008B/2324